THE
GOOD HOUSEKEEPING
ILLUSTRATED BOOK OF
PREGNANCY
& BABY
CARE

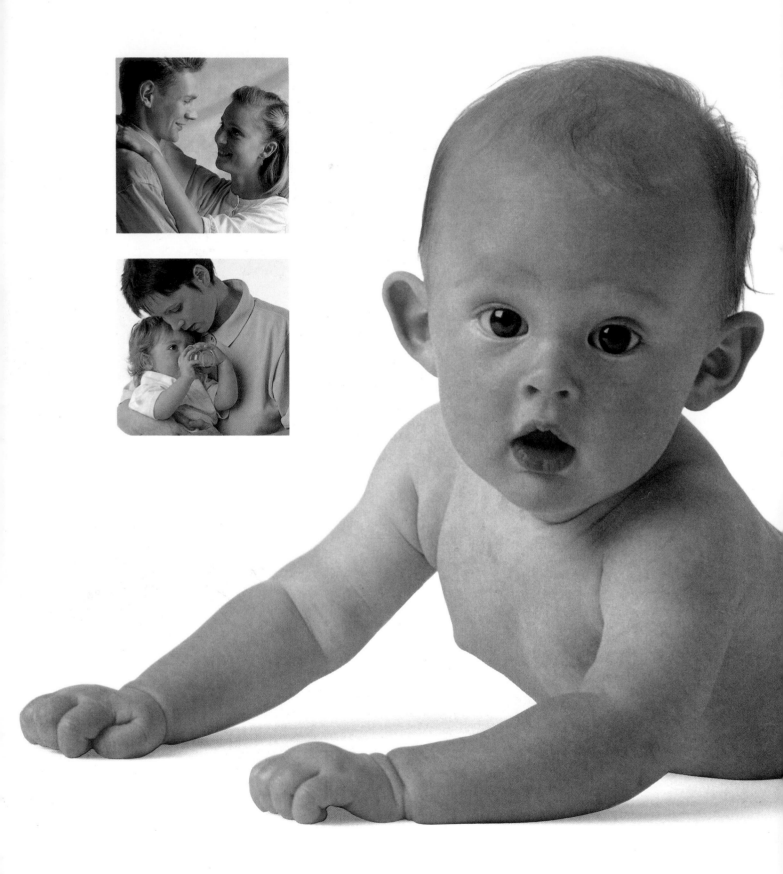

THE
GOOD HOUSEKEEPING
ILLUSTRATED BOOK OF
PREGNANCY
& BABY
CARE

HEARST BOOKS • NEW YORK

GOOD HOUSEKEEPING

Editor-in-Chief John Mack Carter
Institute Director Amy Barr

Infants and Children Laboratory
Director Mary Ann Littell
Associate Jennifer A. Flagg

HEARST BOOKS

Project Editor Maryann Bucknum Brinley
Consultant Sanford J. Matthews, M.D.,
American Academy of Pediatrics

Publisher's note
Throughout this book, the pronouns "he" and "she" refer to both
sexes, except where a topic applies specifically to a boy or a girl.

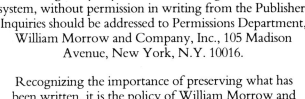

A Dorling Kindersley Book

Copyright © 1990
by Dorling Kindersley Limited, London

Library of Congress Catalog Card Number:
90-81176
ISBN 0-688-09667-0

Printed in the United States of America
First Edition
34456789 10

FOREWORD

We hope this book will show you in a very practical way how to care for your child. Having a baby opens up a whole new and exciting world—but it can be a terribly unfamiliar one, too. Most of us know very little about pregnancy and baby care at first, and we quickly find that there's seldom a "right" or a "wrong" way of doing things. But there's often an easy way. So what we have tried to do is show you what mothers have found worked best, and what makes life easiest.

Every pregnancy is special. Even though it's an experience that has happened countless times, to countless couples, it will still be momentous for you. This book guides you through your pregnancy stage by stage, showing you how to make it a happy, healthy time for yourself and how to give your baby the best possible start in life.

Every baby is special too, a personality in his or her own right from the moment of birth. By showing you all the basics of baby care, by offering practical solutions to common problems and plenty of reassuring advice, this book will help you look after *your* baby, and find out all there is to know about his or her own particular character.

We hope you will quickly discover that parenthood, for all its responsibilities, can be fun. You don't have to aim to be the "perfect parents"; if you and your baby can learn to love each other and get along together, then you can be assured that you are the perfect parents for your child.

CONTENTS

1 PREGNANCY
AND BIRTH
8–73

THINKING ABOUT PREGNANCY **10**

A PREGNANCY CALENDAR **12**

PRENATAL CARE **32**

COMMON COMPLAINTS **40**

KEEPING FIT AND RELAXED **43**

EATING FOR A HEALTHY BABY **50**

PRACTICAL PREPARATIONS **54**

LABOR AND BIRTH **56**

YOUR NEW BABY **68**

GETTING BACK TO NORMAL **71**

2 BABY CARE
74–171

THE FIRST WEEKS OF LIFE **76**

HANDLING YOUR BABY **82**

FEEDING YOUR BABY **87**

BREAST-FEEDING YOUR BABY **90**

BOTTLE-FEEDING YOUR BABY **98**

INTRODUCING SOLID FOOD **108**

CRYING AND YOUR BABY **117**

SLEEP AND YOUR BABY **120**

CLOTHES AND DRESSING **128**

BATHING AND WASHING YOUR BABY **134**

DIAPERS AND DIAPER CARE **146**

GIVING UP DIAPERS **154**

TAKING YOUR BABY OUT **156**

GROWING AND LEARNING **158**

BECOMING A PERSON **168**

3
HEALTH CARE
172–245

THE FIRST THREE MONTHS **174**

DIAGNOSIS GUIDE **180**

FIRST SIGNS OF ILLNESS **182**

GOING TO THE HOSPITAL **185**

THE CHILD WITH A FEVER **186**

ALL ABOUT MEDICINES **189**

CARING FOR A SICK CHILD **192**

COLDS AND FLU **194**

HAVING YOUR CHILD IMMUNIZED **196**

INFECTIOUS ILLNESSES **197**

EYE PROBLEMS **202**

EAR PROBLEMS **204**

MOUTH INFECTIONS **206**

THROAT INFECTIONS **207**

COUGHS AND CHEST INFECTIONS **208**

STOMACH PAIN **212**

CONSTIPATION, VOMITING,
AND DIARRHEA **213**

BLADDER, KIDNEY, AND GENITAL
PROBLEMS **216**

SKIN PROBLEMS **218**

FAINTING, DIZZINESS,
AND CONVULSIONS **225**

YOUR CHILD'S SAFETY **226**

FIRST AID **229**

GROWTH CHARTS **246**

INDEX **250**

ACKNOWLEDGMENTS **256**

1

PREGNANCY
AND
BIRTH

■ ■ ■ ■ ■

*An illustrated guide to a healthy and happy
pregnancy, incorporating practical
advice for labor and birth.*

THINKING ABOUT PREGNANCY

To give any pregnancy the best possible start, it's a good idea to plan ahead. There are a number of steps you can take, which will not only increase your chances of conception, but will also be your best guarantee of having a normal, healthy baby. Ideally, you and your partner should talk about pregnancy at least three months before you conceive. It is in the first few weeks, when you may not even know you are pregnant, that a baby's development can be most easily affected. So keeping fit and eating well will insure that you have done as much as you can to nourish and protect a baby in your womb. There may be other things to consider, too; perhaps there are hazards at work, which could affect the fetus's health, or maybe you were never vaccinated against German measles as a child.

Planning for pregnancy gives you the time you need to consider these kinds of risks and, if necessary, to do something positive about them.

CHECKLIST FOR PREGNANCY

USE THESE QUESTIONS as a checklist if you want to have a baby or have just discovered that you are pregnant. A few may not apply to you, but it's important to ask yourself all of them. Talk to your partner too, because some of the questions relate directly to him. If any frighten you, see your doctor.

Are you immune to German measles?
German measles, or rubella, can cause serious defects in the baby if you develop it in pregnancy, especially early pregnancy, when the baby's internal organs are forming. So before you become pregnant, ask your doctor for a blood test to make sure that you are immune to the disease. If you are not, your doctor can vaccinate you. Arrange for the test right away because you shouldn't try to become pregnant for at least three months after a vaccination.

Do you or your partner have a family history of inherited disease?
Some medical conditions, such as hemophilia and cystic fibrosis, are inherited. If either you or your partner have a close relative with an inherited disease, there is a chance that it might be passed on to your baby. See your doctor before trying to become pregnant, and if necessary he may refer you to a genetic counselor who can assess the level of risk that you will be taking. It's reassuring to know that, in most cases, it takes both partners carrying the gene to cause a real risk of inheriting the disease.

Do you have a long-standing medical condition?
If you have a medical disorder, such as diabetes or epilepsy, you should talk to your doctor before trying to become pregnant. Your doctor may want to change your drug treatment, either because the drugs you are on might affect the baby, or because they might make it more difficult for you to conceive.

QUESTION & ANSWER

"What is generally the best age to have a baby?"
This is probably in your twenties, although more women are deciding to start a family later in life, when they feel emotionally and financially ready for a baby. Risks of a difficult pregnancy do increase when the mother is over 35, but they are reduced if you are fit and healthy. You are also more likely to have a Down's syndrome baby. Women under 18 run a greater risk of having a stillborn or small baby, but regular visits to the obstetrician and keeping healthy minimize this.

Are you, or have you been, on the pill?
It is best to stop taking the pill several months before you want to conceive, to allow your body time to return to its normal cycle. Wait until you have had three menstrual periods before trying to become pregnant. (Meanwhile, find an alternative means of birth control.) If you conceive before the regular rhythm of your periods has been established again, it may be difficult to predict your due date with reasonable accuracy.

Does your work bring you into contact with any risks?
If you or your partner has a job that involves working with chemicals, lead, anesthesia or X-rays, this may affect your chances of conceiving, or involve a risk to the baby, so talk to your doctor. If possible, consider changing to a safer job before you become pregnant, or at least avoid the risk as much as possible. Once you are pregnant, you should take further steps to protect yourself. Your doctor may also advise you to change jobs if yours involves heavy lifting. Computer VDTs (visual display terminals) are now believed to cause no harm to the developing baby.

How much do you weigh?
Ideally, your weight should be normal for your height for at least six months before conceiving, so if you are seriously over- or underweight, see your doctor for advice on attaining the right weight. Unless you have a serious weight problem, never diet in pregnancy, because you may deprive your body of vital nutrients.

Are you eating a balanced diet?
You will increase your chances of conceiving, and of having a healthy baby, if you eat a properly balanced diet, with plenty of fresh foods.

Do you smoke or drink?
Both you and your mate should stop smoking and drinking as soon as you decide to become pregnant, because tobacco and alcohol can affect fertility in men as well as women. Smoking and drinking can also harm the growing baby (see page 13).

Are you exercising regularly?
To keep fit, aim for at least 20 minutes of exercise each day. Walking or swimming are great before and during pregnancy.

"We planned for pregnancy together; it seemed the natural thing to do."

A PREGNANCY CALENDAR

This month-by-month calendar charts the progress of one pregnancy. If you are pregnant, it will show the changes in your body and emotions as it follows the baby's development from conception to the last days in the womb. There is advice on what to do at each stage, as well as reassuring answers to questions and worries you might have. Each month explains at least one additional relevant aspect of pregnancy, such as options for prenatal classes or measuring yourself for a nursing bra. Every pregnancy varies, so don't be surprised if some of the changes don't happen to you exactly as they are described here. Your weight gain, for example, may differ from the one shown. The calendar begins on day one of pregnancy which is the first day of your last menstrual period, so two weeks after conception, you are already four weeks pregnant.

BECOMING PREGNANT

IF YOU ARE THINKING of becoming pregnant, make sure your lifestyle involves nothing that might harm the baby. All the major organs of his body are formed during the first three months, and it is then that his development can be harmed most easily. Once you have conceived, you will probably know or suspect that you are pregnant because of a number of different signs, such as heavy breasts, or feeling nauseous. Most of these changes are set off by the increase in hormone levels during the early weeks, as your body prepares to nurture the baby. The discomforts often lessen or even disappear completely around week 12.

EARLY SIGNS OF PREGNANCY
One or more of these changes can signify that you are pregnant. You may not notice any of them at first, but still instinctively know you are pregnant because you "feel" different.
■ A missed period—but if your periods are normally irregular, or you are anxious, busy, or ill, this may not be a reliable guide. It is also possible after you have become pregnant to have slight bleeding around the time you would normally expect your period.
■ Enlarged, tender breasts, which may tingle a little.
■ A strange metallic taste in your mouth.
■ Tiredness, not just in the evening, but during the day.
■ Feeling faint, and perhaps dizzy.
■ An increase in normal vaginal discharge.
■ Nausea and perhaps vomiting; this may happen at any time of day.
■ A strong dislike of some things, such as alcohol, coffee, and cigarette smoke, and a craving for others.
■ Feeling unusually emotional (because of hormone changes).
■ A frequent need to urinate.

CONFIRMING THE PREGNANCY
Have the pregnancy confirmed as soon as possible. Your doctor or a family planning clinic can test a urine sample. About two weeks after your first missed period, a hormone will appear in your urine, and this confirms the pregnancy. Alternatively, buy a home pregnancy testing kit from a drugstore and do the test yourself. Your gynecologist may examine you internally to confirm the pregnancy.

HOME PREGNANCY TESTING KITS
All kits contain a chemical solution that you mix with a few drops of urine. Some suggest that you do the test immediately after rising in the morning. Various indicators, such as a color change, will suggest whether or not you are pregnant. These tests are fairly accurate if you follow the instructions carefully, but they can give a false result either way, so always ask your doctor to confirm whether or not you are pregnant.

CALCULATING YOUR DELIVERY DATE

Pregnancy lasts about 266 days from conception to birth. The most likely time of conception is when you ovulate. In a normal 28-day cycle, this happens about 14 days before the next period is due, so to calculate your approximate delivery date, count 280 days (266 plus 14) from the first day of your last period. Remember, this is only a guide. While the average pregnancy is 40 weeks, a normal pregnancy can be anywhere from 38 to 42 weeks long.

WHAT TO AVOID

Avoid smoking, alcohol, and any form of medication, unless confirmed as safe by your doctor, throughout pregnancy but especially in the first three months, when the baby's organs are forming.

Smoking

This deprives the baby of oxygen. Babies of mothers who smoke are more likely to be premature and have a low birthweight. Smoking also increases the chances of having a miscarriage, a stillbirth, a malformed baby, or a baby that dies right after birth. The more you smoke, the greater the risk to the baby, so stop smoking completely. If you really can't give it up entirely, cut down in every way you know how: switch to a low-tar brand, ration the number of cigarettes you smoke, don't inhale, and stub out your cigarette when you've smoked half of it. Doctors now believe that the smoke you breathe in from other people's cigarettes can harm the baby, so encourage your partner to stop smoking, too.

Alcohol

Drinking heavily in pregnancy can seriously affect the developing baby. No one knows what a "safe" level of drinking is, so it's best not to drink at all while pregnant. At any rate, drink no more than two units of alcohol once or twice a week (a unit of alcohol is equivalent to a glass of wine or eight ounces of beer). Avoid hard liquor.

Medication

Many drugs can have harmful or unknown effects on the baby, so avoid taking medication in pregnancy, unless it is prescribed by a doctor who knows you are pregnant. This includes many of the remedies you would normally take for minor complaints, such as aspirin. If you need medication to control a condition such as diabetes, your doctor may have to alter your dose.

Other risks

Cats' and dogs' feces, and raw meat, may contain a parasite called toxoplasma, which can seriously harm the unborn baby. Avoid emptying cat-litter boxes (if you really have to, wear gloves and wash your hands well afterward). Wear gloves for gardening. Wash your hands well after handling raw meat.

THE START OF LIFE

DURING THE FIRST EIGHT WEEKS of pregnancy, the baby develops from a single cell at conception to a fetus that is starting to look human.

CONCEPTION TO WEEK FOUR

1 Ovulation

Around day 14 of your menstrual cycle, a ripe egg is released from one of your ovaries, and fertilization becomes possible. The egg is caught by the fingers at the end of the Fallopian tube, and drawn into it. The egg can survive for up to 24 hours; if it isn't fertilized, it passes out of the vagina with the lining of the womb in your next monthly period.

The swim of the sperm

During orgasm, a man may ejaculate between 200 and 400 million sperm into a woman's vagina. Many spill out again, or are lost along the way, but some swim through the mucus secreted by the cervix (the neck of the womb), which becomes thin and soft around ovulation, and cross the womb into the Fallopian tube. If an egg hasn't been released, the sperm can survive in the tube for up to 48 hours.

Position of the womb

5 Implantation

The fertilized egg begins to embed itself in the soft, thick lining of the womb at about the end of week three. This is called implantation. When the egg is securely attached to the lining of the womb, conception is complete.

Sponge-like fingers from the outer cells of the embryo start to burrow into the lining, to link up with the mother's blood vessels. These later form the placenta. Some of the cells also develop into the umbilical cord, and the membranes that protect the baby. The inner cells divide into three layers, which develop into the different parts of your baby's body.

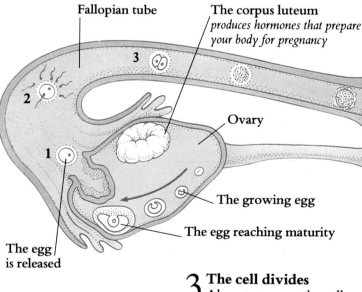

Fallopian tube

The corpus luteum *produces hormones that prepare your body for pregnancy*

Womb

Ovary

The growing egg

The egg reaching maturity

The egg is released

The embryo *embeds itself deep into the womb lining*

The cervix *becomes thin and soft around ovulation, so that sperm can pass through it more easily*

2 Fertilization

Sperm carry a substance that can dissolve the outer covering of the egg, so that one of them can penetrate it. As soon as the successful sperm enters the egg, no other sperm can get through. The sperm loses its tail and its head begins to swell. It fuses with the egg, forming a single cell.

3 The cell divides

Almost at once, the cell starts to divide. It continues to divide into more and more cells as it travels down the Fallopian tube.

4 Reaching the womb

On about the fourth day after fertilization, the egg reaches the cavity of the womb. It has developed into a ball of about 100 cells with a hollow, fluid-filled center, but it is still too small to be seen by the naked eye. For the next few days, it floats around in the womb cavity.

About week six

About week seven

About week eight

WEEKS FIVE TO SIX

■ The embryo is floating in a fluid-filled sac.

■ It has a simple brain, spine, and central nervous system.

■ Four shallow pits have appeared on the head, which will later become the baby's eyes and ears.

■ The embryo has the beginnings of a digestive system, a mouth, and a jaw.

■ The stomach and chest are developing. The heart can be seen as a large bulge at the front of the chest; by the end of the week it will start beating.

■ A system of blood vessels is forming.

■ Four tiny limb buds have developed.

Length: The embryo is now ¼in. (6mm.), about the size of an apple seed.

WEEK SEVEN

■ The head looks large and is bent on to the chest. A face is forming, though the eyes are on the sides of the head and still sealed. Black pigment can be seen under the skin overlying the eyes.

■ The arms and legs are clearly visible, with clefts at the end, which become fingers and toes.

■ The heart starts to circulate blood around the embryo's body.

■ The outline of the baby's nervous system is already nearly complete.

■ Bone cells are beginning to develop.

■ The embryo has lungs, an intestine, a liver, kidneys and internal sex organs, but all are not yet fully formed.

Length: The embryo is now ½in. (1.3cm.), about the size of a small grape.

WEEK EIGHT

■ The embryo can now be called a fetus, which means "young one."

■ All the major internal organs have developed, although they are still in a simple form, and may not be in their final position.

■ A face is recognizable: the nose seems to have a tip, the nostrils have formed, and the two sides of the jaw have joined to make a mouth. A tongue has already formed.

■ The inner parts of the ears, responsible for balance and hearing, are forming.

■ The fingers and toes are becoming more distinct, though they are joined by webs of skin.

■ The arms and legs have grown longer, and shoulders, elbows, hips, and knees are detectable.

■ The baby moves around a lot, although you can't feel him yet.

Length: The baby is now 1in. (2.5cm.), about the size of a strawberry.

TWINS

About one in 80 pregnancies results in twins. If twins run in your family, your chances of having them are greater. **Fraternal twins** occur when two separate eggs are fertilized by two separate sperm. They are three times as common as identical twins. The twins each have their own placenta, may or may not be the same sex, and are no more alike than any other brothers or sisters. **Identical twins** are produced when the egg that is fertilized divides into two separate halves, each of which develops into an identical baby. The twins share a placenta, are always of the same sex, and have the same physical characteristics and genetic makeup.

QUESTION & ANSWER

"Can I do anything to influence the baby's sex?"
The baby's sex is determined by the man's sperm. Research suggests that male sperm swim faster but don't survive as long as female sperm, so you may increase your chances of having a boy if you make love when you are most fertile (about 14 days before your period is due); and your chances of having a girl are greater if you have intercourse up to three days *before* you next expect to be fertile.

WEEK 12

THE BABY LOOKS much more human, although his head is still large in proportion to his body, and his limbs, although fully formed, are small. The discomforts of early pregnancy may begin to wear off. Make sure you have scheduled an appointment with an obstetrician or midwife by now.

Get into the habit *of always standing straight, to help you in later pregnancy*

Position of the womb

SEE ALSO:
Prenatal checkups
pages 34–36
Prenatal exercises
pages 45–47
Healthy eating
pages 50–53
Frequent urination
page 41
Morning sickness
page 41
Pregnancy bra
page 23
Protecting your back
page 44

■ CHANGES IN YOU ■

- If you've been feeling nauseous because of morning sickness, this should start to ease.
- You will probably find that you don't need to urinate as often as you did in the early weeks of pregnancy.
- You may still be emotional, and easily upset by little things, because of hormone changes.
- Constipation may be a problem, because bowel movements tend to slow down in pregnancy.
- The volume of blood circulating in your body is increasing, so your lungs, kidneys, and heart have to work harder.

Your breasts *will feel heavier, and may be tender*

Your shape *is probably still much the same as usual*

The top *of the womb can be felt just above your pubic bone*

The external ears *are well developed*

Tiny fingers *and toes have formed*

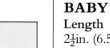

YOUR WEIGHT GAIN		YOUR BABY
The first three months		**Length** 2½in. (6.5cm.)
If vomiting has not been a problem for you, you may have gained 2¼lb. (1.2kg.), about 10% of total pregnancy weight gain. Model's total weight gain at week 12: 4½lb. (2kg.)	10%	**Weight** ⅝oz. (18g.)

PRENATAL CLASSES

START THINKING about the type of class that will best suit you and your partner. You might find an introductory class now—on ways to stay healthy during pregnancy, for example—but prepared childbirth classes themselves start eight to ten weeks before the baby is due. Prenatal exercise classes can continue throughout pregnancy.

CHOOSING A CLASS

Prepared childbirth classes are run by hospitals, individual instructors, as well as various organizations and local groups such as the YWCA. To find one, start by checking the professional advertising section of a newspaper geared for your neighborhood, or any community bulletin boards you see regularly. Ask your doctor, midwife, or friends for recommendations. Make sure that you reserve a spot early in your second trimester even if classes won't begin until you are 28 to 32 weeks pregnant. Most feature a weekly two-hour session, scheduled over a six- to eight-week period. To find the one that suits your feelings about pregnancy, labor, and delivery best, you might want to observe a session before you sign up.

Basics of babycare
It's fun and helpful to learn how to take care of your baby in a class.

What will you learn?

Though the course content may vary according to the philosophy of the instructor, all childbirth classes teach couples basic information about pregnancy, the stages and pain of labor and delivery, stress relaxation techniques, physical exercises, medication and anesthesia, and everything you might need to know about different hospital procedures and policies. In fact, a tour of the hospital is often part of the curriculum. Childbirth classes can be invaluable for first-time mothers and fathers, and even in a second or third pregnancy the review is almost always worthwhile. Most emphasize the close working relationship a woman will want to have with the person she chooses to have by her side during the birth, her labor partner. If your baby's father isn't going to be able to be there, a relative or close friend can join in the preparation. Some classes cover the postnatal period and will include tips on caring for a newborn, breast-feeding, postpartum depression, and exercises for getting back into shape.

Tips for labor
Massage is one of the techniques you and your partner may be taught to help you cope with labor.

WHAT TO DO

- Buy a bra that will support your breasts well.
- Make sure you are eating a varied diet of fresh foods.
- Guard against constipation by drinking plenty of water and eating high-fiber foods.
- Make an appointment with your dentist for a checkup.
- Tell your employer that you are pregnant, so that you can adjust your work schedule.
- Find an obstetrician and arrange for your first checkup.
- Bring along any insurance company identification and ask the nurse or receptionist how benefits and payments will be handled during the pregnancy.
- Practice prenatal exercises. Go swimming or walking.
- Enroll in prenatal exercise classes if you want to.
- Find out about other prenatal classes in your area.

YOUR GROWING BABY

- All of the internal organs are formed, and most are working, so the baby is far less likely to be harmed by infections or drugs.
- The eyelids have developed, and are closed over the eyes.
- The baby has earlobes.
- The limbs are formed, with fingers and toes.
- Miniature fingernails and toenails are growing.
- Muscles are developing, so the baby moves much more. He can curl and fan his toes. He can make a fist.
- He can move the muscles of his mouth to frown, purse his lips, and open and close his mouth.
- He can suck, and he swallows the fluid that surrounds him. He can urinate.

WEEK 16

NOW INTO the second three months of pregnancy, you should be feeling healthier and more energetic than in your first trimester. You will begin to look pregnant and will need looser clothes. Your baby is fully formed, and has been nourished by the placenta since week 14. Over the remaining weeks, he will grow and mature so that he will be capable of independent life at birth.

Moles and freckles *may become darker with the increase in skin pigmentation*

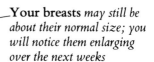

Position of the womb

SEE ALSO:
AFP test page 37
Amniocentesis page 37
Healthy eating pages 50–53
Relaxation and breathing pages 48–49
Skin color page 21
Smoking page 13
Supplements page 52
Ultrasound page 37

■ CHANGES IN YOU ■

- Morning sickness may stop.
- There will be a growing feeling of excitement and anticipation.
- Your nipples and the surrounding skin may darken, and a dark line (the linea nigra) may appear down the center of your stomach. This fades after birth.
- Your appetite will increase.
- Your ordinary clothes will probably be too tight, but you may not be quite ready for maternity clothes.
- Sleeping on your side is probably best for you and your baby from now on.

Your breasts *may still be about their normal size; you will notice them enlarging over the next weeks*

You will *start to lose your waistline*

Your pregnancy *starts to show as a gentle rounding of the stomach*

His head *looks too large for his body*

The baby *has a neck now*

His fingers *have their own unique fingerprint pattern*

YOUR WEIGHT GAIN
The second three months
During the next three months you can expect to gain about 11–15$\frac{1}{2}$lb. (5–7 kg.), 50 to 60% of total pregnancy weight gain. Model's total weight gain at week 16: 5$\frac{1}{2}$lb. (2.5kg.)

60%

YOUR BABY
Length
6in. (16cm.)
Weight
4$\frac{3}{4}$oz. (135g.)

- Give up smoking if you have not already done so. Encourage your partner to do the same.
- Don't use any increase in your appetite as an excuse to eat the wrong kinds of foods; eat nutritiously and watch weight gain.
- Start to take iron and folic acid supplements if they have been prescribed by your doctor. Take supplements on a full stomach.
- Obstetrical visits are scheduled once a month now. An ultrasound scan and an AFP blood test may be done if your doctor needs to pinpoint your due date or clear up any worries. Amniocentesis is also done now if there is any chance of the baby being abnormal.

■ YOUR GROWING BABY ■

- The eyebrows and eyelashes are growing, and the baby has fine downy hair on his face and body (known as lanugo).
- His skin is so thin that it is transparent; networks of blood vessels can be seen underneath.
- Joints have formed in his arms and legs and hard bones are beginning to develop.
- His sex organs are sufficiently mature for his sex to be evident, but this is not always detectable by an ultrasound scan.
- The baby makes breathing movements with his chest.
- He can suck his thumb.
- He moves around vigorously, but you probably won't be able to feel him yet.
- His heart is beating about twice as fast as your own; the doctor or midwife can now hear it with a special listening device after week 14 of your pregnancy.
- The baby grows rapidly during this month.

MIXED FEELINGS

YOU AND YOUR PARTNER are bound to have mixed emotions about the pregnancy, so don't be surprised if as well as feeling elated and excited, you sometimes feel anxious or sad. Try to tolerate and understand any negative feelings; they are normal emotions.

COMMON WORRIES

The best way to dispel any worries that you may have about the baby or parenthood is to talk about them frankly with each other. It also helps to find out as much as you can about pregnancy, so you understand the changes taking place.

You

It's only natural for your feelings of excitement and anticipation to be clouded sometimes by negative thoughts. You may worry about loving the baby, but once he's born and you get to know each other, love will grow. You may also feel depressed about your changing shape, and even resent the baby for putting your body through such strains. But most major bodily changes disappear after birth, and with some gentle exercising your shape will return.

Your partner

The baby may become a reality for the first time when you see him on an ultrasound screen. Up to now you may have felt left out, and perhaps jealous of all the attention your mate and the baby have been receiving. If you're worried about money and having enough to support your new family, try to plan and budget.

Both of you

It's normal to feel excited about the new baby, yet to worry that you're not yet ready for parenthood. If you're anxious about labor and birth, learn all about them, and practice techniques, such as deep breathing, so you can feel more confident and in control when the time comes.

QUESTION & ANSWER

"How can I be sure the baby will be all right?"
The chances of the baby being abnormal are very small. Most abnormalities occur in the first weeks, and end in an early miscarriage. By week 13 the baby is fully formed and very little can go wrong. Make sure that your lifestyle involves nothing that could harm him, and you can reduce the risk even further.

WEEK 20

YOU WILL PROBABLY have a strong sense of well-being during the middle months of pregnancy. Some women look and feel radiant because of noticeable improvements in skin and hair. If you're feeling well, it's often a good idea to take a vacation. You should have had the excitement of hearing the fetal heartbeat and feeling the baby move by now.

■ CHANGES IN YOU ■

■ Any skin pigmentation problem may become more noticeable, but it will return to normal after birth.

■ Your breasts may produce colostrum, a thin cloudy fluid that will provide all the nourishment your baby needs in the first days. Wipe it away with a tissue; don't try to squeeze more out.

■ You may be suffering from some of the common problems of pregnancy, such as bleeding gums and an increase in vaginal discharge. The joints and ligaments of your body have relaxed, so you are more likely to suffer from back trouble and other aches and pains.

Position of the womb

You will first feel *your baby moving as faint flutterings inside your abdomen, like bubbles rising*

SEE ALSO:
Common complaints
pages 40–42
Healthy eating
pages 50–53
Essentials for the baby
page 27
Protecting your back
page 44

Your nipples *become darker during pregnancy*

Your breasts *will probably have increased dramatically in size by now*

The top *of the womb is level with your navel*

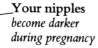

The baby *can grip firmly with his hands*

His legs *are in proportion to the rest of his body*

YOUR WEIGHT GAIN
at around week 20 of pregnancy
During this month you can expect to gain about 1lb. (0.5kg.) a week. Take extra care to eat nutritious foods now: the next few weeks mark the period of maximum growth for the baby and maximum weight gain for you.
Model's weight gain to date: 6½lb. (3kg.)

YOUR BABY
Length
10in. (25cm.)
Weight
12oz. (340g.)

QUESTION & ANSWER

"Is a long trip advisable?"
There's usually no reason you shouldn't travel during pregnancy, but don't go alone, especially on a long car trip. Wear loose, comfortable clothes, and break any drive up by walking around for a few minutes every two hours, to help your circulation. If you are flying or on a train, get up and stretch your legs in the aisles every couple of hours.

■ YOUR GROWING BABY ■

■ Hair appears on the baby's head.
■ Teeth are developing.
■ Vernix, the white greasy substance that protects the baby's skin in the womb, forms.
■ The baby's arms and legs are well developed.
■ Protective substances may be transferred to the baby through your blood to help him resist disease in the first weeks.
■ The baby is very active; you should have felt his movements for the first time as a faint fluttering. He may even react to noises outside the womb, but don't worry if he doesn't move around much; it's fairly common for babies to have quiet periods.

LOOKING GOOD

YOU MAY LOOK and feel your best during the middle months of pregnancy, with lustrous hair, rosy cheeks, and smooth, healthy skin. But not everyone blooms; the high hormone levels can have less flattering effects on skin, nails, and hair, though any adverse changes usually disappear after birth.

HAIR
Thick, shiny hair is often a bonus of pregnancy. However, not all hair improves: oily hair may become more oily, and dry hair, drier and more brittle. You may lose more hair than usual. Facial and body hair also tends to darken.

Have *your hair cut into a style that is easy to take care of*

Your skin *may become smooth and blemish-free*

What to do If your hair is dry and ends split easily, use a mild shampoo and conditioner, and don't brush it too often or too vigorously. Wash oily hair frequently to keep it shiny. Hair is unpredictable in pregnancy, so avoid perms or having it colored now.

SKIN TEXTURE
Your skin may improve in pregnancy: blemishes can disappear, and skin texture sometimes becomes smooth and silky. However, you may find that your skin becomes very dry, oily, perhaps blotchy.
What to do Cleanse thoroughly. If it is dry, gently rub moisturizer over the dry areas, and add bath oil to your bath water. Use as little soap as possible.

NAILS
You may notice that your nails split and break more easily than usual.
What to do Wear gloves for household chores and gardening.

SKIN COLOR
An increase in skin pigmentation is normal during pregnancy. Moles, birthmarks, scars, and freckles usually darken and grow in size, and a brown line often appears down the center of your stomach. You may notice a brownish patch, or "butterfly mask," across your face and neck. Don't worry—this disappears soon after the birth.
What to do Avoid strong sunlight because it can make pigmentation problems worse, but if you go out in the sun, use a sunscreen with maximum protection. Don't bleach the mask; if you want to disguise it, try makeup or a blemish covering stick.

WEEK 24

THIS IS OFTEN the best month of pregnancy. You will probably look well, and feel happy and contented. If you have not gained much weight so far, you'll start to put on pounds this month. You'll be visibly pregnant—finally!

Extra weight *on your upper arms or shoulders may be the result of water retention*

Position of the womb

SEE ALSO:
Prenatal exercises
pages 45–47
Pregnancy clothes
page 25
Relaxation and breathing
pages 48–49

■ CHANGES IN YOU ■

■ Loose-fitting clothes will be more comfortable now.
■ Sweating may be a problem because when you are pregnant, your body temperature is slightly higher so you feel the heat more. Drink lots of water, and avoid wearing clothes made of synthetic fabrics that don't "breathe."

Your face *may look puffy because your body retains extra water*

Your areolas, *the dark areas around your nipples, may become more prominent*

Your belly *is enlarging rapidly*

His skin *is becoming thicker*

His eyes *bulge because his face is thin*

YOUR WEIGHT GAIN at around week 24 of pregnancy	YOUR BABY
You will probably continue to gain weight at the rate of about 1lb. (0.5kg.) a week, although if you were underweight when your pregnancy began you might gain at a faster rate than this. Model's weight gain to date: 10lb. (4.5kg.)	**Length** 13in. (33cm.) **Weight** 1¼lb. (570g.)

THE BABY IN THE WOMB

WHILE THE BABY is developing physically, he is also on the way to becoming an aware, responsive person with feelings. He lies tightly curled up in the womb, cushioned by the bag of waters that surrounds him, entirely reliant on your placenta for food, oxygen, and the disposal of his waste products. However, he looks and behaves much the same as the baby he will be at birth.

SIGHT
His eyelids are still sealed, but by week 28, they become unsealed, and he may see, and open and close his eyes.

HEARING
He can hear your voice, and if he's asleep can be awakened by loud music. He may prefer some types of music, and show this by his movements. He jumps at sudden noises.

FACIAL EXPRESSIONS
He frowns, squints, purses his lips, and opens and closes his mouth.

LIFE-SUPPORT SYSTEM
The baby is nourished by the placenta and protected by warm amniotic fluid, which can change every four hours. It regulates the baby's temperature, and protects against infection and sudden bumps.

MOVEMENTS
He kicks and punches, and sometimes turns somersaults. He can make a fist.

SLEEPING PATTERNS
He sleeps and wakes randomly, and will probably be most active when you are trying to sleep.

PERSONALITY
The part of the brain concerned with personality and intelligence becomes far more complex during the seventh month, so his personality may soon be developing.

SUCKING, SWALLOWING, AND BREATHING
He sucks his thumb, and swallows the warm water (the amniotic fluid) that surrounds him, passing it out of his body as urine. Sometimes he drinks too much of the fluid and hiccups. He makes breathing movements with his chest, practicing for life outside the womb.

TASTE
His taste buds are forming, and by week 28 he can respond to sweet, sour, and bitter tastes.

The placenta *supplies all the nutrients the baby needs; almost anything entering your body, good or bad, is filtered through to him*

The umbilical cord, *a rope of three blood vessels, links the placenta to the baby*

WEEK 28

YOU ARE NOW entering the home stretch, with only three months to go. If you are feeling huge and clumsy, it's because your baby is gaining weight in the form of fat. This makes his skin tone change from red to a flesh color. His activity may startle you when he moves and your midriff shifts dramatically. If he were born now, he could survive with special care.

Stand tall *to avoid developing a swayback as you grow larger*

Position of the womb

Weight gain *can be on your buttocks and thighs, as well as your stomach*

SEE ALSO:
Common complaints pages 40–42
Protecting your back page 44
Stretch marks page 42

■ CHANGES IN YOU ■

■ Some of the common problems of pregnancy may be troubling you, such as heartburn, indigestion, and muscle cramps.
■ You may notice red stretch marks on your stomach.
■ Faint Braxton Hicks, or false, contractions are sometimes felt now. They are not usually painful.
■ You may be having vivid dreams about the birth and the baby. This is normal; the dreams can be caused by discomfort in bed, the baby's movements, or very real anxiety. They do not indicate that there is anything wrong with your baby.

The veins *on your breasts will probably become more noticeable*

The top *of the womb is about halfway between your navel and breastbone*

His eyes *have become unsealed*

His face and body *are covered with vernix, which waterproofs the skin*

Hearing *is well developed*

YOUR WEIGHT GAIN
The third three months
During the final months you will probably gain about 9lb. (4kg.), 30 to 40% of total pregnancy weight gain. Model's total weight gain at week 28: 19lb. (9kg.)

30%

YOUR BABY
Length
14½in. (37cm.)
Weight
2–2¼lb. (900g.–1kg.)

YOUR PREGNANCY WARDROBE

▪ YOUR GROWING BABY ▪

▪ His skin is red and wrinkled, but fat is accumulating beneath it, making it more flesh-colored.

▪ There have been dramatic developments in the thinking part of the brain. It's now bigger and more complex. A seven-month-old fetus can feel pain and respond much like a full-term baby.

▪ Research has shown that the baby has more taste buds than he will have at birth, so his sense of taste is acute.

▪ His lungs are still not fully mature, and need to develop a substance called surfactant, which stops them from collapsing between each breath.

▪ You can feel the baby move if you put your hand on your stomach. You may even see the shape of a foot or bottom as the baby kicks and turns.

UNTIL THE FIFTH or even sixth month of your pregnancy, many of your normal clothes may be wearable if they fit loosely or you use a little creativity. However, new outfits may greatly improve your morale. You don't always have to buy special maternity wear. Look for loose-fitting clothes that are attractive, comfortable, and easy to care for from the regular departments in the stores.

Loose tops
Baggy T-shirts, blouses, sweat shirts and sweaters look and feel good, and can be worn after the birth. Make sure that the top is large and long.

Loosen *the cord as the bulge gets larger*

Stretchy bottoms
Sweatpants with a drawstring waist are comfortable and unrestricting; adapt the waistline by replacing any elastic in the waist with a plain cord.

Dressing up
A jumper is basic and a good buy. Slip a blouse or T-shirt underneath on cool days; wear it like a sundress when it's warm. See if there's enough fabric in the hem so you can adjust the length in front as you grow larger. Maternity dresses are usually 1in. (2.5cm.) longer in the front.

WHAT TO CHOOSE
You tend to feel the heat more during pregnancy, so look for lightweight, loose-fitting clothes made of cotton or other natural fibers. If it's cold, put on layers. Avoid anything tight at the waist or that restricts blood flow in your legs, such as tight knee-high socks.

Comfortable, low-heeled shoes are essential, although completely flat heels may not be as comfortable as ones with a slight lift. It may soon be difficult to lean over to tie shoes or sneakers that lace up.

Choose *a style with plenty of room under the arms and across the chest, because your breasts will grow*

A low *front opening is practical for breast-feeding after the birth*

Make sure *there isn't a restricting waist or belt*

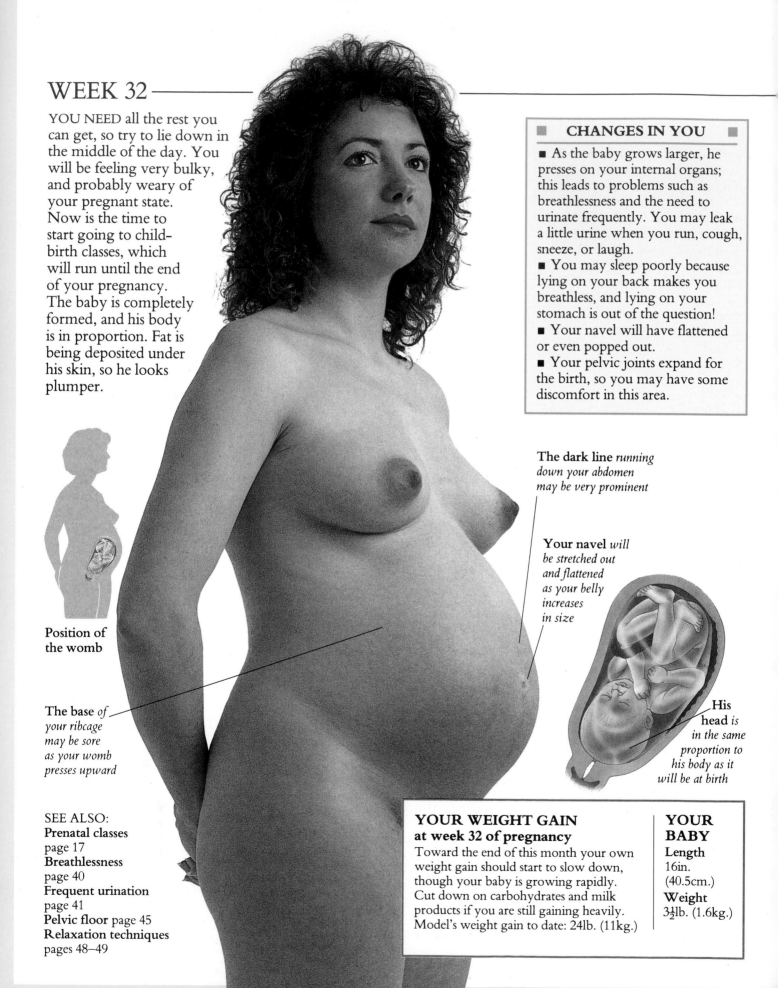

WEEK 32

YOU NEED all the rest you can get, so try to lie down in the middle of the day. You will be feeling very bulky, and probably weary of your pregnant state. Now is the time to start going to child-birth classes, which will run until the end of your pregnancy. The baby is completely formed, and his body is in proportion. Fat is being deposited under his skin, so he looks plumper.

Position of the womb

The base *of your ribcage may be sore as your womb presses upward*

SEE ALSO:
Prenatal classes
page 17
Breathlessness
page 40
Frequent urination
page 41
Pelvic floor page 45
Relaxation techniques
pages 48–49

■ CHANGES IN YOU ■

■ As the baby grows larger, he presses on your internal organs; this leads to problems such as breathlessness and the need to urinate frequently. You may leak a little urine when you run, cough, sneeze, or laugh.
■ You may sleep poorly because lying on your back makes you breathless, and lying on your stomach is out of the question!
■ Your navel will have flattened or even popped out.
■ Your pelvic joints expand for the birth, so you may have some discomfort in this area.

The dark line *running down your abdomen may be very prominent*

Your navel *will be stretched out and flattened as your belly increases in size*

His head *is in the same proportion to his body as it will be at birth*

YOUR WEIGHT GAIN
at week 32 of pregnancy
Toward the end of this month your own weight gain should start to slow down, though your baby is growing rapidly. Cut down on carbohydrates and milk products if you are still gaining heavily. Model's weight gain to date: 24lb. (11kg.)

YOUR BABY
Length
16in.
(40.5cm.)
Weight
3½lb. (1.6kg.)

WHAT TO DO

- Break up the day by putting your feet up for an hour or two if possible.
- If you have difficulty sleeping, practice relaxation techniques before going to bed, and sleep on your side, with one leg bent and your stomach supported on a pillow. Try not to worry if you can't sleep; some insomnia is normal at this stage. All the adverse symptoms can conspire against you at night. Don't toss and turn—get up and do something.
- Keep up with your pelvic floor exercises; this is especially important if you leak urine.
- Start attending prenatal classes if you haven't already.

QUESTION & ANSWER

"I'm worried about harming the baby during intercourse. Is there any danger of this?"

This is a common worry, but an unnecessary one if your pregnancy is normal. The baby is protected and cushioned by the bag of fluid surrounding him, so he can't be harmed when you make love. The doctor or midwife will warn you if there are any dangers, such as a low placenta.

YOUR GROWING BABY

- The baby looks much the same as at birth, but his body still needs to fill out more.
- He can now tell the difference between light and dark.
- Because there is less room in the womb, he may have turned into a head-down position by now, ready for birth.

ESSENTIALS FOR YOUR BABY

Choose *a style of suit with snaps up the front and around the thighs and crotch*

BUY THE FOLLOWING basic items for your new baby. You can always add items after the birth.

EQUIPMENT
You will need:
- a carriage, crib, or bassinet for your baby to sleep in
- appropriate bedding
- a soft blanket
    - bottle-feeding equipment if you are going to bottle-feed
    - baby bathtub
    - two soft towels
    - changing mat or table
    - diaper-changing equipment and diapers
- an infant car seat, if you have a car; some can double as infant seats.

CLOTHES
These should be marked "newborn." You will need:
- six undershirts
- eight stretchsuits
- two sweaters
- two infant sleeping or drawstring gowns
- two pairs of soft socks or bootees
- sun hat or woolen hat.

ENJOYING SEX

MAKING LOVE is often particularly enjoyable during pregnancy. Some women become aroused more easily as a result of the increase in hormone levels. And there are no worries about contraception.

OTHER WAYS OF LOVING
There may be times when you lose interest in sex, especially in the first and last weeks. This doesn't mean that you have to stop loving each other physically. Even if you feel too tired or heavy to make love, find other ways to show your affection, such as kissing, cuddling, stroking, and touching.

A CHANGE OF POSITION
In the last weeks of pregnancy, you may find the traditional man-on-top position difficult. Experiment with other positions; perhaps try sitting on your partner's lap, kneeling with him behind, or both lying side by side.

WEEK 36

BY NOW you should have started to wind your life down in preparation for the birth. You may be longing for the pregnancy to be over, yet feeling apprehensive about labor, birth, and becoming a parent. In fact, your emotions can swing wildly. The baby takes up all the space in the womb, so he kicks and punches rather than shifting his body. If he were born now, he would have a high chance of survival.

Position of the womb

The baby's head *may have dropped even further into your pelvis*

SEE ALSO:
Essentials for the baby page 27
Frequent urination page 41
Preparing for the birth pages 54–55
Protecting your back page 42
Relaxation techniques pages 48–49
Swollen ankles page 42
Varicose veins page 42

■ **CHANGES IN YOU** ■

■ Heartburn, indigestion, and breathlessness should lessen once the baby's head drops into the pelvis.
■ Your bladder is under pressure, so you may need to urinate even more frequently.
■ You may be feeling tired but frustrated because your "nesting instinct"—that impulse to clean and straighten your home—may be at its height. Don't tackle every drawer and closet, or try to wallpaper the baby's room by yourself. You'll put yourself and your unborn baby in danger.

Your growing belly *is really altering your usual weight distribution, so concentrate on good posture*

The baby's shape *is more rounded because fat is being stored.*

His skin *is pink*

His hair *may have grown as much as 2in. (5cm.)*

YOUR WEIGHT GAIN
at week 36 of pregnancy
The rate of gain will have slowed, and by week 38 may stop. If the total is less than 28½lb. (13kg.), you should easily return to your pre-pregnancy weight.
Model's weight gain to date: 26lb. (12kg.)

YOUR BABY
Length
18in. (46cm.)
Weight
5½lb. (2.5kg.)

RESTING IN LATER PREGNANCY

DURING THE LAST WEEKS, you will probably become tired very easily. You may not be sleeping as well as usual, and you will also feel exhausted by the extra weight you have been carrying around. It's important not to fight this tiredness, but to rest and relax as much as possible.

TO AVOID TIRING YOURSELF

Put your feet up whenever you need to during the day. Think of quiet things to do while you rest: practice gentle relaxation exercises, listen to soothing music, read a book or maga-zine, or perhaps knit something for the baby. It also helps if you try to do things at a slower pace than usual, so that you don't become overtired.

QUESTION & ANSWER

"Should I have my partner with me during labor?"
Most hospitals and childbirth experts actively encourage this. Labor can be a long process, and a lonely one unless you have someone close to share it with. The natural choice is your baby's father. But if he really doesn't want to be there, it's unfair to put too much pressure on him. It's quite acceptable to have a relative or a good friend there instead.

■ YOUR GROWING BABY ■

■ If this is your first baby, his head will probably have descended into the pelvis, ready for birth.
■ Soft nails have grown to the tips of his fingers and toes.
■ In a boy, the testicles should have descended.
■ The baby will gain about 1oz. (28g.) every day for the remaining four weeks in the womb.

YOUR NURSING BRA

IF YOU WANT to breast-feed your baby after birth, you will need at least two front-opening nursing bras. To make sure these are the right size, it's best to buy them no earlier than week 36.

WHAT TO LOOK FOR

There are two main types of bra: one has flaps, which open to expose the nipple and surrounding breast; the other fastens in front between the cups, so you can expose the whole breast. The front-opening kind is best, because it allows the baby to feel and touch as much of the breast as possible. This helps your milk letdown reflex (see pages 93 and 96). Look for plain cotton and wide straps.

MEASURING YOURSELF

Take the measurements while wearing one of your ordinary pregnancy bras. If you're in any doubt about the right size of bra to buy, ask a salesperson to help you.

1 Using a standard dressmaker's tape measure, measure under your breasts for the bra size.

2 Measure around the fullest part of your breasts for the cup size.

WEEK 40

AT THIS FINAL count-down, you may experience waves of doubt and fear mixed with exhilaration. Your body's ungainly proportions don't help your mood either. If you haven't decided on a baby's name yet, this is a wonderful way to preoccupy your mind.

■ CHANGES IN YOU ■

■ Every movement takes a great deal of effort.
■ You will have a feeling of heaviness in your lower abdomen.
■ Your cervix will be softening in preparation for labor.
■ Braxton Hicks contractions may be so noticeable that you think you are in labor. If they aren't regular, it's not true labor.

Your skin *will feel stretched and taut across your abdomen, and may be itchy*

Your belly *will be so large that you have difficulty getting comfortable in bed*

His fingernails *may be so sharp that he scratches himself with them*

Position of the womb

You may have *pins and needles in your legs*

He looks *much plumper*

SEE ALSO:
Braxton Hicks contractions
page 56
Breathing techniques
page 49

YOUR WEIGHT GAIN
at week 40 of pregnancy
In the final two weeks you may actually lose a little weight. This is a sign that your baby is fully mature, and you can expect labor to start within 10 days.
Model's weight gain: 26lb. (12kg.) same as at week 36.

YOUR BABY
Length
20in. (51cm.)
Weight
7½lb. (3.4kg.)

BEFORE BIRTH

- Rest as much as possible, and enjoy these last baby-free days.
- If you don't feel at least ten movements from your baby during the day, ask your doctor or midwife to check his heart because he may be in distress.
- If you're having Braxton Hicks contractions, use them to practice breathing techniques.
- Don't worry if your baby doesn't arrive on time; it's perfectly normal for a baby to be born two weeks on either side of the expected delivery date.

TOTAL WEIGHT GAIN

The average amount of weight gain during pregnancy varies between 22 to 27lb. (10 and 12kg.), but you may put on more or less weight. The total weight gain is made up as follows:

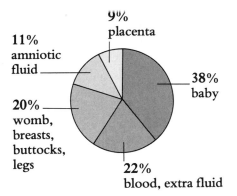

9%
placenta

11%
amniotic
fluid

38%
baby

20%
womb,
breasts,
buttocks,
legs

22%
blood, extra fluid

YOUR UNBORN BABY

- Most of the lanugo hair has disappeared, though there may still be a little on his shoulders, arms, and legs.
- He may still be covered in vernix, or just have traces left in his folds of skin.
- A dark, tar-like substance called meconium gathers in the baby's intestines; this will be passed in his first bowel movements after birth (see page 146).

AFTER THE BIRTH

AFTER ALL the weeks of preparation and planning, you can now hold your baby in your arms. You may feel overwhelmingly protective yet tentative toward this tiny person, so dependent on you for everything.

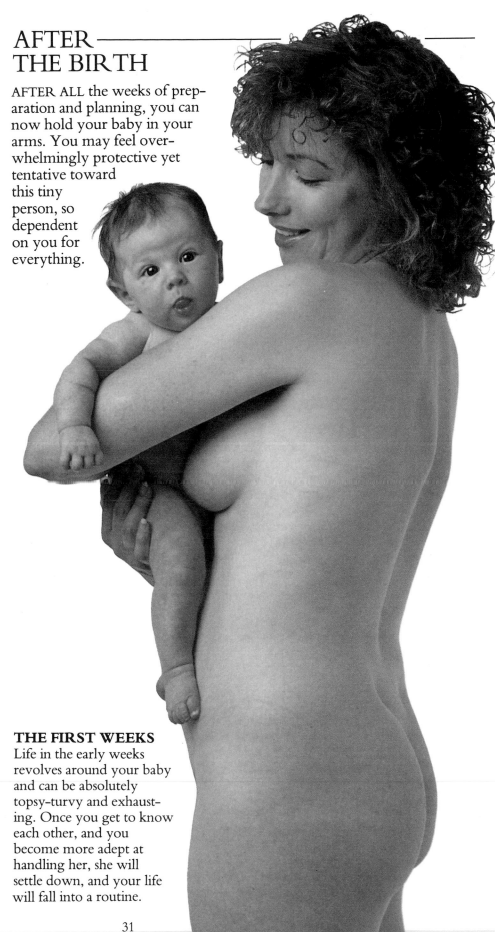

THE FIRST WEEKS

Life in the early weeks revolves around your baby and can be absolutely topsy-turvy and exhausting. Once you get to know each other, and you become more adept at handling her, she will settle down, and your life will fall into a routine.

PRENATAL CARE

Taking good care of yourself and your growing baby during pregnancy is critical. Soon after you miss your first period or your pregnancy is confirmed using an at-home test kit, your prenatal care should begin. This modern system of regular visits to the physician or midwife who will eventually deliver your baby offers mothers-to-be reassuring checks, tests, and a constant source of answers to those troubling questions. Some women stay with their regular physician, others want to find a new specialist. Talk to friends who have recently given birth and ask for recommendations. The more information you can gather, the better your birth experience will be. The important thing is to start your prenatal care early.

WHERE TO HAVE YOUR BABY

ONE OF THE FIRST DECISIONS you will need to make is where to have your baby. Most babies today are born in a hospital. Some hospitals now feature birthing rooms, which are more homelike than typical labor and delivery settings. There are also childbirth centers usually staffed by midwives. And, occasionally it is possible to have your baby at home, providing your obstetrician or midwife is agreeable.

HOSPITAL BIRTH
A hospital offers all the equipment and expertise available for giving pain medication, for monitoring the baby's progress, for intervening in the birth to help you and the baby if necessary, and for providing emergency care to you both. After the birth, a few days in the hospital may give you the rest you need to cope at home later; the average stay is about 48 hours, but you may have the option of staying as long as ten days. If you are a first-time mother, you may also find the support of staff and other mothers reassuring.

Take a hospital tour
Because hospital policies regarding labor and delivery vary tremendously across the country, some women decide to tour nearby medical centers before arranging their first prenatal visit with an obstetrician. Not all doctors are on staff or affiliated at all hospitals in a geographical area.

Call ahead and ask if you and your mate can see the obstetrical unit to learn all about family-centered births, special labor and delivery rooms, and visiting hours for husbands or siblings. Seek recommendations from women who have recently become mothers; word-of-mouth tips are often the best. After you settle on a hospital, you can gather the names of physicians whose patients deliver there.

Birthing rooms
In a traditional hospital birth, a woman labors in one room, and immediately before her baby is ready to be born, she is moved to a special delivery or operating room. However, in recent years, more hospitals have realized that moving a patient at that critical moment in giving birth is not always appropriate. As family-centered births have become more popular, birthing rooms have popped up on many a medical center scene.

Designed for women who are in a low-risk category and expect to deliver their babies normally, these rooms are often more homelike than typical operating rooms, and expectant couples can remain together in an informal setting. A birthing bed, one with a split frame that separates the bottom half from the head of the bed at the time of delivery, is often available, too. Ask about these options; sometimes if you don't inquire you won't be put on a birthing room reservation list.

BIRTHING CENTERS
These are small out-of-hospital facilities where normal, low-risk births can be handled. They are fairly new on the American childbirth scene and are staffed by midwives and nurses, with obstetricians usually on call for special assistance. Checkups, childbirth classes, and some routine prenatal tests as well as normal childbirth are available at these centers.

For the one nearest you, contact the American College of Nurse Midwives, 1522 K Street NW, Suite 1000, Washington, D.C. 20005. Send a self-addressed stamped envelope to speed your reply.

HOME BIRTH
If you are healthy, under 35, and your pregnancy is progressing normally, you may feel that you would be more relaxed and able to cope during labor with your family and familiar objects around you.

It may be difficult arranging a home birth, though. Most doctors are unwilling to deliver a baby at home, especially if there is any likelihood of complications. If your obstetrician can't help, write to the American College of Nurse Midwives (see address above). Explain that you would like a home birth and ask them to refer you to a midwife who has delivered babies at home.

CHOOSING AN OBSTETRICIAN

The American College of Obstetricians and Gynecologists can provide you with a list of specialists in your area. Their resource center is located at 409 Twelfth Street SW, Washington, D.C. 20024. There are other physicians who can manage your pregnancy, too, such as family practitioners. What is crucial for you is to find someone you feel comfortable with and who really understands your needs. You should never be made to feel stupid or that your problems are insignificant. Go to an initial appointment with a written list of questions and be prepared to participate in your prenatal care. Ignorance is never bliss when it comes to having a baby.

PRENATAL-CARE OPTIONS

Group practices Some physicians prefer to work in a group. They relieve each other in a specialty that can demand full concentration 24 hours a day. This may mean that you will see various doctors during your pregnancy. Even if the same doctor treats you at each prenatal visit, try to get to know all the group members. There are group practices as small as two and as large as six or even eight obstetricians.

Hospital midwife programs Midwives, graduate registered nurses who have completed training programs and are certified by the American College of Nurse Midwives, are becoming more popular. Some are associated with hospital maternity units. They handle low-risk cases and an obstetrician is

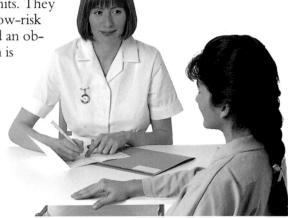

generally on call for backup assistance. If you have no signs of complications, a midwife may be able to monitor your pregnancy and deliver your baby. The letters, C.N.M., alongside the name, indicate the professional qualifications.

QUESTIONS TO ASK

HOSPITAL POLICIES vary, so discuss any issues that are important to you with your obstetrician. It's natural to have preconceived ideas about labor and birth, but the reality is often quite different. Even though you may be dead set against pain medication, for example, keep an open mind. In an emergency or under severe strain, you may need it. This list covers some of the questions you might like to ask.

ABOUT LABOR

Can my partner or a friend stay with me throughout labor? Will he or she ever be asked to leave the delivery room? **Will** I be able to move around during labor? **What** is the hospital policy on pain medication, routine fetal monitoring, and drugs to induce labor (see pages 64, 65 and 66)? **What** kind of pain relief will I be offered; are epidural anesthesia or tranquilizers (see pages 64 and 65) available?

ABOUT THE BIRTH

Will I stay in my labor room or be moved to a delivery area?
Can I give birth in any position I choose to? Are chairs or special birthing beds available?
What is the hospital policy on episiotomies and Cesareans (see pages 66 and 67)?

AFTER THE BIRTH

How long will I stay in the hospital after the delivery?
Is "rooming-in" available?
What are the visiting hours?
Is there a special care baby unit? If not, where will my baby be taken if special treatment is needed?

A TYPICAL PRENATAL VISIT

YOUR FIRST VISIT to the obstetrician should take place soon after you miss your period. You will probably be going once a month until 28 weeks. Visits become more frequent after this; usually every two weeks until you are 36 weeks pregnant, and every week in the last month. Routine tests are carried out by the doctor or midwife at every visit, to make sure that the pregnancy is progressing normally.

URINE SAMPLE every visit
This will be tested for:
- traces of sugar, which, if found repeatedly, could be a sign of diabetes (see page 38)
- traces of protein, which could indicate that your kidneys are not working properly. If protein is found in your urine later in pregnancy, this could be a sign of preeclampsia (see page 38).

HEIGHT first visit
Your height will be measured, as this is a guide to the size of your pelvis; a small pelvis can sometimes mean a difficult delivery. If you are over five feet tall, you are unlikely to have difficulties, unless you are carrying an unusually large baby.

WEIGHT every visit
You will be weighed at each visit to check that you are gaining weight properly (see Calendar, pages 16–31). Don't worry if you lose some weight during the first three months because of morning sickness. Pregnancy weight gain isn't always as predictable or as easily controlled as expectant mothers and their doctors would like.

INITIAL APPOINTMENT
At the first visit, the doctor or midwife will ask some questions about you and your partner, to find out whether there is anything that could affect the pregnancy or your baby. Routines and procedures vary from place to place, but you can usually expect to be asked about:
- personal details, such as your date of birth, and what work you and your partner do
- your country of origin: some forms of anemia are inherited and affect only certain ethnic groups (see Blood tests, opposite)
- your health: serious illnesses or operations you may have had, whether you are being treated for any disease, and whether you have any allergies, or are taking any drugs
- your family's medical history: whether there are twins or any inherited illnesses in your family or your partner's family
- the type of contraceptives you and your partner used before you became pregnant, and when you stopped using them
- your periods: when they began, whether they are regular, when the first day of your last period was, and how long your cycle is
- any previous pregnancies, including miscarriages and abortions.

BLOOD TESTS first visit

Some blood will be taken from your arm to check:
- your blood type and your rhesus, or Rh, factor (see page 38)
- that you are not anemic (see page 38)
- that you are immune to German measles (see page 10)
- that you do not have a sexually transmitted disease, such as syphilis, which must be treated before week 20 if it is not to harm the baby
- for sickle cell trait, if you and your partner are of West Indian or African descent, and thalassemia, if your families come from the Mediterranean, or the Middle and Far East. These forms of anemia are inherited, and could put the baby's health at risk.

GENERAL EXAMINATION
first visit

The doctor or midwife will examine you physically, and listen to your heart and lungs. Your breasts will be checked for lumps and inverted nipples (see page 23). You will probably be asked about your dental health, and encouraged to go for a checkup.

ASKING QUESTIONS

There are bound to be things that puzzle or worry you, or even just interest you, during your pregnancy. Your prenatal visits are your chance to ask about them. It is a good idea to write down any questions before seeing the doctor. Under pressure, it is easy to forget them. Not all doctors are good at explaining medical matters in nonmedical terms, so if you don't understand the answer you have been given, ask again, and again if necessary, to clear up any anxieties you may have.

BLOOD PRESSURE every visit

Your blood pressure is slightly lower in pregnancy, and it is measured regularly to detect any sudden rises and keep them under control. Normal blood pressure is about 120/70, and there will be cause for concern if your blood pressure rises above 140/90.

Raised blood pressure can be a sign of a number of problems, including preeclampsia (see page 38). However, the stress of a prenatal examination, and waiting for test results, can also cause a higher than normal reading so your blood pressure may be taken again later on during the visit. Ask the doctor or nurse to tell you what your blood pressure is, if she does not automatically do so. It should be written on your chart.

LEGS, ANKLES AND HANDS **every visit**

The doctor or midwife will look at your lower legs, ankles, and hands, and feel them to make sure there is no swelling or puffiness (edema). A little swelling in the last weeks of pregnancy is normal, especially at the end of the day, but if it's excessive it may be a sign of preeclampsia (see page 38). Your legs will also be checked for varicose veins (see page 42).

Internal examination

INTERNAL EXAMINATION **first visit**

The doctor may give you an internal examination, to confirm the stage of the pregnancy, to check your pelvis for abnormalities, and to make sure that the entrance to the womb (the cervix) is tightly closed. You may also have a cervical pap smear at the same time to check for abnormal cells; ask for the result at your next visit.

The examination won't hurt you or the baby, and needn't be uncomfortable if you relax. You will be asked to lie on your back with your legs bent and your knees comfortably apart. The doctor will put two fingers of one hand into the vagina, and press your abdomen gently with the other hand.

LISTENING TO THE BABY'S HEARTBEAT **every visit (after week 14)**

From early in pregnancy, this may be done with an electronic instrument (see below), which amplifies the baby's heartbeat so you can hear it, too. After week 28, the doctor or midwife may listen with a standard stethoscope.

FEELING THE ABDOMEN **every visit**

Your abdomen will be felt gently to check the position of the top of the womb, which provides a good clue to the rate of the baby's growth. Later in pregnancy, these physical examinations can tell the position of the fetus. In the final weeks, the doctor will want to see if the head is dropping into the pelvis (engaging).

EXTRA TESTS

YOU MAY be scheduled for an AFP blood test or an ultrasound scan as a part of prenatal care. Some tests are offered only in certain circumstances. If you are over 35 years old, amniocentesis will be recommended, for instance. When problems are detected early enough, intervention may be a possible option.

ULTRASOUND SCAN
week 16 (and sometimes later)

This is an exciting test to have, because it enables you to "see" your baby, often moving around, for the first time. If you are scheduled for an ultrasound scan, ask the hospital staff if you can bring your partner with you. The baby becomes a fascinating reality when you both see him on the screen. You will probably be offered a photograph of the scan, too.

Ultrasound does not always show the baby's sex, but it can be used to:
■ make sure the fetus is growing and developing normally
■ determine the fetus's age and expected delivery date
■ check the position of the baby and the placenta, for example, before amniocentesis, or later in pregnancy to make sure the placenta is not blocking the neck of the womb
■ detect some abnormalities, such as problems with the brain and spine
■ find out whether you are carrying more than one baby.

If you are having the test early in your pregnancy, you will be asked to drink plenty of water and arrive with a full bladder, so that the womb is clearly visible on the screen. The procedure takes about ten minutes, and is safe and painless.

A thin layer of jelly or oil is rubbed over your stomach, and a hand-held instrument, a transducer, is passed over it. This beams and receives sound waves, which are built into an image on the screen.

ALPHA FETOPROTEIN (AFP) TEST weeks 15–18

This blood test measures the amount of alpha fetoprotein, a substance that is produced by the baby in the womb and passes into your bloodstream. A higher-than-normal level of AFP can indicate twins, that the pregnancy is more advanced than you thought, or that the baby has an abnormality. The most common abnormality causing a raised level of AFP is a neural tube defect, such as spina bifida.

If the test shows you have a raised level of AFP, you will have an ultrasound scan and then possibly another blood test. If an abnormality still hasn't been ruled out, you will probably be offered an amniocentesis. Hospital units that have sophisticated ultrasound equipment may not use AFP screening.

AMNIOCENTESIS
weeks 14–18 (and sometimes later)

Amniocentesis can be used to detect some abnormalities in the baby, such as Down's syndrome and spina bifida. It is not offered routinely, because there is a risk of miscarriage in about one woman in 100.

Your doctor may suggest the test if:
■ you are over 35, because your risk of delivering a Down's baby rises with your age
■ you have a family history of inherited disease
■ you had a raised AFP level.

An ultrasound scan is done to check the position of the baby and the placenta. A hollow needle is inserted through the wall of the stomach into the womb, and a sample of the fluid that surrounds the baby, and contains some of his cells, is taken. The cells are then tested for abnormality. The test results for amniocentesis can take three weeks.

CHORIONIC VILLUS SAMPLING (CVS) weeks 6–8

Some inherited disorders can be detected very early in pregnancy, by examining a small piece of the tissue that later develops into the placenta. The sample is usually removed through the entrance to the womb.

The advantage of CVS is that it can be done early in pregnancy. The miscarriage rate for the test is slightly higher than for amniocentesis.

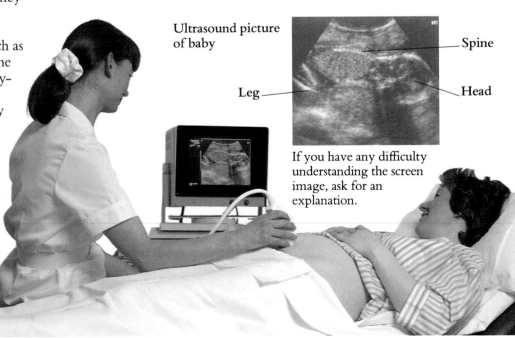

Ultrasound picture of baby

Spine

Leg

Head

If you have any difficulty understanding the screen image, ask for an explanation.

HIGH-RISK PREGNANCIES

NEARLY ALL PREGNANCIES are straightforward, but occasionally there are circumstances that alert your doctor to possible complications. You might have a general medical condition that puts you into a high-risk category. Or sometimes symptoms develop that warn the doctor that special care is needed.

ANEMIA

Many women are slightly anemic before they become pregnant because they lack iron. Anemia simply means a deficiency in the quality and quantity of your red blood cells. But it's important to correct this, so that you can cope with the increased demands of pregnancy. Being anemic can make you feel tired.

Treatment Try to prevent the problem in the first place by eating a varied diet, with plenty of iron-rich foods (see page 52). If blood tests show you are anemic, the doctor can prescribe iron supplements. Some doctors do as a matter of course. Take iron tablets right after meals, with plenty of fluid, because they can irritate the stomach and cause constipation, diarrhea, or nausea.

Anemia Eating foods that are a good source of iron, such as spinach, liver, and red meat, will help guard against the problem.

DIABETES

Diabetes must be carefully controlled during pregnancy and your blood sugar level constantly monitored. If this is done, there's no reason the pregnancy shouldn't be normal and straightforward.

Treatment It's imperative that your blood sugar level remain stable, so the doctor may adjust your insulin intake for the pregnancy. Pay special attention to diet. You may need to visit the doctor more often. Some women develop a mild form of the disease for the first time during pregnancy. This nearly always disappears soon after the birth of the baby.

INCOMPETENT CERVIX

In a normal pregnancy, the cervix (neck of the womb) stays closed until the beginning of labor. When miscarriages frequently occur after the third month of pregnancy, it could be because the neck of the womb is weak. Under the pressure of a growing pregnancy, it opens up and expels the baby.

Treatment Your doctor may suggest minor surgery to stitch the cervix closed at the beginning of your pregnancy. The stitch is then removed toward the end of pregnancy, or as you go into labor.

PREECLAMPSIA

A common but serious problem in late pregnancy, this is a combination of the following symptoms: raised blood pressure above 140/90; excessive weight gain; swollen ankles, feet, or hands; and traces of protein in the urine. If you develop any of these, the doctor will monitor you very carefully.

If blood pressure rises untreated, it could progress to the extremely dangerous condition of eclampsia, where convulsions may occur, putting you and your baby at risk.

Treatment Your doctor will probably advise bed rest. To lower blood pressure, you may be given a drug, or advised to cut down on salt. If the signs are severe, you will be admitted to the hospital, even though you might be feeling perfectly healthy. Labor may be induced (see page 66).

RHESUS NEGATIVE MOTHER

Your blood is tested at the first prenatal visit to see if it is rhesus positive or rhesus negative. About 15 per cent of people are rhesus, or Rh, negative, and if you are one of these, you will only have a problem in pregnancy if you give birth to a rhesus, or Rh, positive baby. When your blood types are incompatible like this, it won't harm a first baby, but could cause complications in later pregnancies.

Treatment If your first baby is Rh positive, and you're a Rh negative mother, you will probably be given an injection of anti-Rh immunoglobin (Rhogam) after birth. This will prevent problems in future pregnancies. The anti-Rh injection stops your immune system from creating antibodies that could hurt your baby.

■ EMERGENCY SIGNS ■

Call for emergency help immediately if you have:
▲ a severe headache that won't go away
▲ misty or blurred vision
▲ severe, prolonged stomach pains
▲ vaginal bleeding
▲ a leakage of fluid, which suggests that your water has broken early
▲ frequent, painful urination (drink plenty of water in the meantime).

Consult your doctor within 24 hours if you have:
▲ swollen hands, face, and ankles
▲ severe, frequent vomiting
▲ a temperature of 101°F (38.3°C)
▲ no movement, or fewer than ten kicks, from your baby for 12 hours after week 28.

MISCARRIAGE

A miscarriage is the ending of a pregnancy before 28 weeks, and this may happen to about one in five pregnancies. Most miscarriages occur in the first 12 weeks, often before the woman even knows she is pregnant, and usually because the baby is not developing normally. Bleeding from the vagina is usually the first sign. Call your doctor immediately and lie down.

Threatened abortion

If bleeding is mild and painless, the pregnancy can often be saved. Your doctor will probably recommend bed rest, the bleeding may stop, and if you take things easy for a few days, the pregnancy may proceed, without any increased risk of abnormality in the baby. You may be given another pregnancy test or ultrasound scan (see page 37) to confirm that all is well.

True miscarriage

If the bleeding is heavy and you are in pain, it probably means that the baby has died. You may have to go into the hospital for a D. and C., dilation and curettage, during which your womb is cleaned out.

Your feelings

Even if you miscarry early in pregnancy, you will feel an intense sense of loss. Other people don't always understand that you need to mourn your baby. Worry about whether you can ever have a normal, healthy baby is common. You may feel guilty too, though you should never blame yourself; it really isn't your fault. It's quite safe to try to get pregnant again as soon as you like, although some doctors suggest waiting until at least three menstrual cycles have passed. Unless you have had a string of miscarriages, there is no reason at all why you shouldn't have a successful pregnancy next time.

VAGINAL BLEEDING

If you notice bleeding from your vagina at any time in pregnancy, call your doctor without delay and go to bed. Before 28 weeks, it can be a sign of an impending miscarriage. After this time, it may mean that the placenta is bleeding. This can happen if the placenta has started to separate from the wall of the womb (placental abruption) or if the placenta is too low in the womb and covering, or partially covering, the cervix (placenta previa).

Treatment The placenta is the baby's lifeline, so if the doctor thinks that there is any risk to it, you will probably be admitted to the hospital immediately, where the position of the placenta can be checked. You may stay in the hospital until after the birth. If you have lost a lot of blood, you may be given a blood transfusion, and the baby will probably be delivered as soon as possible, by inducing labor or by Cesarean section (see pages 67 and 66). But if bleeding is only slight and occurs several weeks before the baby is due, the doctor may wait for labor to start naturally, while observing you closely.

"SMALL FOR DATES" BABIES

A baby who doesn't grow properly in the womb and is small at birth is called a "small for dates" baby. This is not a premature baby and it may happen because the expectant mother smokes or eats a poor diet, or because the placenta isn't working properly. (A general medical condition, such as maternal diabetes can be at fault.)
Treatment If tests during pregnancy show your baby is small, you will be monitored very closely to check his health, and match the flow of blood to the placenta. If the baby stops growing or appears to be distressed in any way, he will be delivered early, either by inducing labor or Cesarean section (see pages 66 and 67).

TWINS

Your pregnancy and labor will progress normally, although you will have two second stages in labor, and you may go into labor prematurely. There's a greater likelihood of complications such as anemia, preeclampsia, and of the babies lying abnormally in the womb. You may also find that all the common disorders of pregnancy are exaggerated, especially in the last few months.
Treatment Regular prenatal visits are essential if you are expecting twins, so that any complications can be spotted immediately. A multiple pregnancy puts great strain on your body so watch your posture and rest as much as possible, especially in the last few weeks. To avoid problems with your digestion, eat small amounts of fresh, unprocessed food at frequent intervals.

Twins You may find this position comfortable to rest in.

COMMON COMPLAINTS

You may suffer from a variety of discomforts in pregnancy that unnerve and exasperate you, but your aches and pains are probably perfectly normal. Many are caused by hormonal changes, or because your body is under extra pressure. A few symptoms, however, should be taken more seriously. Call the doctor if you have any of the signs listed in the box on page 38.

■ COMPLAINT ■	■ SYMPTOMS ■	■ WHAT TO DO ■
Bleeding gums 1 2 3★ The gums become softer and more easily injured in pregnancy. They may be inflamed, allowing plaque to collect at the base of the teeth. This can lead to gum disease and tooth decay.	Bleeding from the gums, especially after brushing your teeth.	▲ Floss and brush your teeth thoroughly after eating. ▲ See your dentist—but you shouldn't have X rays or general anesthesia.
Breathlessness 3 Late in pregnancy, the growing baby puts pressure on the diaphragm, and prevents you from breathing freely. The problem is often relieved about a month before the birth, when the baby's head engages. Breathlessness can also be caused by anemia.	Feeling breathless when you exert yourself, or even when you talk.	▲ Rest as much as possible. ▲ Try crouching if there's no chair around and you feel breathless. ▲ At night, use an extra pillow. ▲ If the problem is severe, consult your doctor or midwife.
Constipation 1 2 3 The pregnancy hormone progesterone relaxes the muscles of the intestine, which slows down bowel movements, making you more likely to become constipated.	Passing hard, dry stools at less frequent intervals than usual.	▲ Eat plenty of high-fiber foods and drink lots of water. Go to the bathroom often. ▲ Exercise regularly. ▲ Take any iron supplements you have been prescribed on a full stomach, with plenty of fluid. ▲ See your doctor if the problem persists. Avoid laxatives.
Cramps 3 May be caused by a calcium deficiency.	Painful contractions of muscles, usually in the calves and the feet, and often at night. Commonly started by a leg stretch with the toes pointed down.	▲ Massage the affected calf or foot. ▲ Walk around for a moment or two once the pain has eased to improve your circulation. ▲ See your doctor and ask about calcium and vitamin D supplements.
Feeling faint 1 3 Your blood pressure is lower in pregnancy, so you are more likely to feel faint.	Feeling dizzy and unstable. Needing to sit or lie down.	▲ Try not to stand still for too long. ▲ If you feel faint, sit down and put your head between your knees. ▲ Get up slowly from a hot bath, or when sitting or lying down. Turn to one side first when you are getting up after lying on your back.

★ The numbers after each complaint relate to the trimester in which you are most likely to suffer from the problem.

Backache see page 44
Skin pigmentation see page 21

Breathlessness
Crouching helps if you suddenly feel out of breath halfway up the stairs. Hold on to the banister.

Cramps
Pull your foot up toward you with your hand, and massage the calf vigorously, to help relieve painful cramps.

■ COMPLAINT ■	■ SYMPTOMS ■	■ WHAT TO DO ■
Frequent urination 1 3 Caused by the womb pressing on the bladder. The problem is often relieved in the middle months of pregnancy.	You need to urinate often.	▲ If you find yourself getting up in the night to go to the bathroom, try drinking less in the evenings. ▲ See your doctor if you feel any pain because you could have an infection.
Heartburn 3 The valve at the entrance to your stomach relaxes in pregnancy because of hormonal changes, so stomach acid passes back into the esophagus (the tube leading to your stomach).	A strong burning pain in the center of the chest.	▲ Avoid large meals, highly spiced or fried foods. ▲ At night, try a warm milk drink, and use extra pillows to raise your head. ▲ See your doctor, who may prescribe medication to treat stomach acidity.
Leaking urine 3 Caused by weak pelvic floor muscles (see page 45), and the growing baby pressing on your bladder.	Leakage of urine whenever you run, cough, sneeze, or laugh.	▲ Urinate often. ▲ Practice your pelvic floor exercises regularly. ▲ Avoid constipation and heavy lifting.
Morning sickness 1 Often one of the first signs of pregnancy, which can occur at any time of day. Tiredness can make the problem worse. Nausea usually disappears after week 12, but sometimes returns later.	Feeling sick, often at the smell of certain foods or cigarette smoke. Most women find there is a particular time of day when this happens.	▲ Try eating something to keep the nausea at bay. ▲ Avoid foods and smells that make you feel sick. ▲ Have small, frequent meals throughout the day.
Hemorrhoids 2 3 Pressure from the baby's head causes swollen veins round the anus. Straining to empty the bowels will make the problem worse. Mild hemorrhoids usually disappear, without treatment, after the baby is born.	Itching, soreness, and possibly pain or bleeding when you empty your bowels.	▲ Avoid constipation. ▲ Try not to stand for long periods. ▲ An ice pack held against the hemorrhoids may ease itching. ▲ If hemorrhoids persist, tell the doctor or midwife, who may give you ointment.
Rash 3 Usually occurs in women who are overweight and who perspire freely. Can be caused by hormonal changes.	Red rash, which usually develops in sweaty skin folds under the breasts or in the groin.	▲ Wash and dry these areas often. Use unperfumed soap. ▲ Soothe the skin with calamine lotion. ▲ Wear loose cotton clothes.
Sleeping difficulty 1 2 3 You may have a problem because the baby is kicking, you have to go to the bathroom frequently, or the sheer size of your baby makes it difficult to get comfortable in bed.	Having trouble going to sleep in the first place, and finding it hard to get to sleep after waking. Some women find they have very frightening dreams about the birth or the baby. Don't worry about dreams; they do not reflect what will happen.	▲ Reading, gentle relaxation exercises, or a warm bath before bedtime may help. ▲ Experiment with extra pillows. If you sleep on your side, put a pillow under your top thigh.

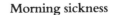

Heartburn and sleeplessness
This piled-up arrangement of pillows is comfortable if you suffer from heartburn, or are unable to sleep.

Morning sickness
To counteract nausea, try eating dry crackers, toast, or fruit. Eliminate fried or highly seasoned foods and drink lots of water.

■ COMPLAINT ■	■ SYMPTOMS ■	■ WHAT TO DO ■
Stretch marks 2 3 These form if your skin stretches beyond its normal elasticity. Excess weight gain can also cause them. The marks may disappear, but are more likely to fade to thin silvery streaks.	Red marks that sometimes appear on the skin of the thighs, stomach, or breasts in pregnancy.	▲ Try not to put on weight too rapidly. ▲ Rubbing moisturizer into the skin may feel cool and soothing, although creams and ointments won't prevent or heal stretch marks.
Sweating 2 3 Caused by hormonal changes, and because blood flow to the skin increases in pregnancy.	Perspiring after very little exertion, or waking up in the night feeling hot and sweaty.	▲ Wear loose cotton clothes. Avoid manmade materials. ▲ Drink plenty of water. ▲ Open a window at night.
Swollen ankles and fingers 3 Some swelling (edema) is normal in pregnancy, because the body holds extra water. This is usually no cause for concern.	Slight swelling in the ankles, especially in hot weather and at the end of the day. This shouldn't cause pain or discomfort. You may also notice stiff, swollen fingers in the morning, and that your rings don't fit.	▲ Rest with your feet up often. ▲ Try gentle foot exercises. Hold your hands above your head; flex and stretch each finger. ▲ See your doctor or midwife. Marked swelling could be a warning sign of preeclampsia (see page 38).
Yeast infections 1 2 3 Hormonal changes of pregnancy increase the chances of developing yeast infections. It is important to treat these before the baby is born, because they can affect his health. Washing with some soaps can worsen the problem.	A thick white discharge and severe itching. There may also be soreness and pain when you urinate.	▲ Keep the genital area as dry as possible. ▲ Wear only cotton or cotton-crotch underpants. ▲ Avoid panty hose, tight jeans, and vaginal deodorants. ▲ See your doctor, who may be able to prescribe treatment.
Tiredness 1 3 Caused by the extra demands that pregnancy makes on your body. Sometimes the result of worry.	Feeling weary, and wanting to sleep in the day. Needing to sleep longer at night.	▲ Rest as much as possible and practice relaxation exercises. ▲ Go to bed earlier. ▲ Don't overexert yourself.
Vaginal discharge 1 2 3 You may notice some increase in the amount of mucus produced by the vagina because of the hormonal changes of pregnancy.	Slight increase in clear or white discharge, without soreness or pain.	▲ Avoid vaginal deodorants and perfumed soap products. ▲ Wear a light sanitary pad. ▲ See your doctor if you have any itching, soreness, colored or foul-smelling discharge.
Varicose veins 1 2 3 You are more likely to develop them in a second or third pregnancy, if you are overweight, or they run in your family. Standing for too long, or sitting cross-legged, can worsen them.	Aching legs; the veins in the calves and the thighs become painful and swollen.	▲ Rest with your feet up often. Try raising the foot of your bed with pillows under the mattress. ▲ Support stockings may help. Put them on before getting up in the morning. ▲ Exercise your feet.

Swollen ankles and varicose veins
Gently circle your ankles and feet to improve circulation.

Varicose veins
Rest with your feet well elevated on at least two cushions if you suffer from this problem. Tuck another cushion into the small of your back.

KEEPING FIT
AND RELAXED

Pregnancy, labor, and birth will make great demands on your body, so the more you can prepare yourself physically, the better you will feel. You will also find it easier to get back into shape after the baby is born. Learning relaxation exercises is just as important; they will help you calm down and cope far more effectively during labor, and they are invaluable for relieving stress and for increasing blood flow to the placenta. Even if you normally hate the idea of exercise, try the exercises on the following pages. They are specially designed to make your joints and muscles more supple, in preparation for labor and birth. You can begin special prenatal exercises as soon as the pregnancy is confirmed, or earlier if you wish. Practice at home or sign up for an exercise class designed for expectant mothers. Don't worry, though, if you are well into pregnancy by the time you begin; it's never too late to start. Build up gradually until you are exercising for 20 minutes every day.

EXERCISING SENSIBLY

If you're athletic, and have always been so, pregnancy shouldn't slow you down. But there are cautions:
■ Pregnancy is not the time to launch into a fitness blitz; just continue with what your body is used to. If you want to keep on going to your dance or exercise class, make sure that the teacher knows you are pregnant.
■ Don't exercise to the point where you get very tired or out of breath.
■ Avoid any sports where there is a danger of hurting your abdomen, such as riding, skiing, and water-skiing.

■ Be extra careful in the first and last weeks of pregnancy, because you may overstretch ligaments.

Swimming
This is excellent and perfectly safe; the water supports your body.

TAKING CARE OF YOUR BODY

DURING PREGNANCY, your posture can make a real difference in your overall health. You're far more likely to suffer from backache because the weight of the baby pulls you forward, and you'll have a tendency to lean slightly backward to compensate. This strains the muscles of the lower back and pelvis, especially toward the end of pregnancy.

Be aware of your body, whatever you are doing. Avoid heavy lifting, and try to keep your back straight whenever possible. Wear low heels, because high heels throw your weight even further forward.

PROTECTING YOUR BACK

To avoid back trouble, it's important to be aware of how you use your body when doing everyday activities such as gardening, lifting a child, or carrying heavy bags. The hormones of pregnancy stretch and soften the muscles of the lower back, so these are more easily strained if you bend over, get up too suddenly, or lift something awkwardly or in the wrong way.

Lower yourself
Do as much as you can at floor level, kneeling down to garden, clean, make a bed, or dress a child, instead of bending over.

Take it easy getting up
Always turn on your side when getting up and on your feet again after lying down. Move into a kneeling position. Use your thigh strength to push yourself up; keep your back straight.

Drop *your shoulders and keep them back*

Hold *your back straight*

Tuck in *your bottom*

Stand *with your feet a little way apart*

STANDING TALL

Take a good look at the way you normally stand in front of a full-length mirror. Straighten your back, so that the weight of the baby is centered and supported by your thighs, buttocks, and stomach muscles. This will help prevent backache, and tone up your abdominal muscles, making it easier for you to regain your figure after the birth.

Lift *your chest and ribs*

Tighten *your stomach muscles*

Bend *your knees slightly*

Poor posture
This is common during pregnancy. As the baby grows, its weight throws you off-balance, so you may overarch your back and thrust your abdomen forward.

Lifting and carrying
When lifting an object, bend your knees and keep your back as straight as possible, bringing the object close in to your body. Try not to reach for heavy objects on high shelves, because you may lose your balance. When you're carrying heavy bags, divide the weight equally on each side.

Keep *your back straight*

Position *your weight around the object, and face it squarely*

THE PELVIC FLOOR

THIS IS A HAMMOCK of muscles that supports the bowel, bladder, and womb. During pregnancy, the muscles go soft and stretchy, and this, together with the weight of the baby pushing down, weakens them, making you feel heavy and uncomfortable. You may also leak a little urine whenever you run, sneeze, cough, or laugh. To avoid these problems, it's essential to strengthen the pelvic floor.

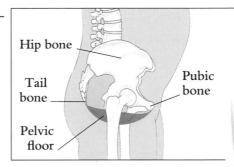

Hip bone
Tail bone
Pubic bone
Pelvic floor

The pelvic floor
This forms part of the pelvis, a bony area, which cradles and protects the baby in the womb. The baby has to pass through it at birth.

Practice *the exercise standing*

STRENGTHENING THE PELVIC FLOOR

Practice this exercise at least three or four times a day: you can do it anytime, anywhere, lying down, sitting, or standing. You will find it useful in the second stage of labor. Knowing how to relax the muscles reduces the risk of a tear, because you can ease the passage of the baby through the pelvis without pushing too fast or frantically.

Lie on your back, with your knees bent and your feet flat on the floor. Now tighten the muscles, squeezing as if stopping a stream of urine. Imagine you are trying to pull something into your vagina, drawing it in slightly, then pausing, then pulling, until you can go no further. Hold for a moment, then let go gradually. Repeat ten times.

Practice *the exercise sitting*

DO THIS WHEN:
- waiting for a bus or train
- ironing or cooking
- watching TV
- having intercourse
- you have *emptied* your bladder.

PELVIC TILT

THIS EXERCISE helps you move the pelvis with ease, which is good preparation for labor. It also strengthens the stomach muscles and makes the back more flexible. It is especially helpful if you suffer from backache, and when you are in this all-fours position, your partner can rub the base of your back to soothe any pain. You can do the tilt in any position; remember to keep your shoulders still.

1 Kneel on the floor on your hands and knees. Make sure that your back is flat. (At first it helps to use a mirror to check this.)

2 Pull in your stomach muscles, tighten your buttock muscles, and gently tilt the pelvis forward, breathing out as you do so. Your back should hump up. Hold this position for a few seconds, then breathe in and let go. Repeat several times, so that your pelvis is rocking in and out of the position.

DO THIS WHEN:
- lying on your back
- standing
- sitting
- kneeling
- you are listening to music.

TAILOR SITTING

THIS STRENGTHENS the back and makes your thighs and pelvis more flexible. It also improves blood flow in the lower part of the body, and will encourage your legs to fall apart naturally at birth. The main position below is easier than it looks, because your body is more supple in pregnancy.

Straighten *your back*

SITTING WITH CUSHIONS
If you find tailor sitting difficult, put a cushion under each thigh, or sit against a wall for support. Remember to keep your back straight.

Stretch *your inner thighs by pressing outward with your elbows*

SITTING WITH CROSSED LEGS
You may find it more comfortable to sit like this. Make sure you change the front leg occasionally.

Keep *your feet close to your body*

THIGH STRENGTHENER
Sit with your back straight, the soles of your feet together, and your heels close to your body. Grasp your ankles, and press your thighs down with your elbows. Hold them there for 20 seconds. Do this several times.

■ **WARNING** ■

When you are doing any exercises, remember these guidelines.
▲ Don't push yourself beyond your own limits.
▲ Never exhaust yourself.
▲ If you feel any pain, stop immediately.
▲ Don't lie flat on your back in late pregnancy.

SQUATTING

THIS MAKES your pelvic joints more flexible, and strengthens the back and thigh muscles. It can protect your back, if you squat down instead of bending over, and is comfortable if you have a backache. Squatting is also a good position during labor.

You may find it difficult to do a full squat at first, so try holding on to a firm support, such as a chair or window ledge, and place a rolled-up rug or blanket under your heels. Get up slowly, or you may feel dizzy.

Clasp *your hands*

Lengthen and straighten *your back*

Press *your elbows against your thighs*

Try to keep *your heels flat on the ground*

Turn *your feet out slightly*

WITH A CHAIR
Stand facing a chair with your feet slightly apart. Keeping your back straight, open your legs and squat down, using the chair to support you. Stay in this position as long as it is comfortable to do so. If you find it difficult to keep your feet flat on the ground, place a folded blanket under your heels.

DO THIS WHEN:
- breathless on the stairs
- picking up an object
- taking something from a low drawer
- on the telephone
- there's no chair around.

UNSUPPORTED
Keeping your back straight, open your legs and squat down, turning your feet out slightly. Try to keep your heels flat on the ground and stretch your inner thighs by pressing them outward with your elbows. Stay in this position for as long as you find it comfortable.

RELAXATION AND BREATHING

THESE EXERCISES are among the most useful you can learn. They are invaluable during labor, when knowing how to breathe properly and relax the muscles of your body will help you cope with contractions and save vital energy. Practice them regularly so that they become a natural response during labor. Relaxation will also help you unwind at any time you feel tense or anxious.

HOW TO RELAX
At first it's best to practice this exercise in a warm room where you won't be disturbed. Later you should find it easy to relax anywhere.

Relax your body
Make yourself comfortable, lying on your back, fully propped up by pillows, or on your side, with one leg bent and supported on cushions. Now tense and relax the muscles of each part of your body in turn, starting with the toes and working upward. After doing this for eight to ten minutes, let your body go limp. Try to feel heavy, as though you are sinking into the floor.

Lying on your side
You may be more comfortable, especially during later pregnancy, lying on your side with one leg bent and supported on cushions. Don't place too many pillows under your head, because this is bad for your spine.

> ### ■ WARNING ■
> Don't lie flat on your back in the late stages of pregnancy. You can restrict the flow of oxygen to the baby in this position, and you yourself may feel faint.

Tilt *your head from side to side, then hold still*

Screw up *your eyes, open, then close*

Pull in *your stomach muscles, then relax*

Arch *the small of your back, then let go*

Clench *your hands, then open*

Squeeze *your buttock muscles, then let go*

BREATHING FOR LABOR

Practice the different levels of breathing with a partner or a friend, so that you are relaxed and calm during labor, and can even control your body during contractions.

Light breathing

This level of breathing will help you at the height of a contraction. Breathe in and out of your mouth, taking air into the upper part of your lungs only. A partner or friend should put her hands on your shoulders and feel them move. Practice making the breaths lighter and lighter, but take an occasional deeper breath when you need one.

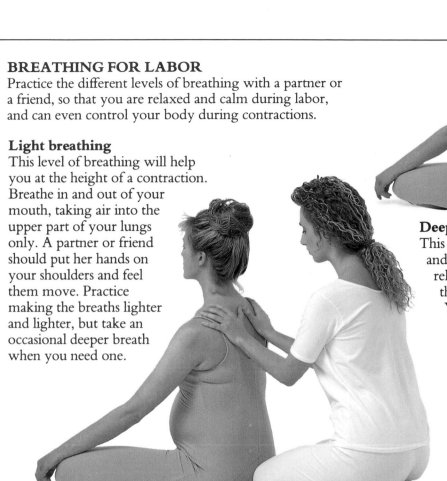

Deep breathing

This has a calming effect, helpful at the beginning and end of contractions. Sit comfortably and as relaxed as possible. Breathe in deeply through the nose, right to the bottom of your lungs. Your partner or friend should place her hands just above your waistline and feel your ribcage move. Now, concentrate on breathing slowly and gently out. Let the next in-breath follow naturally.

Panting

After the first stage of labor, you will want to push, even though the cervix may not be fully opened. You can resist this by taking two short breaths, and then blowing a longer breath out: say "huff, huff, blow" to yourself.

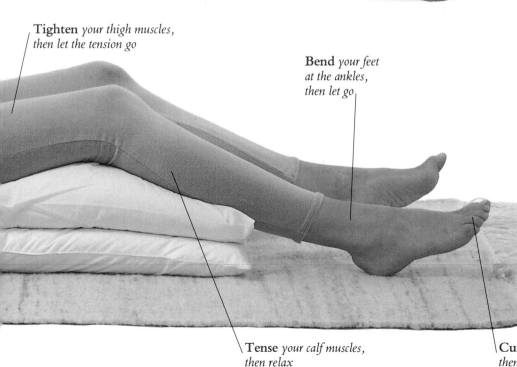

Tighten *your thigh muscles, then let the tension go*

Bend *your feet at the ankles, then let go*

Tense *your calf muscles, then relax*

Curl *your toes, then relax*

Relax your mind

While relaxing your body, try to calm and empty your mind. Breathe slowly and evenly, sighing each breath out gently. Do not breathe too hard.

Alternatively, repeat a word or sound silently to yourself, or concentrate on some pleasant or peaceful image. Try not to follow any thoughts that arise.

EATING FOR A HEALTHY BABY

A baby has only one source of food—you. During pregnancy, more than at any other time, it is essential that you have as varied and balanced a diet as possible. You do not need to plan this specially, nor do you have to eat for two. All you have to do is eat a variety of fresh, unprocessed foods from the selection below, to insure that you get all the nutrients you need. Once you are, or know you want to become, pregnant, think about foods you have been eating regularly. Do you eat or drink anything that might harm the baby? Increase your intake of raw vegetables and fresh fruit, and cut down on sugary, salty, and processed foods.

ESSENTIAL NUTRIENTS

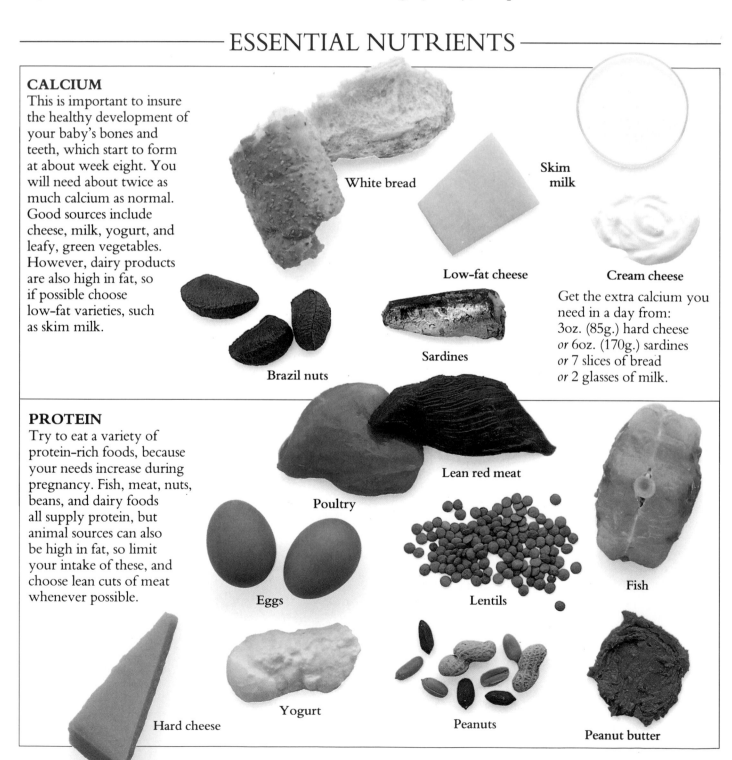

CALCIUM

This is important to insure the healthy development of your baby's bones and teeth, which start to form at about week eight. You will need about twice as much calcium as normal. Good sources include cheese, milk, yogurt, and leafy, green vegetables. However, dairy products are also high in fat, so if possible choose low-fat varieties, such as skim milk.

White bread

Skim milk

Low-fat cheese

Cream cheese

Brazil nuts

Sardines

Get the extra calcium you need in a day from:
3oz. (85g.) hard cheese
or 6oz. (170g.) sardines
or 7 slices of bread
or 2 glasses of milk.

PROTEIN

Try to eat a variety of protein-rich foods, because your needs increase during pregnancy. Fish, meat, nuts, beans, and dairy foods all supply protein, but animal sources can also be high in fat, so limit your intake of these, and choose lean cuts of meat whenever possible.

Lean red meat

Poultry

Eggs

Lentils

Fish

Hard cheese

Yogurt

Peanuts

Peanut butter

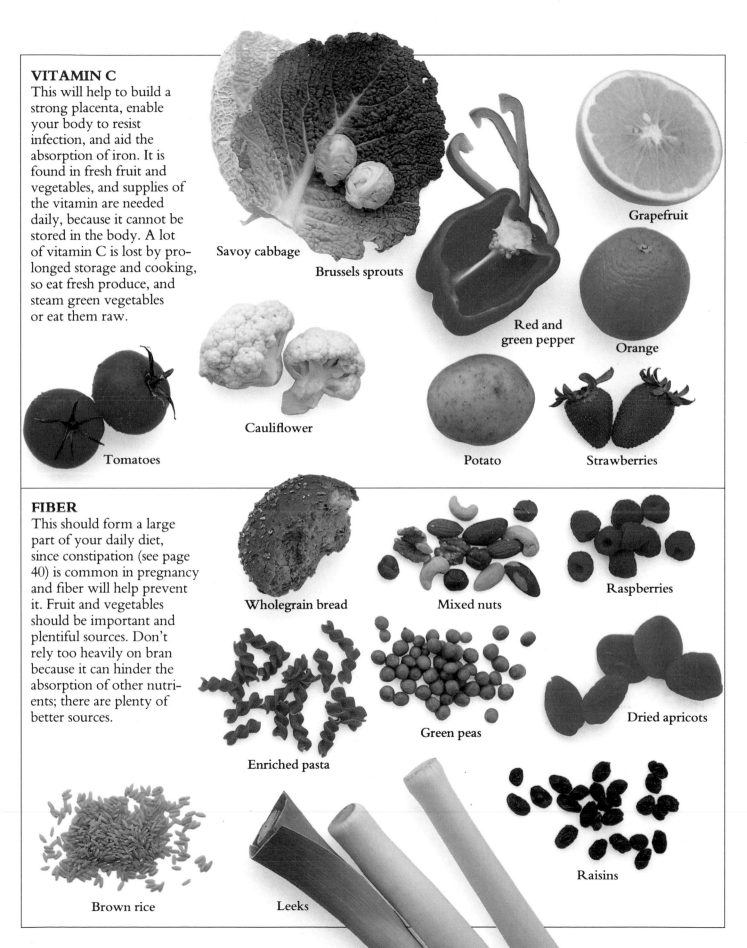

VITAMIN C

This will help to build a strong placenta, enable your body to resist infection, and aid the absorption of iron. It is found in fresh fruit and vegetables, and supplies of the vitamin are needed daily, because it cannot be stored in the body. A lot of vitamin C is lost by prolonged storage and cooking, so eat fresh produce, and steam green vegetables or eat them raw.

Savoy cabbage

Brussels sprouts

Grapefruit

Red and green pepper

Orange

Cauliflower

Tomatoes

Potato

Strawberries

FIBER

This should form a large part of your daily diet, since constipation (see page 40) is common in pregnancy and fiber will help prevent it. Fruit and vegetables should be important and plentiful sources. Don't rely too heavily on bran because it can hinder the absorption of other nutrients; there are plenty of better sources.

Wholegrain bread

Mixed nuts

Raspberries

Enriched pasta

Green peas

Dried apricots

Brown rice

Leeks

Raisins

FOLIC ACID

This is needed for the development of the baby's nervous system, especially in the first few weeks. The body cannot store this nutrient, and during pregnancy it excretes several times the normal amount, so it's essential to have a daily supply. Fresh dark green, leafy vegetables are a good source of folic acid, but steam or eat them raw because a lot of the vitamin is destroyed by cooking.

Broccoli

Spinach

Hazelnuts

Peanuts

Wholegrain bread

IRON

Iron is needed in increased amounts. The baby will need to build up stores of iron for after the birth, and the extra blood your body produces needs iron to carry oxygen. Iron from animal sources is absorbed more easily than from foods such as beans and dried fruit, so if you do not eat meat, combine iron-rich foods with those rich in vitamin C to allow maximum absorption.

Lean red meat

Tuna fish

Liver

Spinach

Dried apricots

VEGETARIAN DIET

If you eat a variety of protein-rich foods and fresh fruit and vegetables every day, you should provide the baby with all that he needs. The only nutrient you may lack is iron; the body has great difficulty absorbing iron from plant sources, so you may be given supplements of the mineral to compensate. If you have also eliminated dairy foods from your regular diet, you may be prescribed calcium, and vitamins D and B12.

SALT

Most people have too much salt in their diet. During pregnancy, it is even more important to reduce the amount of salt you eat, because too much can cause problems such as excess swelling and preeclampsia (see pages 42 and 38).

FLUID

This is essential during pregnancy for keeping your kidneys healthy and avoiding constipation. Water is best; drink as much as you like.

TOP FOODS

These foods are excellent sources of at least one nutrient. Try to eat some of them every day.
■ Cheese, milk, yogurt: calcium, protein.
■ Dark green, leafy vegetables: vitamin C, fiber, folic acid.
■ Lean red meat: protein, iron.
■ Liver: protein, iron.
■ Oranges: vitamin C, fiber.
■ Poultry: protein, iron.
■ Fish such as flounder, tuna, salmon, or bluefish: protein.

■ Wholegrain bread: protein, fiber, folic acid.
■ Enriched pasta and brown rice: fiber.

VITAMIN AND MINERAL SUPPLEMENTS

If you eat a balanced diet, with plenty of fresh foods, you probably won't need vitamin or mineral supplements—though they may be prescribed. If you are anemic they'll be essential (see page 38). Some doctors routinely prescribe iron and folic acid supplements.

PROTECTING YOUR BABY

ALMOST EVERYTHING you consume during pregnancy—both good and bad—can make its way to your baby via the placenta.

PROCESSED FOODS

Avoid convenience foods that have been highly processed. Some processed foods have excess sugar and salt added, and may contain a lot of fat, as well as unnecessary preservatives, artificial flavors and colors. Read the labels carefully and choose products that are free from artificial substances or that feature them low on the ingredients list. Also check the product's date of expiry.

Eat *a variety of fresh, unprocessed foods*

FOUR FOOD GROUPS

Plan your meals around the basic food groups: meat or other protein alternatives; fruits or vegetables; breads or cereals; and dairy products. Use vegetable oils high in polyunsaturated fats such as corn oil and sunflower oil.

Stay away from processed luncheon meats, salted nuts, soy sauce, excess mustard and ketchup. Synthetic fruit drinks don't always contain very much of the listed fruit so buy pure, 100 percent juice brands.

COFFEE, TEA, AND HOT CHOCOLATE

Caffeine, a substance that is found in all these drinks, has a harmful effect on the digestive system. Limit your intake to no more than three cups of caffeinated drinks a day, and if possible cut them out altogether. Drink plenty of water instead.

HERBAL TEAS

If you want to drink herbal teas in pregnancy, it is sensible to check first with your doctor. Most prepackaged teas won't harm the baby— raspberry leaf tea, for example, is a traditional remedy to ease labor—but some may have unwanted effects.

SUGAR

Sugary foods, such as cakes, cookies, candies, sodas, and colas are low in essential nutrients, and can put excess weight on you. Get your energy from starchy carbohydrates, such as wholegrain bread, and cut down on the sweets.

CRAVINGS

It's common in pregnancy to find that you suddenly develop a taste for certain foods, such as pickled onions or ice cream. If you long for a particular food, go ahead and indulge yourself within reason, provided it isn't fattening and doesn't cause indigestion.

ALTERNATIVES TO ALCOHOL

Any alcohol that you drink during pregnancy is passed through the placenta into your baby's bloodstream, and can be harmful. So it's best to cut out alcohol altogether and make your own fresh fruit cocktails, milkshakes, and sparkling fruit juice drinks, using pure, additive-free ingredients.

Even beers, and wines that claim to be alcohol free or low in alcohol may not necessarily be free from additives and chemicals that may harm your baby. Check with your obstetrician before you make them a regular part of your diet.

Sparkling orange
Orange juice diluted with sparkling water or club soda, a simple, but refreshing, drink. Try other varieties of fruit juice for a change.

Banana milkshake
This tastes delicious and is high in calcium and protein. Make it by mixing together a banana and 2 cups of milk. A blender or food processor works best.

Fresh fruit cocktail
Experiment with mixing different varieties of fruit juice to make a range of healthy, thirst-quenching drinks. Garnish with an orange slice, or pieces of fruit on a cocktail stick.

PRACTICAL PREPARATIONS

About a month before your delivery date, make sure that everything is ready for your baby's homecoming. For instance, go food shopping and start planning for meals and other essentials that will make your life easier after the birth. It's not too soon to pack for your trip to the hospital or birthing center either. Put your open suitcase on the floor of your bedroom and start assembling the things you'll want when you are away from home. Some hospitals or doctors offer mothers-to-be a list of what to bring. Buy or borrow the equipment for your new baby.

HELPFUL THINGS FOR LABOR

ALL THE ITEMS below may be useful in labor and immediately after birth. Don't put them into your suitcase. Pack them separately, because you will want them during labor.

Deodorant

Small, natural sponge
Moisten it, and suck on it if your mouth is dry.

Talcum powder
To smooth your back during a massage.

Cosmetic bag, toothbrush and toothpaste, lip balm

Also:
- books, magazines, camera, a radio or stereo with headphones
- food and drink for your partner
- phone numbers of relatives and friends
- coins for the telephone
- anything else that you have practiced with during prenatal classes and would like to use during labor.

Warm socks
You may become cold in the later stages of labor.

Baggy T- shirt or nightgown
Hospital gowns aren't as comfortable as your own familiar clothes. You may be able to wear your own.

Hot water bottle

Aids for labor
Tennis balls, or a hot water bottle, that your mate can press against your lower back may help to ease backache during labor.

GOING TO THE HOSPITAL WHEN YOU ARE IN LABOR
It's always a good idea to make trial runs to the hospital or birthing center long before you feel those first pains of labor. When you and your mate are under the stress of imminent childbirth or you are counting contractions, you certainly don't want to get lost or stuck in unfamiliar territory. Knowing which door to enter when you arrive at the hospital and where you'll be headed inside can be a relief. Ask about the preliminary papers you'll need to fill out. And, if you'll be using a big city hospital, you ought to have a good idea of what rush hour traffic conditions might be like. In the last few weeks of pregnancy, make sure your car always has enough gas to get you there. Put money or tokens for road tolls or emergency calls in your car ahead of time.

If you aren't going to be driving in your own car, keep the name and phone number of a 24-hour taxi service posted by your telephone. Or if someone has volunteered to drive you, make sure that they will be expecting a call and will be able to respond at any hour of the day or night, and post their phone number in a handy location by your telephone.

FOR AFTER THE BIRTH

THIS CHECKLIST will help you as you pack; if you go into labor unexpectedly and haven't packed your suitcase, here are items your mate should assemble. The hospital will probably provide all the essentials for the baby during your stay.

Brush

Comb

Shampoo

Also:
- tissues
- hairdryer
- note paper and pen
- hand mirror for freshening up at bedside.

Breast pads
Slip these inside your bra to absorb leaking milk. Shaped ones are best.

Nipple cream
This relieves sore nipples.

One box *should be super-absorbent for the first few days*

Two boxes of belt-free sanitary pads

Front opening, *to allow your baby to feel as much as possible of your breast; one cup unzips at a time*

Wide *support straps*

Two or three nursing bras
Or pack the bras that you have been wearing throughout pregnancy, if you are not going to breast-feed.

6 pairs of underpants
Buy cotton pants. You may go through several pairs a day so pack a pile.

Two to three machine-washable nightgowns and a bathrobe
These should be made of cotton because it is the most comfortable fiber.

Front opening, *with buttons that undo well below the breasts, if breast-feeding*

Low-heeled slippers

COMING HOME
Choose an outfit for your partner to bring when it's time for you to be discharged. Don't pick anything too tight fitting; you may not be back to your pre-pregnancy size. The baby needs clothes for coming home, too, so set aside:
- two diapers (don't forget a pin and plastic pants if you're not using disposables)
- undershirt
- stretchsuit or nightgown
- sweater and hat
- receiving blanket or a warm blanket for cold weather.

LABOR AND BIRTH

At last the long weeks of waiting are over. Labor and delivery are the culmination of your pregnancy, and the moment when you first see your baby is now only a matter of hours away. You may be excited, yet apprehensive about how well your labor will go. If you have prepared yourself and understand what is happening to your body and your baby at each stage, it won't be so frightening. Stay calm and you'll save energy. The pain of labor can be intense or mild but you should never be made to feel like a failure. There are no perfect standards for having a baby, so even as you practice your breathing and relaxation techniques, don't be too hard on yourself. This is not a race you are going to win or lose but a little human being you are bringing into the world.

KNOWING YOU ARE IN LABOR

EVERY WOMAN'S EXPERIENCE is different, but first-time mothers often worry that they won't recognize true labor. In late pregnancy, you may be plagued by short, irregular pains, called Braxton-Hicks contractions, and there's always the possibility of confusing these with the real thing.

SIGNS OF LABOR
A show
The plug of thick, blood-stained mucus that blocks the neck of the womb in pregnancy usually passes out of the vagina, either before or during the early stages of labor.
What to do The show may happen a few days before labor starts, so wait until you feel regular pains in your stomach or back, or your water breaks, before calling the doctor or midwife.

Your water breaks
The bag of fluid that surrounds the baby can break at any time during labor. It may be a sudden flood, but it's far more common to notice a trickle of fluid. When the baby's head engages, it may stem the tide.
What to do Call the doctor or midwife immediately. You need to go to the hospital even if you don't have contractions, because there is a risk of infection. Meanwhile, wear a sanitary napkin.

Contractions
These may start off as a dull backache, or you may have shooting pains down your thighs. As time goes by you will have contractions in your stomach, rather like bad menstrual cramps.
What to do When the contractions seem to be regular, time them. If you think you are in labor, call the doctor or midwife. Unless contractions are coming very frequently (every five minutes), or are very painful, there is no need to go to the hospital immediately. A first labor usually lasts about 12 to 14 hours, and it is often better to spend several hours of this time at home. Move around gently, resting whenever you need to. Perhaps relax in a warm bath, if your water hasn't broken, or eat a light snack. The hospital will probably suggest that you wait until the contractions are quite strong and occurring every five minutes or so before you leave home.

FALSE STARTS
Throughout pregnancy, the womb contracts. In the last weeks, these Braxton-Hicks contractions become stronger, so you may think you are in labor. However true labor contractions occur very regularly, and grow stronger and more frequent, so you should be able to tell when the real thing begins.

Occasionally contractions start and then die away. If you stay active, they may begin again.

TIMING CONTRACTIONS

10 minutes — Contraction
20 minutes
15 minutes — Interval between contractions
15 minutes

Time contractions for an hour, noting when each one starts and ends. They should become stronger and more frequent, and last for at least 40 seconds. The diagram shows intervals between contractions in early labor.

THE FIRST STAGE

DURING THIS STAGE, the muscles of your womb contract to open up the cervix (neck of the womb) to allow the baby to pass through at birth. It takes an average of ten to twelve hours for a first baby.

Don't be surprised if at some time in the first stage you suddenly feel panic-stricken. However well prepared you are, the feeling that your body has been taken over by a process that you can't control can be frightening. Stay calm and try to go with your body. It is now that you will most appreciate having your partner or a good friend by your side, especially if they understand labor, and have gone to prenatal classes.

After admission
When initial checks are over, some hospitals allow a shower.

ADMISSION TO THE HOSPITAL

Your obstetrician or midwife will probably call the hospital ahead of you to let them know you will be arriving. This helps with red tape tremendously. It's also critical to have a partner alongside you all the way. He or she can act as a kind of intermediary between you and the medical staff, which will help when you don't feel like talking.

Once you reach the hospital, a nurse or technician will carry out several routine admission procedures.

Checking you

After you have changed into the hospital gown or the clothes you brought for the birth, the nurse may take your blood pressure, temperature, and pulse, and give you an internal examination to check how far the neck of the womb has opened. You will also give a urine sample, to be tested for traces of protein and sugar.

Checking the baby

The nurse or midwife will check the baby's position by feeling your abdomen, and she will listen to his heartbeat with an obstetric stethoscope or a special instrument (see page 65).

The nurse or doctor may attach an external or internal fetal monitor to record the baby's heartbeat. It will indicate that your baby is getting enough oxygen during contractions.

Necessary hospital routines?

Many hospitals routinely administer enemas to women in labor in preparation for delivery. This "prep" is something you should question. It can be a personally demeaning way to begin your childbirth experience, and studies say it has little effect on the progress of labor.

Another "prep" that is still quite common is shaving the pubic area of the expectant mother. It is done to make the perineum area clear during birth, but if you don't want to be shaved, tell your obstetrician. When pubic hair is growing back after birth it can make you feel itchy and uncomfortable.

INTERNAL EXAMINATIONS

The doctor may give you regular internal examinations to check the position of the baby, and how much the cervix is dilating (opening up). Ask for progress reports if you are not told. It is encouraging to find that the cervix is widening, but it may not happen at a steady rate.

The examination is usually done between contractions, so tell the nurse if you feel one coming. You may be asked to lie on your back, propped up with pillows, but if this is uncomfortable, try your side. Relax as much as possible. Don't pressure yourself to be perfect. Getting through labor can be tough.

THE CERVIX IN LABOR

This is normally kept closed by a ring of muscles. Other muscles run from the cervix up and over the womb. These contract during labor, drawing the cervix into the womb, and then stretching it so it is wide enough for the baby's head to pass through.

Cervix

1 The tough cervix is gradually softened by hormonal changes.

2 Gentle contractions then efface (thin) the cervix.

3 Once it is fully effaced, stronger contractions dilate it.

POSITIONS FOR THE FIRST STAGE

Try a variety of positions in the first stage. Different positions will probably be comfortable at different times. Practice these positions beforehand, so that you can follow your body's natural cues with ease.

You may find that you want to lie down during the first stage. Rest on your side, not your back, with your head and upper thigh supported by cushions.

Staying upright

During early contractions, support yourself on a nearby surface, such as a wall, chair seat, or the hospital bed. Kneel down if necessary.

Sitting forward

Sit facing the back of a chair. Put a cushion or pillow over its back and lean on it. Rest your head on your folded arms. Keep your knees apart. Cushion the seat of the chair, too.

WHAT YOUR PARTNER CAN DO

■ During contractions, give her plenty of praise, comfort, and support. Don't worry if she becomes annoyed with you; you are important.
■ Remind her of the relaxation and breathing techniques she has learned (see pages 48–49).
■ Mop her brow, give her sips of water, hold her hand, massage her back, suggest a change of position, or do anything else that seems to help. Learn beforehand where and how she likes to be touched and massaged.
■ Act as a mediator between your partner and the hospital staff. Support her decision, for example, on pain medication.

Resting on your partner

As you move around in early labor, it may help to lean against your partner during contractions. He can massage your back, or gently stroke your shoulders.

Massage *her lower back*

Have *your feet comfortably apart*

Kneeling forward

Kneel down, legs apart, and relax forward on a pile of pillows. Stay as upright as possible because you want the baby to move down. Sit to one side between contractions.

On all fours

Kneel down on your hands and knees on the floor (you may find a mattress more comfortable), and tilt your pelvis up and down. Do not arch your back. Between contractions, relax forward and rest your head in your arms.

BACK LABOR

When the baby is facing toward your abdomen, instead of away from it, his head tends to press against your spine, causing backache. To relieve pain:
■ lean forward with your weight supported, such as on all fours, to take the baby's weight off your back, and rock your pelvis up and down (as shown above); move around between contractions
■ ask your partner to massage your back, or hold a hot-water bottle to the base of your spine between contractions.

> **BREATHING FOR THE FIRST STAGE**
>
> Deep even breaths   Light breaths   Deep even breaths
>
> At the beginning and end of a contraction, breathe deeply and evenly, in through the nose and out of the mouth. When the contraction peaks, try a lighter, shallower kind of breathing. Both in and out breaths should be through your mouth. Don't do this for too long, because you may feel dizzy.

HOW TO HELP YOURSELF

■ Keep moving between contractions; this helps you cope physically with the pain. During contractions, take up a comfortable position.
■ Try to stay as upright as possible, so the baby's head sits firmly on the cervix, making your contractions stronger and more effective.
■ Concentrate on your breathing, to calm you and take your mind off contractions.
■ Relax between contractions (see pages 48–49) to save energy for which you need it.
■ Sing, or even moan and groan, to release pain.
■ Look at a fixed spot or object to help take your mind off a contraction.
■ Take one contraction at a time, and don't consider the contractions to follow. Think of each contraction as a wave, which you have to ride over to reach the baby.
■ Urinate often, so a full bladder doesn't get in the way of the baby.

Lower back massage

This will relieve backache, calm, and reassure you. Your partner should massage you at the base of the spine, using the heel of his hand to make firm, circular movements. Talcum powder can help prevent friction.

TRANSITION

THE MOST DIFFICULT time in labor is often at the end of the first stage, when contractions are strongest. They last about a minute, and may be only a minute apart, so there is little time to rest after one before the next is upon you. This phase, which often lasts about half an hour, is known as transition. You will be tired, and may feel disheartened, tearful, excitable, or just bad-tempered. You will probably lose all sense of time and doze off between contractions. Nausea, vomiting, and shivering are common, too.

Eventually, you should have a strong urge to push. If you do this too early, the cervix can become swollen. Tell the doctor you are ready to push. She may examine you to determine whether your cervix is fully dilated.

To stop yourself from pushing
If the doctor says you are not fully dilated but you feel the urge to push, say "huff, huff, blow" (see above, right) to yourself and adopt this position. Kneel down and lean forward, resting your head in your arms; stick your bottom in the air. This reduces the urge to push, and also makes pushing more difficult.

BREATHING FOR TRANSITION

Short breaths   Short breaths   Short breaths
IN

OUT   Blow   Blow   Gently out

If you want to push too early, say "huff, huff, blow" to yourself, taking two short in- and out-breaths, and blowing a longer breath out. When the need to push fades, give a slow, even breath out.

WHAT YOU CAN DO AS A PARTNER
- Try to relax her, encourage her, and wipe away any perspiration; if she doesn't want to be touched, stay back.
- Breathe with her through contractions.
- Put thick socks on her legs if they start to shake, and hold them still.
- If she wants to push, call the doctor at once.

THE CERVIX IN LABOR

Cervix

At 2¾in. (7cm.), the doctor can feel the cervix stretched out around the baby's head.

When the doctor can't feel the cervix—at about 4in. (10cm.) dilated—you are fully dilated.

THE SECOND STAGE

ONCE THE CERVIX has dilated and you can push, the second stage of labor has begun. This is far more rewarding than the first stage, because you now add your own efforts to the powerful contractions of the womb, and help push the baby out.

Even though the contractions are stronger, they may not feel as bad as before. Pushing is hard, but if you find the most comfortable position for this and work together with your partner, it will go faster. Your obstetrician or midwife can guide you so you push when it's most needed. Some women experience a sense of satisfaction when pushing. The second stage usually lasts about an hour for a first baby.

BREATHING FOR THE SECOND STAGE

Deep breath   Deep even breaths   Even breaths
IN
     Push   Push

OUT

When you want to push (this may happen several times during a contraction), take a deep breath and hold it for a short time as you bear down, if this helps the push; it's important to do what your body tells you. Between pushes, take a few deep calming breaths. Relax slowly as the contraction fades.

POSITIONS FOR DELIVERY

Try to be as upright as possible when pushing, so you are working with gravity, rather than against it.

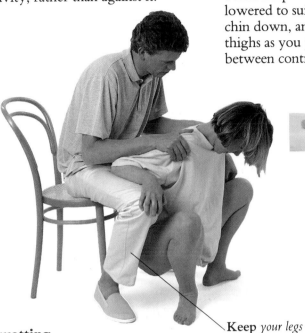

Keep *your legs comfortably apart*

Squatting

This is an excellent position for delivery, because it opens the pelvis wide and uses gravity to help push out the baby. But unless you have practiced it beforehand (see page 47), you may find it tiring after a while.

If your partner sits on the edge of a chair, with his legs apart, you can squat between his knees, resting your arms on his thighs for support.

Kneeling

This may be less tiring than squatting, and is also a good pushing position. A helper on each side will make you feel more stable. You may also find kneeling down on all fours comfortable; keep your back straight.

WHAT YOU CAN DO AS A PARTNER

■ Try to relax her between the contractions, and continue to give encouragement and support.
■ If she is interested, tell her what you can see as the baby's head emerges, but don't be surprised if she doesn't seem to notice you.

Sitting upright

A common delivery position is to sit propped up by pillows at a 45-degree angle. Some hospital beds can be raised and lowered to suit you. Keep your chin down, and grip under your thighs as you push. Relax between contractions.

WAYS TO HELP YOURSELF

■ Push smoothly and steadily during a contraction.
■ Try to relax the muscles of your pelvic floor, so you feel as if you are letting go completely.
■ Keep your face relaxed.
■ Don't worry about trying to control your bowels, or about any leakage of water from the bladder.
■ Rest as much as possible between contractions, so you save all your energy for pushing.

THE BIRTH

THE CLIMAX of labor has now arrived, and your baby is about to be born. This is very exciting, because you may want to touch her head for the first time as it emerges. You'll hold her soon and will probably feel a great sense of physical relief, but there may also be wonder, emotional tears of joy, or perhaps a feeling of overwhelming tenderness toward your baby.

Relax with your partner
Your partner's company may calm you and give you confidence during the long hours of labor and delivery.

1 The baby's head moves nearer the vaginal opening, until eventually there is a bulge where it is pressing against the pelvic floor. Soon the head itself will be seen, moving forward with each contraction, and perhaps slipping back slightly as the contraction fades. Don't be discouraged if this happens; it is perfectly normal.

2 When the head "crowns" (the top is visible), the doctor may ask you not to push, because if the head is born too quickly, your skin might tear. So, relax, and pant for a few seconds. If there is a risk of a serious tear, or the baby is distressed, you will have an episiotomy (see page 66). As the head widens the vaginal opening, there will be a stinging feeling, but this only lasts for a short while, and is soon followed by numbness because the tissues have been stretched so much.

3 The head is born face down. The doctor will probably check the umbilical cord, to make sure it isn't looped around the baby's neck. (If it is, the cord can usually be slipped over the head when the body is delivered.) Then the baby turns her head to one side so that it is in line with her shoulders. The doctor cleans her eyes, nose, and mouth, and if necessary sucks out any fluid from her upper air passages using a tube.

4 The body comes sliding out within the next two contractions. The doctor will usually lift the baby up under her armpits and deliver her on to your stomach, while the cord is still attached. Your baby will probably look rather blue at first. She may be covered in vernix, a sticky, grayish-white substance, and streaks of blood. She may be crying. The umbilical cord is usually clamped and cut at this point. The doctor may clear the baby's airways again to make sure she can breathe easily.

QUESTIONS & ANSWERS

"I'm very worried about damaging the skin or muscles of my vagina during birth. Is there danger of this?"
You won't damage yourself pushing. The vaginal walls are elastic, with many folds, so they can stretch to allow the baby through.

"Should I breast-feed my baby immediately after the birth?"
Try offering your baby the breast but leave it up to her. There will not be any milk, but a newborn baby's urge to suck is often quite strong, and sucking is comforting.

THE APGAR SCORE
Immediately after birth, the doctor will assess the baby's breathing, heart rate, skin color, movements, and response to stimulation, and give her an Apgar score of between 0 and 10.

Most babies score between 7 and 10. The test is done again about five minutes later, so even if the score was initially low, it may improve the second time around.

THE THIRD STAGE
Your birth experience is not complete until the placenta is also delivered. It may take only a few seconds for it to separate spontaneously from the wall of your uterus and contractions will reduce it in size dramatically. Or it might take up to half an hour. You may lose a little blood as this happens. You may also have to push a bit to rid your body of it, but the pushes will be nothing in comparison to what you have just gone through. The doctor may push down gently on your abdomen and tug on the umbilical cord still attached at one end to the placenta. Occasionally, oxytocin is administered to speed up this third stage. The doctor will make sure the placenta is complete because if pieces of it remain in your uterus, they can cause excessive bleeding later.

AFTER THE BIRTH
You will be cleaned up, and the obstetrician will stitch any tears or surgical cuts you've sustained (see page 66). The doctor will weigh and measure the baby, and quickly rule out any abnormalities. Sometimes, the baby is given vitamin K at this time to prevent a rare bleeding disorder.

Becoming a family
After birth, you can relax and spend a few quiet moments alone gently cuddling your new baby.

PAIN RELIEF

ALTHOUGH LABOR is not usually pain-free, the pain does have a purpose; every contraction brings you one step nearer to the birth of your baby. However determined you may be at the start to have a completely natural birth with no pain medication, keep an open mind. Whether you need it or not depends very much on your labor and your ability to deal with pain—and pain is always worse if you try to fight it. You may be able to cope using the self-help methods on pages 59 and 61. But if the discomfort is more than you can bear, ask for pain medication, and don't feel like a failure.

EPIDURAL
An epidural is a type of anesthesia that relieves pain by temporarily numbing the nerves in the lower body. It can be especially good for back labor. Not all hospitals offer epidurals, and they are always administered by a specially trained anesthesiologist.

Epidural or caudal anesthesia numbs you all the way from your waist to your toes. It's an anesthesia that could interfere with your ability to push your baby out and make it more likely that the obstetrician will use forceps at delivery. It can slow the baby's heartbeat and your blood pressure, and take hours to wear off afterward. However, it may also be exactly what you need to get you through a physically difficult experience. Talk to your obstetrician and weigh all the pros and cons, especially if either of you anticipates a difficult labor and delivery.

An epidural may take about 20 minutes to start working. You will be asked to curl in a ball, with your knees tucked up under your chin, so your back is as rounded as possible. The anesthesia is injected through a catheter inserted in your lower back. A tube may be taped in place, so that you can be given additional medication at a later stage. Whenever you opt for an epidural, you will automatically be hooked up to an intravenous (IV) line in your arm, and you will also be monitored continually, so movement is restricted.

If the epidural works properly, you should have no pain, and remain aware of what is happening. Some women feel faint, and have a headache.

SADDLE BLOCK
A saddle block, like an epidural, is a type of spinal anesthesia but is usually used for delivery only and often during a Cesarean section. The numbness can extend up to your ribcage but you'll be wide awake for the delivery. The medication is injected into the spinal fluid of your back.

DEMEROL
Also called meperidine, this is a synthetic narcotic that is often used in the hospital during labor.

With small dosages, you remain awake and able to participate in all aspects of the birth. With an average dose, it takes about 20 minutes for the relaxation to come over you, but it will last up to three hours and it gives some women the strength or willpower to stay on top of difficult contractions. In that brief interval between contractions, you can actually nap. However, some women report that they end up feeling nauseous or disoriented by Demerol.

Unfortunately, narcotics like Demerol do cross the placenta and end up in the baby's system. At birth, this might inhibit the newborn's ability to breathe deeply, but this effect can be minimized by keeping the dosages small. And medication is always available in the delivery room to handle any infant suffering from a drug-induced side effect such as this.

TRANQUILIZERS AND SEDATIVES
Sometimes if you are especially anxious during the early stages of your labor, the doctor may suggest something to take the edge off. These drugs have a soothing effect on your mood and studies show that there is no real effect on the baby. If you are already on an intravenous (IV) drip, then it will simply be added to that fluid, but if not, you may be given an injection. If you don't want it, just say, "No thanks," or have your partner say it for you.

LOCAL ANESTHESIA
These pain inhibitors may be used at various times during labor and delivery. A paracervical block might be injected into the skin next to your cervix during labor to numb it. Another type, the pudendal block,

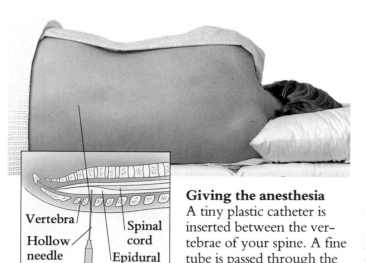

Giving the anesthesia
A tiny plastic catheter is inserted between the vertebrae of your spine. A fine tube is passed through the needle, and a local anesthesia is fed into this.

Vertebra

Hollow needle

Spinal cord

Epidural space

will work on the nerves that supply the vagina and perineum, or that space between your vagina and rectum. Sometimes, these locals are administered because your doctor has decided on a forceps delivery. You'll also have local anesthesia if you've had an episiotomy, when the surgical cut is stitched up.

GENERAL ANESTHESIA
In years past, women in labor were just put to sleep and drugs such as sodium pentothal were given at delivery. This is no longer common medical practice. Unless your baby is suddenly in distress and you are being rushed in for an emergency Cesarean section, you won't have general anesthesia. When that happens, the doctor needs to deliver the baby immediately and can't wait the 20 to 30 minutes necessary for an epidural to take effect. When C-sections can be planned in advance, many mothers now choose to be awake for the delivery.

MONITORING

THROUGHOUT LABOR your baby's heartbeat will be monitored so that any signs of distress can be detected as early as possible. This will be done either with a hand-held standard obstetric stethoscope, an electronic monitor attached to your stomach or an internal fetal monitor inserted into your cervix and strapped to the baby's head.

OBSTETRIC STETHOSCOPE
A nurse or doctor may place the instrument on your stomach at regular intervals throughout labor to listen to the baby's heartbeat.

ELECTRONIC FETAL MONITORING (EFM)
This is a way of recording the baby's heartbeat and your contractions using sophisticated electronic equipment. Some hospitals routinely monitor women throughout labor, others do so only at intervals because:
- your labor was induced
- you are having an epidural
- you have a problem or condition that puts you or the baby at risk
- the baby is distressed at any time.

External or internal EFM is not usually painful, but it does restrict your freedom to move around, which may make your contractions more uncomfortable. In recent years, routine electronic fetal monitoring has come under fire because of the incidences when the machines weren't providing accurate readings. If the doctor suggests continual monitoring for no obvious reason, ask if it is really necessary.

What happens
You will probably be asked to sit or lie on the hospital bed with your trunk supported by pillows, and small pads will be strapped to your abdomen, to monitor the baby's heartbeat and measure your contractions. These appear on a paper printout attached to the monitor. Later in labor, when your water has broken, the baby's heartbeat can be measured directly by clipping an electrode to his head. This internal method is the most accurate way to monitor the progress of labor.

Monitors look for abnormalities in the baby's heart rate. Is the fetus getting enough oxygen? Is the umbilical cord twisted or wrapped around his neck? EFM can help answer such questions.

The pad *measures your contractions*

SPECIAL PROCEDURES

■ EPISIOTOMY ■	■ ASSISTED DELIVERY ■	■ INDUCTION ■
This small cut widens the vaginal opening and prevents a tear. Some hospitals perform episiotomies more often than others, so speak to your obstetrician about routine practices in the hospital you have chosen. To avoid an episiotomy or a tear: ■ learn how to relax your pelvic floor muscles (see page 45) ■ stay upright during delivery.	Sometimes the baby has to be helped out with forceps or by suction. Forceps are used only when the cervix is fully dilated, and the baby's head has engaged, although suction or a vacuum extractor may be used occasionally before full dilation has been reached, if labor is prolonged.	If you are induced, labor is started artificially. Some of the methods may be used to speed up labor if it is going slowly. Hospital policies on induction vary from place to place, so ask your obsterician about his policies on induction.
When used An episiotomy may be needed if: ■ the baby is breech, premature, distressed, or has a big head ■ you have an assisted delivery ■ you are having difficulty controlling your pushing ■ the skin around your vaginal .opening hasn't stretched enough.	**When used** You may have an assisted delivery if: ■ you cannot push the baby out, perhaps because he has a big head ■ you or the baby shows signs of distress during the labor ■ your baby is breech or premature; the forceps protect his head from pressure in the birth canal.	**When used** Labor may be induced if: ■ you are long past the baby's due date, and he shows signs of being distressed or the placenta starts to fail ■ you have high blood pressure, or another problem or condition that puts you or the baby at risk.
What happens Your pelvic floor area will probably be numbed with an injection of local anesthesia, and a small cut is made from the bottom of the vagina, usually slightly out to one side, at the peak of a contraction. Sometimes there is no time for an injection, but the stretching of the tissues also numbs them, so you shouldn't feel any pain. Stitching up after an episiotomy or a tear may take some time, because the different layers of skin and muscle have to be carefully sewn together. It can be painful, too, so ask for more anesthesia if you need some. The stitches will dissolve so they won't have to be removed.	**What happens** ■ **Forceps** You will probably be given an injection of local anesthesia into your pelvic floor area, and an episiotomy. The doctor positions the forceps on either side of the baby's head and gently pulls to deliver it. You can help by pushing. The rest of the body is delivered normally. **Forceps** These form a cage around the baby's head, protecting it from pressure and damage. ■ **Vacuum** A small plastic or metal cup, connected to a vacuum pump, is passed into the vagina and attached to the baby's head. The baby is gently pulled through the birth canal as you push.	**What happens** Induction is always planned in advance, and you will be asked to go into the hospital. Labor may be induced in either of two ways: 1 Breaking your water or amniotomy. The doctor makes a small hole in the bag of fluid surrounding the baby using a special instrument that passes through the cervix. Most women don't feel any pain. Contractions nearly always start soon afterward. 2 Giving you a hormone, pitocin, or oxytocin, which makes the womb contract. This is fed through an IV in your arm at a controlled rate. Ask for the needle to be inserted into the arm you use least. Sometimes, the drug is administered to speed up a labor that has slowed considerably or stopped altogether. The amount given can be electronically calculated with the intravenous drip.
Effects Some discomfort and soreness is normal after an episiotomy, but pain can be severe if an infection develops. The wound should heal within 10 to 14 days, but if you are sore after this time, ask your doctor. There is less pain with a tear.	**Effects** ■ The forceps may leave pressure marks or bruises on either side of the baby's head, but these are harmless and disappear within a few days. ■ The vacuum cup will cause slight swelling, and later a bruise, on the baby's head. This gradually subsides.	**Effects** ■ Amniotomy is usually painless and labor ordinarily begins soon after the membranes have been broken. ■ When artificial hormones like oxytocin or pitocin are used, labor can come on with full immediate force, so you are much more likely to need pain medication.

CESAREAN SECTION

BREECH BIRTH

A breech baby is born bottom, or occasionally feet, first. About four in 100 births are breech. During a normal vaginal delivery, the baby's head puts tremendous pressure on the birth canal, forcing it to dilate. The head itself decreases in diameter during labor, making it easier to emerge at birth. That's why so many newborns have elongated or misshapen heads at first.

In a breech presentation, however, the baby's bottom or feet don't put enough pressure on the birth canal to dilate it sufficiently, and the baby's head doesn't have the chance to change shape during labor so that it will fit through the mother's pelvis without stress. That's why some hospitals automatically suggest C-sections when they see the breech position in sonograms during the later stages of pregnancy.

TWINS

There is always an increased risk of complications when twins are on the way, so they should be born at a hospital. Sometimes, they arrive prematurely or the stress of carrying them brings on preeclampsia. One of the babies may be in a breech or some other awkward position.

A woman carrying twins will go through one first stage, but have two second stages as you push first one baby out, and then the other. The second twin is usually born 10 to 30 minutes after the first.

WITH A CESAREAN birth, the baby is delivered abdominally. You may know you are going to have a Cesarean in advance, or it may be an emergency operation because of problems in labor. If a Cesarean is planned, you can have it under an epidural (see page 64), so you are awake throughout and can hold your baby right away. This may also be possible if you are told in labor that a C-section is imminent. In a real emergency, however, general anesthesia is often necessary so the doctor can deliver the baby quickly.

It's only natural to feel disappointed, and perhaps cheated of a normal delivery, if you need a Cesarean. But these feelings can be minimized if you prepare yourself thoroughly by understanding the reasons for the decision. Ask the obstetrician if your partner can be with you throughout.

WHAT HAPPENS

Your pubic hair will be shaved and you will be hooked up to an IV in your arm. A catheter will also be inserted into your bladder to keep it empty during the surgery. If the Cesarean section was planned, you may have opted for an epidural so you can be awake during the procedure. If it's an emergency because of something that has come up during your labor, you may have to be given general anesthesia that will put you to sleep. There are two types of incisions: a vertical cut from your navel to your pubic hairline or a horizontal ("bikini") cut made near the top of your pubic hairline. The baby's head is delivered first and mucus may be suctioned from his mouth even before his feet are visible. The operation, from start to finish, should take approximately 45 minutes.

The incision
The "bikini" cut is usually made horizontally, just above the pubic hairline, and it is almost invisible when it heals.

Stitching the incision
You or your partner can hold the baby, while the obstetrician stitches up.

AFTER THE OPERATION

You will be encouraged to walk soon after the birth. The incision will be painful for a few days, so ask for pain medication. Moving around won't open it up. Stand tall, and cup your hands over the wound. You may find that it helps to hold your stomach when you laugh, sneeze, or cough. Try using a footstool when you are getting in or out of bed. By about two days after the operation, begin gentle exercises (see page 72), unless advised otherwise by the doctor. The stitches will be removed several days later, unless they're the soluble type, and you will feel much better after a week. Don't strain yourself for at least six weeks. The scar fades, usually within six months.

YOUR NEW BABY

Don't let very first impressions of your newborn shock you. Your baby may look dramatically different from the cherubic pictures of infants you've seen in books. His head may be misshapen from having been elongated to fit through the birth canal. His arms and legs may be a little blue, and he may be covered with a white, greasy substance called vernix. His body is not working efficiently yet, so you may notice spots, blotches, and changes of color, which are perfectly normal. Ask your pediatrician if anything worries you. He can put your mind at ease. You may love your baby immediately. But if you don't feel this way at first, give yourself time. Once you get to know each other as you care for him, and find that he responds to your touch and the sound of your voice, love will grow naturally.

FIRST IMPRESSIONS

VERY FEW BABIES look picture perfect at birth. In fact, blotchy skin, pointy heads, swollen genitals, lots of downy body hair, and the grayish-white vernix covering their little bodies may make you want to delay those first formal portrait sittings.

HEAD
A strange, pointed shape is caused by the pressure of birth. The head should look normal in two weeks.
On the top of the head is a soft spot (fontanelle), where the bones of the skull have not yet joined together. They should fuse by the time the child is 18 months.

EYES
These are blue at birth. True eye color may not develop until the baby is about six months old.
Puffy eyelids are usually caused by the pressure of birth, but ask the doctor or midwife to check your baby's eyes.
Squinting is common. The baby may look cross-eyed at times in the first months.

TONGUE
This may seem anchored to the floor of the mouth, so that the tip looks slightly forked when the baby sticks it out. The tip will grow forward in the first year.

HANDS AND FEET
These may be bluish because the baby's circulation is not working properly. If you move your baby into another position, they should turn pink.
The fingernails are often long at birth.

BREASTS
Your baby's breasts may be swollen and even leak a little milk. This is perfectly normal in both sexes. The swelling should go down within two days; do not squeeze the milk out.

GENITALS
These look large on both male and female babies.
A baby girl may have discharge from her vagina. This is caused by the mother's hormones and will soon disappear.
The testicles of a baby boy are often pulled up into his groin.

The **fontanelle** *cannot be damaged through everyday handling*

Your baby *may have a good head of hair, or he may be bald*

His hands *will be clenched*

Red marks *are caused by pressure from the birth, or because the baby's skin is still immature*

The umbilical cord *stump drops off in about two weeks*

The baby can see *you at birth if you hold him about 8in. (20cm.) away from your face*

SKIN

Spots and rashes are very common, and should vanish of their own accord.

Peeling skin, especially on the hands and feet, should disappear in a few days.

Downy body hair (lanugo) may be noticeable, especially if the baby was born early. This rubs off within two weeks.

Greasy white vernix is the substance that protects the baby's skin in the womb, and may cover him completely. It can be easily wiped off.

Birthmarks usually vanish. These include:

■ red marks often found on the eyelids, forehead, and at the back of the neck; they take about a year to go away

■ strawberry birthmarks can be worrisome because they gradually increase in size. However, they may disappear by the time the child is five

■ blue patches, often found on the lower backs of babies with dark skin

■ port wine stain, a bright-red or purple mark, which is permanent.

STOOL

A newborn baby's first bowel movement contains a dark, sticky substance called meconium. Once he is fed, the stool changes.

The baby's legs
often look bowed because he has been curled up in the womb

CHECKS ON THE BABY

YOUR BABY will be examined many times in the first week. The obstetrician or midwife will do a quick and immediate check right there on delivery while he's lying on your abdomen or in your arms. If you've arranged for your own pediatrician to be at the hospital, that's who will begin the careful weighing, measuring, and reassuring that all is normal.

GENERAL EXAMINATION

The pediatrician will check the baby from head to toe to insure nothing is abnormal.

1 The doctor measures the head and looks for any abnormalities. He checks the fontanelle, and feels the roof of the mouth to make sure it is complete.

2 He listens to the heart and lungs to see if they are normal. An irregular heartbeat is common among newborn babies, and does not usually indicate a defect.

3 By putting his hand on the baby's tummy, the doctor checks that the abdominal organs are the right size. He also feels the pulses in the baby's groin.

4 The genitals are checked for abnormality. If you have a boy, the doctor will be looking to see if both testicles have descended.

5 He gently moves the baby's limbs back and forth, and checks that the lower legs and feet are aligned, that the legs are the right length, and that his reflexes are normal.

6 The doctor checks the hips for any dislocation, by bending the baby's legs up and gently circling them.

SPECIAL TESTS

A blood test is done during your hospital stay to check for a thyroid deficiency or phenylketonuria (PKU), a rare but treatable, metabolic disorder. It involves a small prick on the baby's heel. PKU can cause mental disabilities if it's not detected early in life.

7 He runs his thumb down the baby's back, making sure that all the vertebrae are in place along the spine.

SPECIAL CARE BABIES

SOME BABIES need special care after birth. When an infant is born prematurely (before 37 weeks), or is small for dates (see page 39), she may spend the first days of her life in the intensive care unit because of problems with breathing, feeding, and keeping warm. Life with a baby under intensive care is bound to be hard. Not only will you be separated from her but you will see her surrounded by the intimidating array of equipment. This can be frightening. Helping the hospital staff take care of your baby will calm you and make this difficult bonding go a little better.

Portholes, *so you can touch your baby and talk to her*

You may want *to bring along a soft toy for your baby*

Feeding tube, *which passes into the baby's stomach; you can express your own milk to be fed to the baby*

The baby in the incubator
Your baby needs just as much love and attention as any normal healthy baby.

Tilting tray, *to help with respiration and feeding*

Control, *to regulate the temperature inside the incubator*

GETTING TO KNOW YOUR BABY
It's important to spend as much time with your baby as possible; many hospitals have special rooms for parents. Stay near your baby and take part in her daily care. At first, she may look so small and vulnerable that you worry about touching her. But all babies respond to loving handling, and even if she can't be taken out of the incubator to cuddle, you can still talk to her and stroke her, and perhaps help change her diaper and dress her.

ASKING QUESTIONS
Ask the doctor or nursing staff about anything that worries you. Often parents don't ask questions, because their baby looks so frail that they are afraid of the answers. But with modern medical technology, even babies born before 28 weeks can survive.

FEEDING
If the baby can suck, you may be able to feed her normally. Otherwise, she will be fed through a tube, which is passed through her nose or mouth and down into her stomach.

JAUNDICE
Many newborn babies develop very mild jaundice about three days after birth, which turns their skin and the whites of their eyes slightly yellow. This happens because a baby's liver is still immature, and a pigment called bilirubin accumulates in the blood.

Jaundice usually clears up in a few days of its own accord, although the baby may be more sleepy than usual, so wake her up often, and encourage her to eat. It also helps if her bed is near a window so she is exposed to sunlight. Sometimes jaundice has to be treated with special light (phototherapy). This can usually be done in the newborn hospital nursery. Only in a few severe cases is the baby transferred to intensive care.

STILLBIRTH
When a baby is born dead after 20 weeks of pregnancy, it's commonly called a stillbirth. But it happens only rarely. Because of modern medical techniques, an infant isn't likely to die during labor or delivery. All these positive statistics won't make it any easier for you to bear if your baby is stillborn. Don't turn away physically from your dead baby, however. Hold him, give him a name, and grieve for him. Studies show that you will recover faster emotionally. You will feel angry, and will want to know what went wrong and be anxious to blame. Shame and guilt are also common. Don't carry the burden single-handedly and do find someone with whom you can talk frankly, whether it's an individual therapist or a self-help group.

GETTING BACK TO NORMAL

For the first week after delivery, sleep whenever you can. Don't be tempted to use free moments to catch up on housework or errands. Your postpartum check-up isn't usually scheduled until four to six weeks after the birth, but you should not hesitate to call your obstetrician before that if you have any problems, even what you might consider minor. Your baby's pediatrician can be a storehouse of answers. Get to know him; your worries should never be discounted. You may be aghast when you first see your body after birth. Your familiar belly will be gone, though your stomach will be far from flat. Your breasts will be large, and the tops of your legs will feel heavy. If you feel good and the doctor says okay, start your postnatal exercises from the first day after birth.

HOW YOU WILL FEEL

YOU WILL have some discomfort, and even pain, in the first days after birth. Speak up with your doctor or hospital staff members if anything worries you.

AFTERPAINS
The cramping pains in your stomach, especially when breast-feeding, mean the womb is contracting back to its prepregnant size. This is a good sign that your body is returning to normal. These afterpains may last several days.
What to do If contractions are severe, ask your doctor to recommend a mild pain-killer to ease them.

BLADDER
It's normal to urinate often in the first days, as the body eliminates the extra fluid gained in pregnancy.

What to do Urinating may be difficult at first, because of soreness, but try to do so as soon as possible after the birth.
■ Get up and move around to encourage the flow.
■ Take a long shower as soon as you feel steady on your feet. The warm water will relax your muscles.
■ If you have stitches, try pouring warm water over them as you urinate to stop your skin from stinging.

BLEEDING
You may have vaginal bleeding for anywhere from two to six weeks. This usually stops more quickly if you are breast-feeding. The bright red discharge is heavy at first, but over the next few days it changes color, and gradually becomes brownish. Often the discharge will continue until your first menstrual period.
What to do Wear sanitary pads; don't use internal tampons at this time, as they can cause infection.

BOWELS
You may not need to empty your bowels for a day or more after the birth.
What to do Get up and move as soon as you can: walking around will start your bowels working.
■ Drink plenty of water and eat high-fiber foods to stimulate your bowels.
■ When you need to move your bowels, do so at once, but don't strain or push.
■ It is most unlikely that any stitches will tear when you move your bowels, but holding a clean sanitary pad against the area while you do so may feel good and give you confidence.

STITCHES
These may be very sore until you are healed. Most dissolve in about a week; external ones may fall out.
What to do The following suggestions will help.
■ Practice pelvic floor exercises as soon as possible after birth to speed up healing.
■ Keep stitches clean by relaxing in a warm bath. Dry the area thoroughly afterward; try using a hair dryer set on cool.
■ Soothe soreness by applying an ice pack to the area —try a bag of frozen peas.
■ Lie down to take pressure off the stitches that can come from being on your feet. Sit on a rubber ring.

COPING WITH THE BLUES
Many women feel low a few days after delivery, usually when their breast milk comes in. One cause is the sudden change in hormone levels, another is the feeling of anticlimax that inevitably occurs after birth. These postnatal blues usually vanish. If you feel depressed for more than four weeks, or your depression is very severe, see your obstetrician or talk to your midwife.

Thinking positively
It's easy to to get bogged down in all the work having a newborn entails. Don't lose sight of the joys.

SHAPING UP AFTER BIRTH

WITH SOME GENTLE EXERCISING every day, your figure can return to normal again in as little as three months after the birth, although your stomach muscles may not be as firm as before. Build up slowly at first, because your ligaments are still soft and stretchy, and always stop if you feel pain or tiredness. It's best to exercise in short but frequent spurts.

> ### ■ WARNING ■
> If you have had a Cesarean, you won't be ready to start the exercises for your stomach muscles until much later after birth. When you're ready, begin with the week one routine. Check with your doctor first before practicing any exercises, and stop if you feel pain.

WEEK ONE
You can begin to strengthen the stretched, and possibly weakened, muscles of your pelvic floor and stomach from the first day after birth. The pelvic floor and foot pedaling exercises are also good several weeks after a Cesarean.

PELVIC FLOOR EXERCISE from day one
Practice gentle squeezing and lifting exercises (see page 45) as often as possible every day to stop yourself from leaking urine involuntarily. It's important to do this before you go on to the exercises in week two. If you have had stitches, strengthening the pelvic floor will help heal them.

FOOT PEDALING from day one
This will stop swelling in the legs and improve circulation. Bend your feet up and down at the ankle. Practice hourly if you can find the time.

STOMACH TONER from day one
A gentle way to strengthen these muscles is to pull them in as you breathe out, hold them in for a few seconds, then relax. Try to do this as often as possible.

From day five after birth, if you feel all right, practice the following exercise twice a day:

1 Lie on your back with your head and shoulders supported on two pillows, and your legs bent and slightly apart. Cross your arms over your stomach.

2 Lift your head and shoulders, and as you do this, breathe out and press gently on each side of your stomach with the palms of your hands, as if pulling the two sides together. Hold this position for a few seconds, then breathe in, and relax.
Repeat three times.

WEEK TWO
After about a week, try the following exercises as a daily routine, and continue for at least three months. Repeat each exercise as many times as is comfortable. Begin with the curl-downs, and when you can do these easily, move on to the other exercises. If you find that new exercises strain you, practice the curl-downs for a few days longer. Remember to keep practicing the exercise for your pelvic floor.

CURL-DOWNS
1 Sit up, with your legs bent and slightly apart, and your arms folded in front of you.

2 Breathe out, while gently tilting your pelvis forward, and gradually lean back until you feel the muscles of your stomach tighten. Hold for as long as you comfortably can while breathing normally. Then breathe in and sit up straight.

SIDE BENDS

1 Lie flat on your back with your arms by your side and the palms of your hands resting on the outsides of your thighs.

2 Lift your head slightly, and bending to the left, slide your left hand down your leg. Lie back and rest for a moment, then repeat on your right side. As this becomes easy, try bending to each side two or three times before you lie back and rest.

CURL-UPS

1 Lie flat on your back on the floor, with your knees bent and your feet slightly apart. Rest your hands on your thighs.

2 Breathe out, and lift your head and shoulders, stretching forward to touch your knees with your hands. Don't worry if you can't reach far enough at first; you will succeed with practice. Breathe in and relax.

WHEN THIS IS EASY, TRY:
■ lifting yourself up more slowly and holding the position for longer
■ placing your hands on your chest as you lift your head and shoulders
■ clasping your hands behind your head as you lift yourself up

CHECKING YOUR PELVIC FLOOR
By three months after birth, these muscles should be strong again. Test them by skipping. If any urine leaks, practice the pelvic floor exercises for another month and try again. If leaking is still a problem after four months, see your doctor.

HOW YOUR BODY RECOVERS

YOUR BODY won't be fully recovered for at least six months after the birth, but by the time you have your six-week checkup, it should be getting back to normal. Your womb may have shrunk back to its prepregnant size, and you may have started your periods again. If you have been exercising regularly, your muscles should be in far better shape.

YOUR CHECKUP
Your postpartum checkup with the obstetrician or midwife is usually set four to six weeks after delivery. The visit is a chance to relive the happy moments of the birth, so do ask about aspects you may have missed. These memories are important.

What happens
■ Your blood pressure, weight, and a sample of urine will be checked.
■ Your breasts and stomach will be examined. The doctor will make sure any stitches have healed.

■ You will have an internal examination to check the size and position of the womb, and may be given a cervical pap test.
■ The doctor will discuss contraception; if you wish it, you may be fitted for a diaphragm or IUD.

YOUR PERIODS
The first menstrual period after birth is often longer and heavier than usual. If you are breast-feeding, your periods may not start until after your baby is weaned. If you are bottle-feeding, a period usually comes four to six weeks after the birth.

QUESTIONS & ANSWERS

"When can we resume our sex life?"
The best time to start making love again is when your vagina has healed and you are both ready. For most women, it takes four weeks. But you may feel too sore and tender to resume sex until after your checkup.

When you do resume your sex life, take it slowly. Relax as much as you can, and use extra lubrication, because your vagina may be sore and drier than normal.

"I'm breast-feeding my baby; do we still have to use contraception?"
Even if you are breast-feeding or haven't started your periods again, you need to use contraception. The doctor or midwife can discuss this with you soon after the birth. If you want to go on the pill, make sure the doctor knows you are breast-feeding; if you previously used a diaphragm, you must have a new one fitted because your cervix will have changed shape.

2

BABY CARE

■ ■ ■ ■ ■

*A step-by-step, practical guide to
caring for your baby,
from birth to three years.*

THE FIRST WEEKS OF LIFE

Nothing can really prepare you for the reality of having a child. The first weeks in the life of your baby can seem like a chaotic whirlwind of new experiences and sensations as you get to know this new person in your lives and adapt to the feeling of being a parent. You have so much to learn: how to feed and nourish your baby, how to dress her and care for her skin, what she likes and what she doesn't like. Looking after a new baby involves a combination of warmth, attention, and physical stamina. Although some of this will be instinctive, at other times you may both feel lost. In fact, you'll learn new skills: before long, eating with one hand while nursing or holding a bottle with the other will come naturally. The early phase of adjustment and chaos doesn't have to last long. This chapter tells how one couple and their new baby Amy coped in the first few weeks. Every baby is different, and you will soon find your own way of managing.

"The first weeks weren't easy. You think you're a capable, confident person, then you have a helpless baby to look after and you feel like jelly!"

First days at home
Life with your new baby will take you by surprise. Her apparent vulnerability produces new, powerful feelings within you, while a turmoil of emotions makes you burst into tears for no reason, or become distressed by, say, the television news. Don't fight your feelings; concentrate on the new life that you are nurturing.

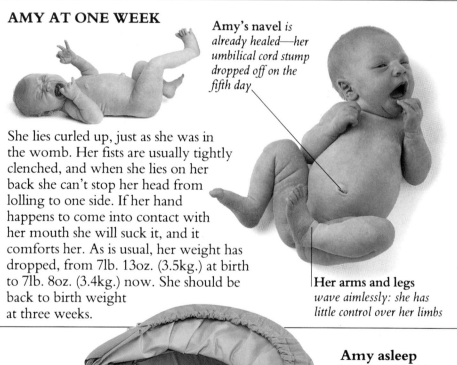

AMY AT ONE WEEK

Amy's navel *is already healed—her umbilical cord stump dropped off on the fifth day*

She lies curled up, just as she was in the womb. Her fists are usually tightly clenched, and when she lies on her back she can't stop her head from lolling to one side. If her hand happens to come into contact with her mouth she will suck it, and it comforts her. As is usual, her weight has dropped, from 7lb. 13oz. (3.5kg.) at birth to 7lb. 8oz. (3.4kg.) now. She should be back to birth weight at three weeks.

Her arms and legs *wave aimlessly: she has little control over her limbs*

Amy asleep
Newborn babies sleep an average of 16 hours a day, but Amy rarely manages that much sleep. Some days she sleeps as little as 10 or 11 hours in total, with a long, stormy period from late afternoon to late at night when she only dozes for short periods. During her times of deep sleep she is totally oblivious to her surroundings. Within five weeks she adopts a more sociable pattern, sleeping longer at night and going to bed earlier.

Becoming a family

Now there are three of you, and everything changes. Your partner is no longer just your lover, he's your companion and ally in this new adventure of parenthood—and she's as much his baby as yours. Your tried and tested family relationships will subtly change too: you're not just a son or a daughter any more, you're a parent, with a new life depending on you. No matter how topsy-turvy your life seems at this time, try to make time for your partner. Often the new father is shell-shocked in the days immediately following the birth, and he needs your support as much as you need his. Let him share in the care of the baby: he may be more nervous than you when handling her floppy body, but, with practice, he will grow more confident.

"The first days were such a tangle of conflicting feelings—elation and overwhelming pride at being a father, anxiety about Ruth, exhaustion from the round-the-clock demands of our new baby, even a tiny regret that our happy, carefree life together seemed to be at an end."

AMY'S DAY

"Amy seemed insatiably hungry. Ruth was good at expressing her milk, so in the evenings when Amy would cry inconsolably for hours at a stretch, I could take over with a bottle. I took over the diaper-changing, too, to give Ruth a break. I was surprised to find I even loved that—it was one way Amy and I built a closeness together. We would play little games, or I would make funny faces, or introduce her to her feet and hands."

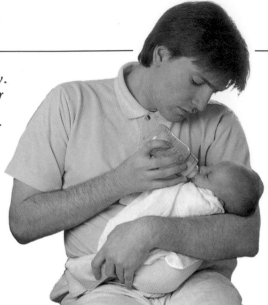

Building a loving relationship

Right from the beginning, your relationship with your new baby is an intense, two-way one that will grow into a real and lasting love. As you bring her up close to talk and coo to her, she will gaze raptly at your face—and eye contact plays a big part when you are falling in love. She will reward your efforts to calm her by quieting down at the sound of your voice when you sing and talk to her. And when she's miserable, she wants you to comfort her.

A TYPICAL DAY AT AROUND THREE WEEKS OF AGE

9 am	**Ruth is awakened** by Amy crying next to her in the bed: she had nursed her there at 5 am, and they both fell asleep together. Amy is breast-fed again.	**1 pm**	**Amy cries** so Ruth nurses her, and afterward they both doze off on the sofa.
10 am	**Ruth takes Amy** into the bathroom to change her diaper and clothes, and sponge bathe her. Then she puts Amy in the infant seat and chats to her while she dresses herself.	**3:30 pm**	**A friend** ringing the doorbell wakes Ruth. She has some advice on how to relieve Ruth's sore nipples, then together they wake Amy and chat to her.
11 am	**Amy falls asleep.** Ruth puts the dirty laundry in the washing machine and straightens up; then she puts her feet up.	**4 pm**	**Her friend** leaves, but Amy is cranky from being awakened, so Ruth feeds her to soothe her.
12:30 pm	**Ruth has** some lunch.	**5:30 pm**	**Ruth puts Amy** in the baby carriage, then she walks to the station to meet Tim. The fresh air and movement put Amy to sleep.

"Rubbing her stomach was a good way to soothe her, provided we rubbed fast and firmly—yet my instincts were to be very gentle. You soon learn how tough babies are."

Amy crying

Crying is your baby's way of expressing her need for love and comfort. Always respond—don't ignore her.

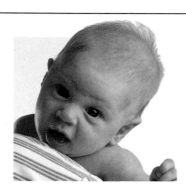

Amy wakeful
Held against your shoulder, your baby has a good view of the world, and will enjoy her wakeful times.

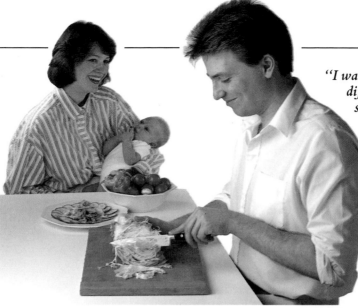

"I was astonished at how difficult it was to get any small job finished during the day. Once Tim got home from work it was up to him to get dinner ready—sometimes I wouldn't even be dressed! It was odd for me to be so disorganized; I wasn't used to having so little time for myself."

6:15 pm	**Home again,** and Amy starts to cry. Ruth feeds her, changes her, then rocks her in her arms. Feeding is the only thing that really soothes Amy at this time of day, but Ruth is sore, so it's painful. Tim catches some sleep	**10 pm**	**Amy is still crying:** she will be soothed for a while, then cry again. Tim and Ruth let her suck, walk her around, or push her in her carriage.
8:30 pm	**Tim wakes up** and he and Ruth take turns carrying Amy around and preparing some food. Amy dozes off for a few minutes at a time, then wakes and cries—so dinner is an erratic affair with Tim trying to bottle-feed and then Ruth breast-feeding Amy.	**2 am**	**Amy falls asleep** at last. Tim and Ruth, exhausted, go to bed.
		4 am	**Amy wakes** and cries, so Ruth takes her into bed to nurse her. Tim wakes up, too, and helps to rock Amy back to sleep after she's been fed.
		7 am	**The alarm goes off** and Tim gets up to go to work —he's had four hours' sleep plus two earlier.

Involving other family members
Your parents, sisters, and brothers will all be eager to meet the new baby; but don't feel guilty about limiting visitors if you want to.

Getting plenty of rest
Every new mother has to learn to cope with too little sleep. Plenty of rest whenever you can catch it is the only answer—and it's especially important if you're breast-feeding. Rest whenever your baby sleeps, even if you don't sleep. Your body isn't strong enough yet for strenuous work, and the housework can go undone for now.

SIX WEEKS OLD

"By six weeks Amy was a real person—nothing like the greedy, screaming bundle of only weeks before. She responded to each of us in her own way: her first, crooked smiles were just for me, usually when I changed her, but at times only Ruth would do. We were lucky, Amy was very perky and she helped us to love her; and you certainly learn fast when you have a new baby relying on you for every need."

PREMATURE BABIES

Your baby's first six weeks at home may be especially difficult if she was born prematurely. She may cry incessantly and refuse to be comforted, or be very sleepy and reluctant to nurse. In addition to your natural anxiety about your baby, you may feel rejected by her: she doesn't make you feel as if she loves you, so it's that much harder to love her in return. Your pre-term baby will need extra care from you: she loses heat quickly, so you need to keep your home warm for her, especially when bathing or changing her; and she will need frequent feeding to help her grow. Even though she may have a small appetite and be a troublesome eater, offer her the breast or a bottle as often as every three hours, letting her take as much as she wants. Concentrate on giving the physical and emotional care she needs: in time she will grow more responsive to you, and you will learn to understand her better.

AMY AT SIX WEEKS

Amy has much more control over her limbs now, and enjoys the sensation of kicking them around in the air. She's no longer curled up, and her fists are unclenched. When she lies on her stomach, she may lift her head momentarily. She doesn't cry as much as before: she has a definite wakeful time during the day, when she will sit happily in her infant seat and be entertained by Ruth and the world around her.

Amy already has *a range of facial expressions*

She has a round stomach *in relation to the rest of her torso*

AMY'S SIX-WEEK CHECKUP

The one-month or six-week checkup is usually the first of the major development exams for a new baby. Your pediatrician or family practitioner will do it in a friendly atmosphere.

1 **General assessment** The doctor discusses Amy's general well-being and demeanor with Ruth. She wakes Amy and talks to her to assess how she responds to the stimulus of a new face. The doctor is looking for that magical early smile, a sure sign that Amy is developing a normal, sociable personality. She checks Amy's sight by moving a rattle across her field of vision. Amy follows it with both eyes, demonstrating healthy eyesight with no sign of a squint.

Amy already *has some control over her neck muscles*

2 Limbs and muscle tone The doctor undresses Amy herself, so she can observe her muscle tone and how she moves her limbs.

3 Control of head The doctor holds Amy in the air to see that she holds her head in line with her body. Then she watches as she pulls Amy into a sitting position.

4 Grasp reflex A baby at birth can grasp hold of a finger put into her palm and hold on strongly. By six weeks it's normal for her birth reflexes to have faded, as Amy's have.

5 Head circumference Amy has her head measured, to check for normal growth. Her head is now 15in. (38cm.).

6 Heartbeat The doctor listens to Amy's heart with a stethoscope: about 120 beats a minute is normal for the first year.

7 Internal organs A good feel around Amy's stomach reassures the doctor that her liver, stomach, and spleen are all growing normally, and none is too big or the wrong shape.

9 Weighing Amy has been weighed in her diaper by Ruth at weekly intervals up to now, and she will be weighed at every visit to the pediatrician's office. Normal weight gain usually means a healthy baby. Amy's weight chart will be an important record for years to come.

8 Hip check Hip dislocation is a possibility still, so the doctor tests the action of the joints with her middle fingers, as she manipulates Amy's legs.

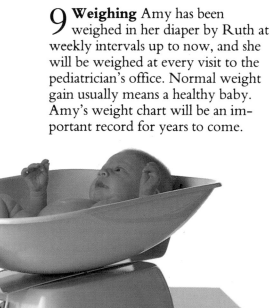

Amy's weight *is recorded on her personal chart*

HANDLING YOUR BABY

From an early age, your baby needs closeness and comfort as well as food, warmth, and sleep. To begin with, you will probably feel quite nervous about handling and cuddling him: your hands seem so clumsy, his limbs so floppy, his head and neck so fragile. Your normal, careful handling won't hurt him; even the soft fontanelle on the top of his head has a tough membrane to protect it. But you may startle him if you pick him up suddenly, making him fling his limbs out.

It frightens him when he senses he may fall. It won't be long before you're both much more confident around each other. As your baby gains control over his muscles, he may enjoy some boisterous games— at four or five months he may love to be swung up above your head, or perched on your shoulders. If he's timid—and some babies are—handle him gently until he is more outgoing. Respond to your baby's moods, and let him set the pace of your physical play.

PICKING UP AND PUTTING DOWN A NEWBORN BABY

TALK TO YOUR BABY as you transfer her from one position to another—your voice is familiar and reassuring. Remember that until she is about eight weeks old she cannot control her head or muscles. You need to support her body all the time, so that her head does not flop or her limbs dangle.

PICKING YOUR BABY UP

1 When your baby is lying on her back, slide one hand under her lower back and bottom.

2 Slide your other hand under her neck and head, going in from the opposite side.

3 Lift her gently and slowly, so that her body is supported and her head can't loll back.

4 Carefully transfer her head to the crook of your elbow or your shoulder, so it is supported.

PUTTING YOUR BABY DOWN

1 Put one hand underneath her head and neck, then hold her under the bottom with the other. Lower her slowly, gently supporting her until the pad or mattress is taking her weight.

2 Slide your nearest hand out from under her bottom. Use this hand to lift her head a little so you can slide out your other hand, and lower her head down gently. Don't let her head fall back on to the surface, or jerk your arm out quickly.

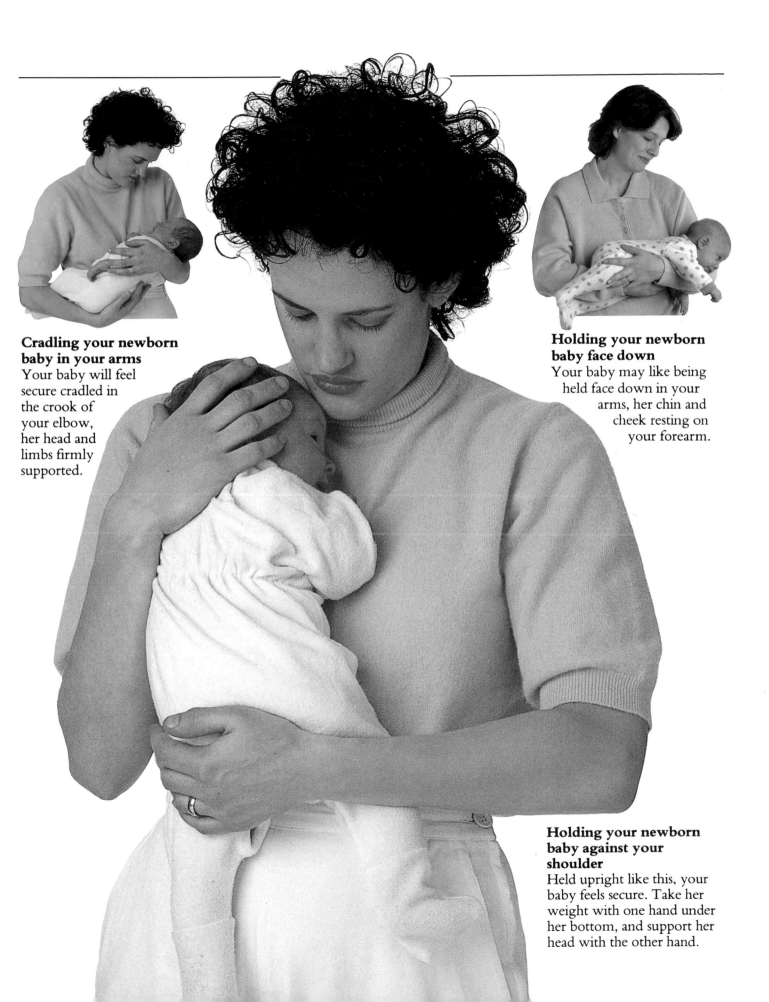

Cradling your newborn baby in your arms
Your baby will feel secure cradled in the crook of your elbow, her head and limbs firmly supported.

Holding your newborn baby face down
Your baby may like being held face down in your arms, her chin and cheek resting on your forearm.

Holding your newborn baby against your shoulder
Held upright like this, your baby feels secure. Take her weight with one hand under her bottom, and support her head with the other hand.

PICKING YOUR BABY UP FROM HER SIDE

1 When asleep in her bassinet or crib, your baby is safest lying on her side. To pick her up, slide one hand under her neck and head, the other under her bottom.

2 Scoop your baby into your arms, making sure her head doesn't flop. Lift her slowly and gently.

3 Hold her against your body, then slide your forearm under her head.

4 Now her head is supported in your elbow, and she feels secure.

PUTTING YOUR BABY DOWN ON HER SIDE

1 When you put your baby down to sleep, lower her to the mattress, keeping her nestled in your arms and her head supported in your elbow.

2 Once she is on the mattress, slide out the hand under her bottom.

3 Lift her head so you can slide your arm out and lower her head gently.

PICKING YOUR BABY UP FROM HER FRONT

1 When your baby is lying on her stomach, slide one hand under her chest so your forearm will support her chin when you lift, the other under her bottom.

2 Lift her slowly, turning her toward you. Bring her up to your body and slide the arm supporting her head forward, until her head nestles comfortably in the crook of your elbow. Put your other hand under her bottom and legs, so she is cradled and secure.

USING AN INFANT CARRIER

AN INFANT CARRIER is an excellent way of carrying your baby around in the first three months: the contact with your body and the motion as you walk will soothe her, and it leaves your arms free. It's not difficult to put one on when there's nobody to help you; take it off using the same method in reverse.

A rigid support *for your baby's head is essential*

Front-carrying *fabric ones are best for small babies*

Wide shoulder *straps will be most comfortable for you*

A machine-washable fabric *is a good idea*

PUTTING ON AN INFANT CARRIER

1 Buckle or tie the carrier belt around your waist: if you find it awkward, do it in front and then twist it around.

2 Pick your baby up and hold her against your shoulder, your hand behind her head.

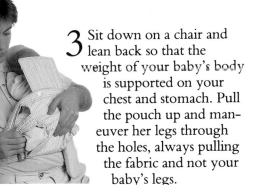

3 Sit down on a chair and lean back so that the weight of your baby's body is supported on your chest and stomach. Pull the pouch up and maneuver her legs through the holes, always pulling the fabric and not your baby's legs.

4 Pull the shoulder straps up and over your shoulders, using one hand to take your baby's weight all the time.

5 As you sit forward the carrier will gradually take her weight.

Have the carrier *at a comfortable height that won't give you backache*

WEARING THE CARRIER

Always put a hand behind your baby's head when you lean forward: the built-in support isn't always adequate for her heavy head.

HANDLING AND PHYSICAL PLAY

LET HER FACE FORWARD
Your alert three-month-old has a good view of the world facing forward. Put one hand between her legs, the other around her chest. She doesn't need you to support her head any more.

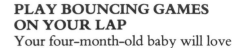

PLAY BOUNCING GAMES ON YOUR LAP
Your four-month-old baby will love the feeling of being jogged up and down on your knees, in time to a favorite rhyme. Hold his arms in case he jerks backward.

SIT HER ASTRIDE YOUR HIP
Your three-month-old can adjust her own position if she's uncomfortable, and will cling to you when she needs extra security.

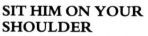

SIT HIM ON YOUR SHOULDER
Sit your six-month-old on your shoulder so he's taller than you are: he will be exhilarated by this new perspective.

EYE-TO-EYE CONTACT
Your baby will love it when you swing her up high. Your face is always the best entertainment of all.

PLAY ROCKING GAMES
Rock her back and forth, going higher and higher if she likes the game. This type of rocking motion is a good way to soothe her, too.

WINDING DOWN
However boisterously you play with your baby, spend a few minutes of gentle, quiet cuddling afterward. Always take your cue from your baby, and forget the roughhousing for today if he's not responding with his usual giggles of pleasure.

FEEDING YOUR BABY

One of the first decisions you and your partner will have to make is whether to breast-feed or bottle-feed your baby. Breast milk meets his needs perfectly and is digested easily; but your baby won't suffer if you do decide to bottle-feed. Feeding your baby should be a pleasure, not a challenge, and it will be no pleasure if you breast-feed from a sense of duty, or bottle-feed with a sense of guilt. If instinctively you think you would prefer to bottle-feed, it's a good idea to put the decision off until after your baby is born. There's no substitute for the colostrum that your breasts produce in the first few days (see page 92), and feeding your baby this will provide him with valuable antibodies to help him fight infection in the early months. You can't switch from bottle-feeding back to breast-feeding because, without the stimulation of your baby sucking, your breasts will have stopped producing milk. But you can stop breast-feeding and go to bottles. Whichever method you opt for, remember that love, cuddling, and attention are just as important to your baby as the milk you give him.

BREAST OR BOTTLE?

YOU MAY KNOW how you want to feed your baby. If you want to breast-feed, then with information and support you will almost certainly succeed. But even if you're sure bottle-feeding is the method for you, it's worth considering the advantages and disadvantages, and listening to the comments other mothers make. It's a decision that will affect you, your partner, and your baby for months to come.

"I knew that by breast-feeding I was giving him the best possible milk he could have. I could tell he was digesting it easily, and I knew it had exactly the right blend of nutrients."

Breast milk contains substances that help protect your baby from disease until his own immune system has matured, and protects against allergies —which is important if there is an allergy in your family. Infant formula can't provide either protection.

"I loved the convenience of breast-feeding my baby: the milk was always there, always sterile, always at the temperature she liked."

"The sheer enjoyment of breast-feeding took me by surprise. It's so intimate, so physically satisfying: her little hand used to come up and stroke my breast, and I could feel her face against my skin. It got better and better, too, as the first year went on."

"The breast was always the best method of soothing my baby when he cried. He wasn't necessarily hungry, he just needed the comfort of sucking."

"The obstetrician told me that the reason I slimmed down to my pre-pregnancy figure so quickly was because I persevered with breast-feeding. So that was an unexpected benefit of listening to her advice."

Breast-feeding is more time-consuming in the early weeks, partly because a breast-fed baby eats more frequently, partly because he likes to suck—in fact sucking is a need and a pleasure quite distinct from the need for food. However, preparing and sterilizing bottles also takes a lot of time, and will soon become a chore when you've done it for several months, while nursing becomes less frequent and quicker as your baby gets older.

"I had always been convinced that I couldn't breast-feed—my bust was so small. But I sailed through. I had plenty of milk, and my baby certainly didn't mind my small breasts."

Traveling is easier if you breast-feed: there's no bottle to warm, and no danger of storing the prepared formula at too high a temperature.

"The only thing I didn't like about breast-feeding was the nursing at night. I didn't enjoy expressing milk, so the whole burden of those nocturnal sessions fell on me. But it was only for a few weeks of our lives."

"I felt that my decision to bottle-feed was the right one when I saw how much my husband enjoyed feeding our baby: they built a very strong relationship right from the start as a result."

"With a bottle, I could always see how much formula my baby had taken—and that was very reassuring after so many miserable weeks trying to get the hang of breast-feeding."

Exhaustion, illness, or stress, which can reduce a breast-milk supply, won't affect the bottle-fed baby's diet.

You may find it harder to trust your baby's own appetite when bottle-feeding, so it is easier to overfeed him and encourage him to be overweight.

A bottle-fed baby is more at risk of picking up microorganisms that could cause diarrhea and vomiting.

ESSENTIALS OF FEEDING

DEMAND FEEDING

Feeding on demand means giving your baby the breast or a bottle when he is hungry, not following timetables.

Hunger is a new sensation for your newborn baby. In the uterus his hunger was being continually "topped up;" now he has to go for long periods without food. His digestive system is too immature to cope with large meals at infrequent intervals; so feed him little and often at first.

There is nothing to be gained by keeping your baby hungry once he has cried to be fed—he will only get so distressed that he may refuse to suck. You will have to comfort and calm him until he'll settle to suck. You're not spoiling your baby by answering his needs. In the early weeks his empty stomach is the usual reason for waking and crying: as his digestive system matures and his stomach grows, he'll take more at each feeding and the intervals between feedings will become longer.

How often will he demand food?

Your baby will demand food whenever he needs it, and in the beginning, this will be often. Newborn babies will have no discernible pattern of feeding. By day three or four, feedings will be about every two to three hours, and there may be eight or so a day with a lot of short ones during the evening. At night, you may be feeding your baby two or three times, because few babies under the age of six weeks are able to sleep more than five hours at a stretch without waking with hunger. Breast-fed babies usually need more frequent feedings than bottle-fed babies, because breast milk is more easily and quickly digested than formula.

By three months your baby will probably be settling to a roughly four-hour feeding routine, with five a day plus one or two at night. If you are bottle-feeding, you will probably be able to establish a four-hour routine more quickly.

SPECIAL CASES

Premature babies Your pre-term baby may have a small appetite but he will need to be fed frequently. He could sleep a lot, and may not wake and demand food even though he needs it, so wake your baby every three hours and offer a feeding.

If you managed to express milk for your baby when he was in the hospital intensive care nursery, you will be able to breast-feed once you get him home. It isn't always easy for a baby to adapt to taking milk from a breast. To help him, express a little milk before you start nursing (see page 94) and rub breast milk over the nipple to give him the taste.

Twins It's perfectly possible to breast-feed twins successfully. Feed them one at a time at first. Then when you are more confident, you'll find it's easy to feed them both at the same time. Tuck their legs under each of your arms, and their heads can lie in your hands.

GAS AND BURPING

Whether your baby is breast- or bottle-fed, give him the chance to burp up any swallowed air when he pauses for a rest; the gas may be making him feel full. If he doesn't burp after about half a minute, give up: he probably doesn't need to bring up any air at that feeding.

Protect your clothes *with a clean cloth diaper*

Your newborn

To help a very young baby bring up gas, put her against your shoulder and rub her back, or lean her forward on your lap, supporting her floppy head under the chin. She's very likely to bring some milk up too, so have a clean cloth diaper or receiving blanket handy.

Hold her face down

At any age, holding your baby face down across your lap or in your arms may help her bring up gas.

Rub or pat her back *gently but rhythmically*

Your older baby

By three months, when your baby can sit up for short periods, jiggling him gently on your lap while you rub his back will help him burp up swallowed air.

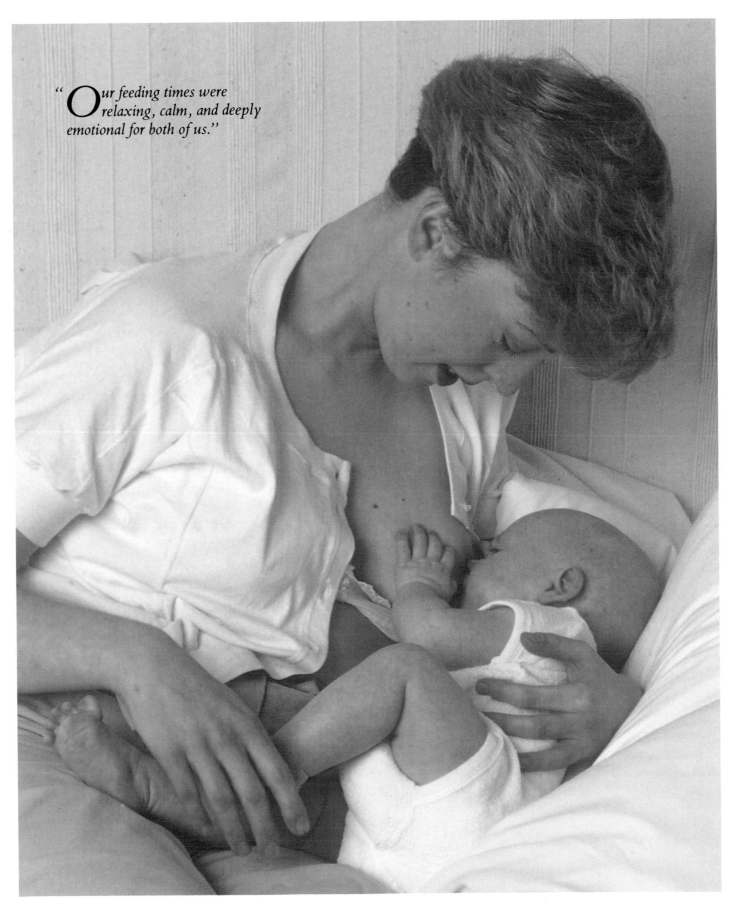

"*Our feeding times were relaxing, calm, and deeply emotional for both of us.*"

BREAST-FEEDING YOUR BABY

Breast-feeding can be a supremely rewarding aspect of caring for your baby, and you'll be giving her the best nourishment nature can provide, so don't be deterred if you encounter a few problems in the early days. You and your baby have to learn this new skill together, so if at first she doesn't seem to know how to suck, or doesn't suck for very long, be patient with her. She doesn't need a lot of food just after the birth, and your nipples need time to toughen up and get used to being sucked on. There will be plenty of friends, relatives, and professionals all keen to offer you advice, and it may take time before you are able to sift out the helpful suggestions and develop a feeling of self-confidence. If you can, get in touch with someone who has breast-fed successfully and listen to her. It's worth persevering. After the first week or so of possible uncertainty and self-doubt, you can look forward to months of successful and satisfying nursing.

SETTLE YOURSELVES comfortably: you may be there for up to an hour. Take a deep breath and relax your shoulders: the more · relaxed you feel to your baby, the easier she will settle down to nurse. Give her plenty of opportunity for skin contact. If you're in private, take your top off: with no clothes in the way, you might find it easier to get her "latched on"— that is, properly positioned on your breast and sucking efficiently.

FINDING THE NIPPLE

1 Your baby has an instinctive reflex that makes her search for your nipple to find food—this is the "rooting" reflex. Until about her tenth day of life, alert this reflex by stroking the cheek nearest to you: she will turn toward your breast and search for your nipple.

————GETTING COMFORTABLE————

The areola *is the large dark circle around your nipple that your baby "milks" when she nurses*

Nursing your young baby
Sit comfortably in an upright position with your back supported. A low chair without arms is ideal, or sit up in bed with plenty of pillows propping your back. If it gives you confidence, put a pillow on your lap to bring your baby to the right level, or raise one knee to support her body. Don't bend your back when you lean forward to nurse her.

A pillow *takes the weight of your baby's body*

Make sure your *baby has a hand free to touch and stroke your breast*

Nursing your older baby
Once you're both adept at breast-feeding, you will find you can nurse in almost any relaxed position. Sitting cross-legged on the bed or floor is excellent, especially if you can lean against pillows or furniture.

2 If your baby doesn't turn her head instinctively, try gently squeezing just behind your areola until a few drops form on your nipple. Touch her lips with this to encourage her to open her mouth.

HOW TO BREAST-FEED

LATCHING ON

3 Bring her head up close to your breast, so her chin is against it and her tongue is underneath your nipple. Guide your breast in.

1 Once latched on, your baby doesn't just suck, she "milks" the breast with her jaws by pressing on the reservoirs of milk at the base of the areola. If your baby just sucks on the nipple, you will get sore and she won't get any milk. If you feel a momentary piercing pain, breathe deeply to help you relax.

2 From your viewpoint, your firmly latched-on baby will have her jaws open very wide and her mouth full of your breast. You can tell she is nursing properly when you see her temples and ears moving, indicating that her jaw muscles are working.

THE LET-DOWN REFLEX

Your baby's sucking action stimulates your breasts to release the milk they have stored. You may feel the warm rush of milk— the let-down reflex—as a tingling sensation soon after your baby has latched on. Not everyone feels it though, so don't be surprised if you don't. If the reflex makes milk leak out of the other breast too, hold a breast pad over your nipple to catch drips.

Talk to your baby *as you feed her: communication is as vital as the milk itself*

Hold your baby *with her head higher than the rest of her body*

TAKING YOUR BABY OFF THE BREAST

1 Let your baby nurse at the first breast until she drains it—your breast will look smaller, and feel lighter, when all the milk has gone. Your baby will often pause when you are nursing her. She may want to keep sucking though. If after several minutes she doesn't take any milk, remove her from the breast to burp her. Don't pull your nipple away—this will hurt. Slip a finger between her jaws to break the suction.

Use your clean *little finger to break your baby's suction*

2 Slip a tissue into your bra on the side your baby has emptied. At the next feeding put her on the other side to begin with, so both breasts get equal stimulation. Sit your baby up to burp her.

OFFERING THE OTHER BREAST

1 After a burp or two, perhaps a short sleep, offer your baby the other breast. She may be hungry enough to drain this one, too, or she may just suck for comfort— which she needs as much as the milk.

2 When your baby's had enough, she will fall fast asleep in your arms and let your nipple slip from her mouth. Don't worry if you don't think she's taken enough milk; you can trust your baby to know how much she wants and needs at any time.

HOW YOUR BREASTS PRODUCE MILK

In the first days after the birth your breasts produce colostrum, a protein-rich food that supplies your baby with valuable antibodies against infection. Once you begin to produce milk around the fourth day, your baby will naturally stimulate your body into producing plenty.

The key to a good milk supply is feeding your baby when she wants to be fed—and in the early days that means nursing at two- or three-hour intervals. Breast milk production works on a supply and demand system: the more often your baby nurses, and the more she takes, the more your breasts will produce.

Supplementary bottles of formula will undermine this system: if your baby's hunger is satisfied by a bottle, she won't be eager to suck and your breasts won't be stimulated.

Breast milk isn't all the same: at the beginning of the feeding your baby takes what is sometimes called the foremilk, which is watery and thirst-quenching. As she nurses, the fat content of your milk rises, and she soon starts getting the hindmilk, rich in calories. This is why it's important to let her suck for at least 10 to 15 minutes on one breast at each feeding: otherwise she will soon be hungry again.

What you need to do
All *you* need to do to produce enough milk is to eat a good, balanced diet with plenty of protein, to drink whenever you are thirsty— have a glass of juice on hand while you nurse—and to rest as much as you can. Your baby's natural appetite will do the rest.

You need a lot of energy to produce breast milk, so this is not a time to diet. Dieting will make you run down and exhausted. Follow your appetite, and make sure you get the extra calories you need from fresh, vitamin-rich foods rather than "empty" carbohydrates.

WHEN YOUR MILK COMES IN

The areola *is swollen, so it may be hard for your baby to grasp; and the nipple is flattened*

Normal breast   Engorged breast

Draw your fingertips down toward the areola

1 On about the fourth day of breast-feeding your breasts start to produce mature milk, rather than the colostrum that you've fed your baby up to now. You may wake up to find your breasts big, hard, and uncomfortable. This is engorgement, and it may last for 48 hours. Your baby will find it hard to latch on because the nipple isn't sticking out, but is flattened by the swollen areola. The following tips should help her to nurse, lessen the engorgement, and ease your discomfort.

2 Before you try to nurse your baby, soften your breasts by laying warm washcloths or hand towels over them for several minutes, or stand in the shower and run warm water over them.

3 Massage your breasts gently with your hands, and try to express some milk to relieve the swelling and help your baby get the nipple in her mouth (see page 94). Don't worry if you can't get the hang of expressing at this stage. You soon will.

4 When you put your baby to the breast, put your free hand on your ribcage under your breast and push gently upward: this should help the nipple to protrude so your baby can get the areola in her mouth. Her sucking will quickly relieve the engorgement and discomfort.

QUESTIONS & ANSWERS

"Joe cries a great deal; could it be that he isn't getting enough milk from me to satisfy his hunger?"
When you are breast-feeding, you can't actually *see* what your baby takes, so it's natural sometimes to worry that he's not getting enough. But as long as you nurse whenever your baby cries, *and* he is gaining weight normally with occasional spurts, you have no need to worry. Remember that your baby will probably *lose* weight during the first days of life, and won't regain his birth weight until he is two or three weeks old.

"Will breast-feeding alter my figure for life?"
Your breasts may be slightly smaller after you've weaned your baby from the breast, because some of the fatty tissue has been replaced by milk glands. Otherwise, you will probably regain your pre-pregnancy figure more quickly if you breast-feed, because the hormones released encourage the uterus to shrink back to normal quickly, and the fat reserves that your body stored during pregnancy are used in the production of breast milk. Your waistline contracts sooner, too.

"Do I have to be as careful about the drugs and medications I take as when I was pregnant?"
What you eat and drink can be passed on to your baby through your milk, so it's still vital that you tell your pharmacist or doctor that you are breast-feeding before they suggest any medicines for you. It's sensible to avoid stimulants such as alcohol and caffeine, too. If your baby doesn't sleep well, it may be worth cutting coffee and tea out of your diet for a few weeks to see if the situation improves—the caffeine may be keeping him awake.

EXPRESSING MILK BY HAND

THE ABILITY to express your own milk gives you great flexibility. You can freeze the milk (keep it for up to one month), and someone else can give it to your baby when you're out: see pages 98–107 for bottle-feeding advice. Expressing by hand is not that difficult. Wash the equipment and your hands. Encourage the flow of milk by having a warm bath, or hold warm washcloths over your breasts. Make yourself comfortable by a high surface, with the bowl in front of you.

■ YOU WILL NEED ■
Large bowl
Clean bottle
Nipple
Plastic funnel

THE FIRST BREAST

Use your *whole hand to massage the breast*

1 Support your breast in one hand and start to massage, working downward from above the breast.

2 Work your way all around the breast, including the underside. Complete at least ten circuits: this helps the flow of milk through the ducts.

3 Stroke downward toward the areola with your fingernails several times. Avoid pressing on the breast tissue.

4 Apply gentle downward pressure on the area behind the areola with your thumbs and fingers.

5 Squeeze thumbs and forefingers together, at the same time pressing backward: the milk should spurt out through the nipple. Keep this up for a couple of minutes.

ALTERNATING BREASTS

1 Repeat the massaging on the other breast.

2 Squeeze some milk out of the nipple.

3 Go back to the first breast and repeat the whole procedure: the production of milk should have been stimulated by now, so you should get more milk out. Alternate between breasts until no more milk flows.

STORING THE MILK

Always use *freshly washed equipment*

Screw *the bottle parts together*

1 Pour the milk through a funnel into a bottle: in the early weeks you may get 2–3fl. oz. (60–80ml.).

2 Seal the bottle tightly and refrigerate, or cool and freeze. Thaw for four hours at room temperature.

EXPRESSING MILK USING A PUMP

EXPRESSING BY PUMP can be quicker and less tiring than hand expressing, but you may find it harder to get a reasonable quantity of milk—and some mothers find it painful. (If you do, express by hand instead.) The "syringe" type of pump is generally more efficient than the bulb type. Choose one with an outer cylinder that converts into a baby's bottle. If you need to express large quantities, ask your pediatrician about renting an electric pump.

Funnel

Inner cylinder

Outer cylinder

Breast pump

2 Keep a tight seal and draw the outer cylinder away from you: the suction draws milk from your breast.

1 Wash and dry all the equipment thoroughly, then wash your hands. Assemble the pump. Soften your breasts in warm water and massage them just as when expressing by hand. Place the funnel of the pump over the areola so that it forms an airtight seal: it needs to press on the milk ducts just as your baby's jaws do.

3 Put the cap on tightly and refrigerate, or cool and freeze until needed.

BREAST-FEEDING PROBLEMS

GET PROFESSIONAL HELP quickly if you have any problems with breast-feeding: struggling alone is discouraging, and something minor like a blocked duct can lead to mastitis if it is not taken care of right away. *Don't stop nursing if you encounter the problems below:* you will only get engorged with milk, making any problem potentially much worse.

Take good care of your breasts. Wear a comfortable nursing bra both day and night in the early weeks: don't wear one that is too tight, as it may constrict the ducts. Be gentle when you massage your breasts, too. Let the air and occasionally sunlight get to your nipples, and wash them with water only. Soap dries the skin, and perfumes can irritate it.

LEAKING BREASTS

Your breasts may leak copiously between feedings in the early weeks before supply has matched demand.
Treatment Breast pads inside your bra will absorb some drips, but change the pads frequently because continually being wet may make your nipples sore. Try using men's 100% cotton hankies, for padding.
To stop leaking If one breast leaks profusely while your baby is nursing from the other, press the heel of your free hand, or even a finger, on the nipple for a minute or two just as you begin breast-feeding and especially during let-down. Applying pressure like this will stop the leak.
Prevention None, but leaking breasts are proof of a good milk supply, and help prevent engorgement. The leaking will diminish as your supply better matches your baby's appetite.

Disposable breast pad
A breast pad will absorb drips and small leaks.

BLOCKED DUCT

A hard, tender, red lump in the breast usually means that one of the milk ducts has become blocked.
Treatment Bathe the breast in hot water and massage it gently, then put your baby to the breast. You may get a moment's intense pain, but the duct should clear. If it doesn't, see your doctor that day.
Prevention Make sure your bra is not too tight, and take care not to press hard on your breast tissue when you nurse your baby or express milk.

MASTITIS

A blocked milk duct may become infected, producing flu-like symptoms. *Seek medical help urgently:* if untreated, mastitis may lead to a breast abscess, which may need surgery.
Treatment Your doctor will prescribe antibiotics, and you must complete the course of medication. Continue to nurse from both breasts as normal to maintain your supply.
Prevention Never let a tender lump in your breast go longer than a day without medical attention.

SORE OR CRACKED NIPPLES

Sore nipples may be the result of your baby not latching on properly, due to poor positioning. Your skin will be red, and it will be painful to nurse. A cracked nipple will give you a shooting pain as your baby sucks. Your skin will soon get tougher as you grow more used to nursing.
Treatment Try the following suggestions:
■ Dry your nipples after nursing: use a hairdryer on a cool setting.
■ Let air get to them for several hours a day. Try sitting in sunlight if you can find a private place where you know you won't be interrupted.
■ Don't nurse but rather express from the worst breast for a day.
■ Change the position in which your baby breast-feeds, so the pressure is applied to different parts of the areola at each feeding.
■ Don't let your baby suck for more than a couple of minutes after she's emptied the breast.
■ Talk to your pediatrician or obstetrician.
Prevention: Make sure that your baby takes the areola into her mouth. Keep your nipples dry between feedings.

Nipple cream
A vitamin E-based cream or oil may help to relieve the soreness.

YOUR EMOTIONS AND LET-DOWN
Your let-down reflex is highly associated with your emotional state of being. When you are embarrassed, irritated, exhausted, anxious, or angry with a colicky baby, your breast milk doesn't always appear like magic. Sometimes, your breasts will begin leaking milk at the very sound of your baby's cry. At other times, though, your own tension and anxiety seem to hinder the let-down: your baby cries all the harder, your temper gets worse, and your milk is even less likely to be let-down. A few minutes of quiet cuddling together in private should help to relax both of you and make you and your baby ready to nurse.

FEEDING THROUGHOUT THE FIRST YEAR

UNTIL THE AGE of about four months, you will be feeding your baby milk alone. But how will your breast-feeding routine change once you start to introduce solids? How long should you keep nursing each day? During the second half of her first year, your baby will need less and less milk from you and will be more willing to take drinks from a cup or bottle. Between the ages of nine months and a year she may wean herself off the breast quite happily, and with no prompting from you: she's reached an age when she's getting her nourishment and her comfort from other sources.

How will my routine develop?
A typical routine for a fully breast-fed baby might be:
■ three months: five feedings a day plus night feedings
■ five/six months: five feedings a day plus some solid food
■ eight months: two breast-feedings a day: early morning and bedtime
■ nine months: bedtime feeding only.

Going back to work
It's perfectly possible to return to work and continue breast-feeding. If your baby is under six or seven months old you will need to express at the times she would normally nurse to keep your milk supply stimulated.
■ Get your baby used to a bottle before you start work. Have someone else give the first bottle-feedings—your baby will associate you with breast-feeding.
■ You need clean bottles and a private place to express milk during the day, plus access to a refrigerator to store it. Transport the milk home in an insulated cooler with ice packs inside (see page 101).
■ Leave bottles of expressed milk for your baby's daytime feedings.
■ Ask your babysitter to delay the late afternoon feeding so your baby will be ready to nurse when you get home.
■ If necessary, boost your supply by nursing extra times during the evening and night.

When should I stop?
You can continue to breast-feed well into your baby's second year if you both want to; or you can gradually wean your baby off the breast at any time in the first year. She may give up the breast of her own accord between nine months and a year. Biting your breast is not a reason to give up feeding: tell her sharply that it hurts, and she will soon learn.

Never give up abruptly. It's important to let your production of milk reduce gradually over a period of weeks, by letting your supply-and-demand system work in reverse. Drop one feeding at a time, waiting at least three days before dropping another (see page 106). Don't express to relieve the full feeling. It hurts but the milk will be gradually reabsorbed in a few days.

Giving up the final feeding
Most babies usually settle down to sleep easier at night after they have nursed quietly, so this is usually the last feeding to be dropped.

Toward the end of the first year, gradually reduce the length of this feeding. Then drop it altogether, and give plenty of attention and love for a few days to make up for it. Offer her a drink in a cup or bottle at bedtime.

What do I give my baby instead of breast milk?
If you give up breast-feeding before six months, you will need to feed your baby formula from a bottle. If you are happy to breast-feed until your baby is at least six months, you can wean her straight on to a cup (see page 113); give formula until nine months, then check with your pediatrician. However, she may settle down better at night if she can suck on a bedtime bottle.

BOTTLE-FEEDING YOUR BABY

In the last twenty years there has been a dramatic increase in the number of new mothers who are breast-feeding their babies. But if you have decided to bottle-feed, the first rule of thumb is: Don't let anyone make you feel guilty about your choice. It's a good one, and your child is just as likely to thrive as the breast-fed baby. What your infant needs is enough to eat and lots of tender loving care. Cuddling, cooing, and holding your baby in the crook of your arm while you feed him will give him the same kind of security and sense of you that a breast-feeding mother might offer. So don't fall into an insecurity trap. Besides, you'll be able to share the feedings with your mate. There is no other baby in the world quite like yours, and what you bring to him through your choice of feeding is your own particular style of mothering. Someone else's way of doing things is not what he needs. It's you that makes the criticial difference in his brand new life, not bottles or breasts. Feeding your baby can be as easy as pouring ready-made formula into a clean bottle and finding a comfortable spot to sit down. With your pediatrician's help, pick a manufacturer's brand, and always follow the directions very precisely when you mix the powder or concentrated liquid kinds.

EQUIPMENT FOR BOTTLE-FEEDING

FOR A FULLY bottle-fed baby you will need at least eight full-size 8oz. (250ml.) bottles. Buy extra nipples, and have them ready in a clean jar in case the one you are using is inadequate. Sometimes the holes are either too large or too small. Some bottles have throw-away plastic liners, which reduce the air your baby swallows: the bag collapses as he sucks, so the nipple doesn't flatten and halt the flow.

BOTTLES

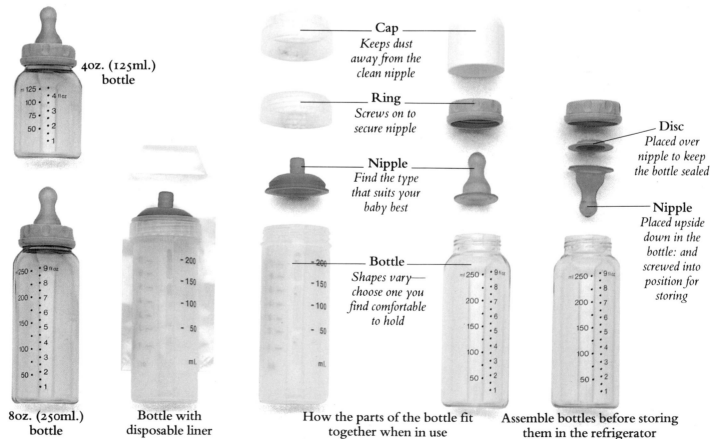

4oz. (125ml.) bottle

Cap *Keeps dust away from the clean nipple*

Ring *Screws on to secure nipple*

Disc *Placed over nipple to keep the bottle sealed*

Nipple *Find the type that suits your baby best*

Nipple *Placed upside down in the bottle: and screwed into position for storing*

Bottle *Shapes vary— choose one you find comfortable to hold*

8oz. (250ml.) bottle

Bottle with disposable liner

How the parts of the bottle fit together when in use

Assemble bottles before storing them in the refrigerator

NIPPLES

The holes *should point toward the roof of your baby's mouth*

Valve in rim *lets air under the nipple and into the bottle*

Nipples for young *babies are sometimes shorter*

Natural-shaped nipple
This nipple most closely mimics the sucking action of feeding from your breast, so it encourages proper development of your baby's palate and jaws. It should go into your baby's mouth with the holes facing up, so the formula sprays over the roof of his mouth.

Universal nipple
The standard shape of a nipple gives a sucking action that is not really like sucking from your breast. Nipples are sold with different rates of flow, but check at each feeding: there should be two or three drops a second. A cross-cut hole gives a better formula flow than a pinhole.

Anti-colic nipple
An anti-colic nipple lets air into the bottle as your baby sucks. This stops the nipple from collapsing, enabling him to get a steady stream without gulping air. Silicone nipples, shown above, last up to a year; latex nipples deteriorate after about one month of heavy use.

Wide-based nipple
This type is not interchangeable among different bottles. As your baby sucks, his lips push against the squashy base and the nipple moves in and out within his mouth, rather like a human nipple. Fit the nipple and ring together before assembling the bottle ready for filling.

OTHER EQUIPMENT

Bottle brush Needed to clean thoroughly inside the bottles. Keep it for this purpose only.

Can opener
For opening cans of formula. Wash well first.

Measuring cup (optional) For mixing powder formula.

Plastic funnel (optional)
Useful for pouring formula into the bottles.

Plastic spoon (optional)
For stirring formula.

Plastic knife For leveling off scoops of powder formula.

STERILIZING BOTTLES
Not all pediatricians agree about the need to sterilize bottles. If you wash them thoroughly using soap and hot water, there may be no need. If you use a dishwasher, the high heat of the drying cycle will kill any potentially dangerous bacteria. However, some doctors do recommend sterilizing, especially for a newborn baby. If this is true for you, you'll need an extra large pot in which to boil your bottles and all your formula-making equipment.

Tongs Useful for gripping hot bottles.

Large pot Choose one big enough to accommodate several bottles.

KEEPING YOUR BOTTLES CLEAN

FORMULA, when it is warm or held too long at room temperature, is an ideal breeding ground for the bacteria that cause gastroenteritis, a disease that can be life-threatening in a young baby. There are a few guidelines that you must follow to keep your baby healthy when bottle-feeding. First of all, make sure that your hands are absolutely clean, then wash everything else that comes in contact with your baby's bottle before filling it. Always keep bottles of formula refrigerated, and use them within 24 hours of their being made up. Check with your pediatrician for his recommendations about sterilization.

WASHING

1 Put all the rinsed out bottles, nipples, caps, rings, discs, funnel, spoon, and knife directly into hot soapy water. Wash each of the individual items extremely thoroughly.

2 Scrub inside the bottles with the bottle brush to remove all traces of formula. Scrub around their necks, and scrub the screw thread, where bacteria can grow, too.

3 By rubbing some salt inside the nipples and moving it around, squeezing and massaging the tip, you can remove any traces of caked-on formula, which can be hard to clean.

4 Rinse the bottles, nipples, and other items of equipment thoroughly under running water. Use a pin that has been heated in a flame to clear the holes in the nipples.

USING A DISHWASHER

Dishwasher-proof nipples *should be put upward within the silverware compartments*

An easy way to wash equipment is to put it in your dishwasher and make sure it goes through the hot drying cycle. The high heat is usually sufficient to kill any bacteria. But be careful—nipples may have to be boiled separately on the stovetop because dishwashers can turn them into unusable sticky blobs.

STERILIZING BY BOILING

All items *must be fully submerged during the boiling period*

Wash the equipment and boil for five minutes. When pediatricians suggest that new mothers sterilize bottles and formula-preparation equipment, this basic boiling method is ordinarily sufficient. Use tongs to remove the hot bottles and fill them when they cool slightly. Don't let the sterile equipment sit around too long on your kitchen counter gathering dust or germs. Store it in the refrigerator or a cupboard. The five-minute boil is the length of time suggested by all major formula manufacturers.

Insulated cooler

Wide-necked thermos

PROTECTING YOUR BABY FROM AN UPSET STOMACH

If you take the precautions below, you should be able to protect your baby from the bacteria that cause upset stomachs or gastroenteritis.

■ Wash or, if your pediatrician recommends it, sterilize feeding equipment before use, especially when it's brand new.

■ If you have no refrigerator, make up each bottle only when you need it.

■ If your baby doesn't finish his formula at a feeding, throw the rest away: don't save it for next time, because his saliva may have contaminated it.

■ Throw away any formula warmed for your baby, even if he doesn't touch it: the process of warming encourages bacteria to grow.

■ Don't keep prepared formula in the refrigerator for longer than 24 hours.

■ Boil the water you are going to use in mixing up any concentrated formula, the liquid or the powder. Tap water in your area may not be as pure as it could be and you'll be protecting your baby from potentially harmful bacteria and chemicals.

■ Remember to wash your hands before preparing your baby's bottles.

TAKING CARE OF NIPPLES

Your baby can only suck happily if the nipple allows him to get the formula at the right rate. When you shake the bottle upside down, you should see two or three drops a second: too small a hole will mean that your baby gets frustrated in his efforts to satisfy his hunger; if the hole is too large the formula will gush out, possibly causing him to choke. Nipples deteriorate and the holes clog up. Have some spare nipples stored in a jar, so you can just swap an imperfect nipple for a fresh one. Throw away nipples if the holes are too large; holes that are too small can be enlarged with a needle. Check the flow again afterward.

When you're away from home

If you're going out for more than a couple of hours, make up several bottles and chill them in the refrigerator. Put these cold bottles into an insulated cooler along with an ice pack. They will keep for up to eight hours like this. Don't pack them when they are still warm. Bring along a separately packed thermos filled with hot water. When your baby is ready for a bottle, warm it by sitting it in hot water poured into the thermos cup.

The needle *must have a very fine sharp point*

Enlarging a hole that is too small

Push the eye of a needle into a cork. Heat the point in a flame until hot, then push into the hole.

If you'll be filling bottles away from home, simplify your life by buying ready-to-feed formula. Take along clean bottles, nipples, and a can opener in a plastic bag and just pour out formula as your baby gets hungry.

FORMULA: WHAT'S IN IT?

Have you tasted your baby's formula? It's sweeter than cow's milk and as close in composition to breast milk as manufacturers can make it. That's because whole milk is not well suited to your baby's needs; it doesn't contain all the nutrients she must have for growth, and it can be very difficult for her to digest because of the concentrations of protein and fat. Most infant formulas are adapted from a cow's milk base but are supplemented with other long-tested ingredients. Vegetable oils are added to replace cow's butter fat, and lactose is used to sweeten the mixture. Some come with additional iron, clearly marked on the cans, and some are based entirely on soy. If your baby vomits after a bottle, has diarrhea, cramps, or excessive gas, wheezes, develops a rash, or is generally irritable, suspect an allergy to cow's milk and call your pediatrician.

MAKING UP YOUR BABY'S BOTTLE

IN THE EARLY WEEKS you need to have a supply of bottles ready in the refrigerator so that whenever your baby cries, wanting to be fed, you can respond quickly and easily. Until your baby is at least nine months old, give him an infant formula. Most are modified cow's milk. Your pediatrician will help you choose a brand. You can upset your baby by switching brands, so never do so without professional advice.

Making up formula

Infant formula is most commonly and cheaply available as concentrated liquid or powder that can readily be mixed up as required.

The instructions on the cans tell you the correct amount of liquid or number of scoops to add to each measure of water. It is very important to maintain these proportions exactly. If you add too much formula, the feeding will be dangerously concentrated: your baby may gain too much weight, and his kidneys may be damaged. If you consistently add too little powder, he may gain weight too slowly and eventually could become malnourished. The only occasion on which it is correct to dilute formula concentrations is when your baby brings up most of his feeding but shows no other signs of illness. Then, for the next few days, dilute the formula (see Vomiting, page 179). If your baby is not vomiting, follow the directions and allow him to take as much as he wants at each feeding.

Always use fresh, cold tap water to make up your baby's formula, and boil it once only. Some types of water should never be used:
■ water that has been repeatedly boiled, or left standing in the kettle for more than an hour or two
■ water from a tap with a domestic softener attached—the extra sodium (salt) can damage your baby's kidneys
■ water from a tap with a domestic filter attached—these filters can trap harmful bacteria
■ mineral water—the sodium and minerals may be harmful.

There are two methods of making up your baby's bottle: mixing the formula directly in the bottles, or mixing it in a container or measuring cup first. Use the cup method if you use bottles with disposable liners.

Ready-to-feed formula

Some brands of infant formula are also available ready-mixed in cans. You need add no water. If the formula you are feeding your baby comes in this form, then you have a very convenient option.

The formula in the cans has been ultra-heat treated (UHT), so it's already sterile. Store unopened cans in a cool place, and do not use after the "expiration" date.

Once opened, the formula can be stored in the refrigerator for up to 24 hours, either in a sterile, sealed bottle, or in the can, which must be covered. But unless you can be sure that you won't forget when you put the can in the refrigerator, it's probably safer to pour all the formula into clean, ready to use bottles. Throw away any he doesn't drink after each feeding.

How much will my baby want?

Babies' appetites vary from day to day. During the first weeks of life put 4fl. oz. (125ml.) of formula into each of six bottles, and see how that matches your baby's appetite. As he gains weight, he will often cry for more at the end of a feeding, so gradually increase the amount you put into each bottle. By the time he is six months old you will be making up bottles of 7fl. oz. (200ml.). As a rough guide, your baby needs about 2½fl. oz. of formula per pound (150ml. per kg.) of body weight every 24 hours. So if a 12lb. (5.5kg.) baby is on six feedings a day, he may take about 5fl. oz. (140ml.) of formula at each feeding.

Demand vs. scheduled bottles

It takes weeks and often months for babies to settle into predictable feeding schedules. At first, your baby may be hungry every half hour, then every two, three, or four hours. In years past, mothers were advised to follow strict four-hour feeding schedules, withholding bottles until the appointed hour had arrived. Nowadays, both pediatricians and mothers take a softer approach and believe that babies should take the lead as far as schedules are concerned. By ten weeks, most babies are close to an eating pattern of every three or four hours. If your baby is cranky right after draining a full bottle or within an hour, try burping her or offering some cool, sterile water in a bottle.

Should I give anything else?

Most bottle-fed babies don't need anything but formula for the first six months of life. Some doctors recommend vitamin and mineral supplements or additional fluoride, but do check first. Too many vitamins can make your baby sick.

The majority of doctors and the American Academy of Pediatrics generally suggest holding off on solid foods until at least five or six months of age. You may be tempted to try some cereal in your baby's diet if he appears not to be satisfied with just formula, but until he can let you know that he wants more or less food, pushing solids can amount to force-feeding, so be patient.

When bottle-fed babies are allergic to formula

Because many commercial formulas are modified cow's milk, some infants do have allergic reactions. Upset stomachs, diarrhea, irritability, and skin rashes will let you know that something isn't quite right. Call your pediatrician if you suspect an allergy; he'll be able to recommend formulas that have no cow's milk (soy-based, for instance) as an alternative.

USING CONCENTRATED LIQUID FORMULA

■ YOU WILL NEED ■
Can of concentrated liquid formula
Bottles and nipples
Can opener

1 Boil water in a kettle. Rinse the top of the can by pouring the boiling water over the lid. Shake the formula can well.

2 Open the can in two places using a clean can opener. Refill the kettle with fresh tap water, boil it, then let it cool for five minutes.

3 Pour the concentrate into a clean bottle until you have half the total feeding amount. Check the amount at eye level.

4 Top off with an equal quantity of cooled boiled water. With the bottle at eye level, make sure you have doubled the amount of concentrate.

Note the measured markings on the side of the bottle. Never guess the quantity of water required

5 Attach the disc and ring to the bottle. Shake the mixture, leaving out the nipple to avoid coating it in milk. Store in the refrigerator.

USING READY-TO-FEED FORMULA

■ YOU WILL NEED ■
Can of ready-to-feed formula
Bottles and nipples
Can opener

1 Rinse the can lid by pouring boiling water over it. Shake the formula can well to ensure the contents are evenly mixed.

2 Open the can using a clean punch-type opener. Then make a second opening very carefully so the formula does not spill.

3 Pour the formula into a bottle. Attach the nipple and ring. Shake the bottle, test the temperature and feed.

MAKING UP POWDERED FORMULA IN BOTTLES

■ YOU WILL NEED ■

Powdered formula
Bottles and nipples
Knife
Paper towels

1 Boil water in the kettle to rinse the freshly washed equipment. Pour the boiled water all over the equipment. Drain everything on paper towels. Dry the knife.

Make sure you **fill** *the bottle to a marked level*

2 Empty the kettle, fill it with fresh, cold tap water, and re-boil. Pour the boiling water into the bottles, filling them to a suitable measure. Check at eye level: the measure must be exact to mix the formula to the right concentration.

3 Open the can of formula and use the special scoop inside. Level each scoop off with the back of a clean knife: *do not* heap the scoop, nor pack the powder down inside it.

4 Drop each scoop of powder into the bottle of water. Add only the number of scoops recommended for that amount of water. The powder will dissolve quickly in the hot water.

5 Put the disc and ring on the bottle—not the nipple at this stage—and screw on tightly to seal. Shake the bottle briskly to mix the formula thoroughly.

MAKING UP FORMULA USING A CUP

■ YOU WILL NEED ■

Powdered formula or concentrated liquid
Bottles and nipples
Knife
Paper towels
Measuring cup
Spoon
Plastic funnel

1 Make sure your equipment is clean and dry. Boil fresh, cold tap water in the kettle. Fill the cup to an exact full measure. Use the scoop inside the formula can. Level each scoop off with the back of a knife.

2 Add scoops of powder or the correct amount of concentrated liquid to the cup. Use only the amount recommended for that measure of water, and never any more.

3 Stir the formula well with a spoon until it is thoroughly mixed. The hot water will help dissolve the concentrated liquid.

4 Pour into bottles through the funnel. Put the nipple in upside down. Cover with the disc and ring. Make up more formula until the bottles are full.

USING DISPOSABLE LINERS

■ YOU WILL NEED ■
Powdered or concentrated liquid formula
Bottles and nipples
Disposable liners
Knife
Paper towels
Measuring cup
Spoon
Plastic funnel

1 Make up the formula in a measuring cup, a pitcher, or any clean container and follow the manufacturer's directions carefully. If you prefer, open a can of ready-to-use formula (see page 103). Wash your hands. Push the nipple into the ring without touching the tip of it. Tear a presterilized disposable liner off its roll.

Touch the outside *of the liner only*

2 Fold the liner in half lengthwise and place in the "bottle"—it's not a real bottle, but a plastic sleeve that supports the liner, nipple, and ring.

3 Make sure the liner folds well down all around the rim—otherwise formula will spill out.

Touch the plastic ring *only, once the nipple is secure*

4 Hold the liner firmly in place so the weight of the formula can't pull it down, and pour formula in through the funnel. Add as much as your baby needs.

5 Screw on the ring with the nipple already secured—this will hold the liner. Pull off the perforated tabs and dispose of them immediately. Put the cap over the nipple of each one and store the bottles in the refrigerator.

STORING THE BOTTLES

1 To store a batch of feedings, put the nipples in upside down after you've shaken the formula, or insert the nipples later.

2 Cool the bottles under the cold tap and store in the refrigerator with the caps on. Use stored formula within 24 hours.

STORING OPENED CANS

If you prefer to make up feedings as your baby asks for them, you can store the cans of unused formula in the refrigerator for up to 48 hours. Always cover the can so bacteria cannot enter. It's easy to forget when you opened the can, so use date labels or mark the date on your calendar. Be very strict with yourself about throwing away any formula opened for longer than 48 hours.

Covering the can
Place plastic wrap over the lid of an opened can and secure with a rubber band.

GIVING YOUR BABY A BOTTLE

FEEDING YOUR BABY is the most important thing you can do for her—but don't make the mistake of thinking that the formula in the bottle is all she needs, or that "anyone" can feed her. Your love, your cuddling, and attention are just as important to your baby as the formula itself. Always hold her close and cuddle her against you, smile and talk to her—just as you would if you were breast-feeding. Never leave your baby alone with her bottle, she may choke.

Right from the beginning, give your baby as much control over feeding as you can. Let her set the pace, pausing to look around, touch the bottle, or stroke your breast if she wants to—feeding may take as long as a half hour if she's feeling playful. Above all, let her decide when she's had enough.

Make yourself comfortable, put a pillow under your arm, and have a cloth diaper ready to burp her.

Dad's turn
Your partner can feed your baby, too. Fathers can be critical in a switch from breast to bottle.

FROM BREAST TO BOTTLE

If you must switch to bottle-feeding for any reason, remember that the transition calls for a gradual approach.

Offering one bottle every third day in place of your breast is the best method. Go slowly. Start with a middle-of-the-day nursing. If your baby resists, don't force it. Try again at the same time the next day. Buy a different type of nipple. Or ask your husband to feed the baby the bottle. Some infants automatically associate breast-feeding with their mothers but will be more daring in their acceptance of a bottle from someone else. Save nighttime nursings for last when you make the switch.

QUESTION & ANSWER

"My baby never seems to finish her bottle: is she getting enough?"
A poor appetite could be a sign of illness, or of a serious problem that needs medical attention. Check how much formula your baby should be getting for her weight (see page 102), and see if that matches what she drinks. It's important to have your baby weighed regularly. Your doctor should plot her weight on a growth chart. A baby who is never interested in her bottle or is not gaining weight at a steady rate is always a cause for concern.

GETTING THE BOTTLE READY

1 Take a bottle from the refrigerator and turn the nipple right side up. Warm in warm water. Don't use a microwave oven, because the formula may get very hot although the bottle still feels cool.

2 Check the flow of formula: it should be two or three drops a second. Too small a hole will make sucking hard, too large will allow formula to gush out. If the nipple isn't right, swap it for another one and test the flow again.

3 Test the temperature by shaking a few drops on the inside of your wrist—it should feel tepid. Cold formula is safe, but your baby may prefer it warm.

4 Unscrew the ring slightly, leaving it on the bottle, but letting a little air in. This simple step will stop the nipple from collapsing as your baby sucks.

GIVING YOUR BABY HER BOTTLE

1 For the first ten days of life, you might want to alert your baby's sucking reflex: stroke the cheek nearest you, and she should turn and open her mouth. If she doesn't, let some drops of formula form on the nipple, then touch her lips with it to give her the taste.

2 During a feeding, hold the bottle firmly so that she can pull against it as she sucks, and tilt it so that the nipple is full of formula, not air. If the nipple collapses, move the bottle around in her mouth to let air back into the bottle.

3 When your baby has finished all the formula, pull the bottle away so she can't swallow too much air. If she wants to suck, offer her your clean little finger or a pacifier.

IF SHE WON'T LET GO

If your baby doesn't want to let go of the empty bottle, slide your little finger between her gums and the nipple to release the suction.

*It's **easier** for your baby to swallow if she lies in a semi-upright position*

Put a bib on your baby before you begin

SLEEPING DURING A FEEDING

If she dozes off during her feeding, she may have gas, which is making her feel full. Sit her up and burp her for a couple of minutes, then offer her some more formula.

INTRODUCING SOLID FOOD

Let's face it, meals are an important part of family life, not just a time to eat. As your baby grows closer to age six months—becoming more of her own little person each day—you may find yourself curious and eager to let her try "real" food. Perhaps she's been watching you from her infant seat while you eat dinner. Or maybe a neighbor has been insisting that she will sleep longer at night if you feed her solids. (Don't believe it! Food isn't the only factor in a sleepless night.) Check with your doctor before introducing anything into her diet because starting solids too soon can cause problems. But if your baby is between five and six months, your pediatrician will probably agree that she is physically capable of taking her first tastes. Learning to eat is a gradual, enjoyable, and messy process for your baby, and it can be a challenge for you, too. Introduce her to as many new foods as you can to vary her diet and tastes, but let her decide how much she eats.

IS YOUR BABY READY?

WATCH OUT FOR the fascinating signs that your baby might be ready for "real" food. By six months, her sucking reflex is much less intense. She may be trying to bite and chew on anything and everything. All her dribbling means that saliva can help her swallow. And she can move food from the front of her mouth to the back now. All these signs mean you'll soon be needing some new equipment for her.

UTENSILS

Plastic bowl

Spoon for first tastes

Spoon and fork

Blade size will give different textures

Hand or electric food mill
Or use an electric blender.

A spout prevents the drink from spilling if the cup tips

Plastic cups

SPILLPROOF BOWL

A plastic bowl with a suction ring on the bottom is difficult for your baby to throw on the floor. This bowl has three food compartments as well as a double shell with a stoppered hole, so that you can fill the cavity with hot water to keep food warm for a slow eater.

BIBS

Plastic and terrycloth bib
This is the best type in the early months. Plastic backing and ties at the sides insure that your child's clothes are protected.

A bib that covers your baby's front and arms is ideal as she gets older

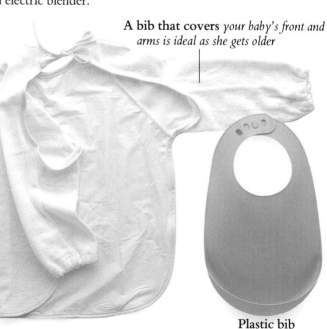

Bib with sleeves

Plastic bib with crumb-catcher

CHAIRS

Some chairs have reclining seats for infants

Make sure the tray *can be wiped clean*

A rim around the edge *of the tray will stop at least some food from falling on the floor*

An easy-care seat cover *is advisable, because food will go everywhere*

The frame must *lock rigid, so your child's fingers can't get pinched*

A restraining strap *or bar is important to stop your baby from slipping down between tray and seat*

A chair that folds *up is useful in a small kitchen*

High chair
Your baby needs a high chair from the age of about six months, or from when she can sit up steadily; before that feed her on your lap and then in her infant or car seat. Strap her into her high chair with a safety harness or belt. Put the chair on a plastic sheet, and involve your child in family mealtimes by setting it next to the table. A footrest is great for toddlers.

Portable seat
A seat that screws or hooks on to a table is excellent when you're away from home—but follow the manufacturer's guidelines carefully, because there are several types of table on which this chair must not be used. Use safety belts when available, and protect the floor underneath.

Booster seat
From the age of about 18 months to two years, your child can reach the level of the table with a booster seat strapped securely to an ordinary chair. Adjust the height by turning the seat over. It's harder to fall off a booster seat than a cushion.

WHY WAIT TO FEED YOUR BABY SOLIDS?

Years ago, parents fed their infants puréed or liquefied solids almost from birth. It wasn't unusual for a two-week-old to be sucking pablum or rice cereal from a spoon. But studies have shown that the digestive tract of a baby that young isn't ready for solid foods. Allergies, indigestion, constipation, and diarrhea are more likely to plague your infant if you start solids too soon. The kidneys and intestines of a young baby are equipped to handle the proportion of fat, protein, and carbohydrates in formula or breast milk, and not much else.

Another reason to hold off on solids is that your baby will be able to let you know when he wants more by leaning forward with an open mouth or that he has had enough by turning his head away. He can't do this until he has gained head, neck, and upper body control.

Should you balance your baby's diet?
Pediatricians often provide a list of suggested first foods with amounts indicated. But you shouldn't worry if your baby rejects solids at first. At six months, the average infant needs only 800 calories a day, and most of them can come from formula or breast milk. There's no real need to be religious about balancing his diet, but do try a wide variety of foods.

WHAT TO FEED YOUR BABY

THE AVERAGE AMERICAN BABY samples a bit of rice cereal mixed with breast milk or formula for her first taste of solid food because rice is less likely to cause an allergic reaction. However, baby diets vary tremendously across the country and around the world, and there are only a few hard rules about where to begin this adventure in eating. In fact, if you happen to like fruit, you may want to start with a little mashed banana, or perhaps some applesauce, puréed apricots, pears, peaches, or plums. Stay away from citrus fruits (including orange juice), tomatoes, fish, berries, egg whites, and spinach; many babies either don't digest these easily or end up with a diaper rash. The key to introducing solid foods is to start with one food at a time and to wait at least 24 hours before adding a new one. If your baby is going to react adversely, you'll know by that time. You may want to make your own baby food using fresh fruits, vegetables, and meats, or you can buy prepared foods in jars at the grocery store, but be sure you select from the correct age range. Always stick with single food jars for the best nutritional value.

MAKING YOUR OWN BABY FOOD

There's absolutely nothing wrong with feeding your child commercially prepared jars of baby food. However, some mothers prefer to rely on home-cooked foods specially prepared for the baby. It does call for extra time in the kitchen but it's usually a little cheaper.

Preparation Wash, peel, and remove all seeds or pits from fruits and vegetables. Slice or chop and then bake, boil, or steam until tender. To purée or mash fruits and vegetables, use a fork, blender, sieve, food mill, or processor for a smooth, lumpless consistency at first. Later, after your baby has learned how to chew and can swallow solids more easily, foods can be minced or whipped to the texture of cottage cheese. You might try mixing a little water, formula, or breast milk into some fruits or vegetables to make them even more liquid.

How to store home-made baby food

Always store puréed or prepared fruits and vegetables in clean containers

Baby rice cereal
Mix with water, breast milk, or formula until liquid.

Puréed carrot
Peeled, cooked, and mashed or from a small jar of baby carrots.

Applesauce
Or puréed pear; either homemade or store-bought are good starters.

Mashed banana
Slice and then mash with a fork.

Minced chicken Try mixing in a little cooked carrot.

Mashed potatoes Try not to overseason with salt or butter.

Finger foods
Shapes of cheese and banana are always popular.

Bread and butter
Keep butter to a minimum.

Plain yogurt
Mix with cooked mashed fruit for an easy dessert.

with lids that fit tightly. Keep them refrigerated for up to 24 hours. Raw fruits or cooked meats will be fine in the refrigerator for up to two days.

Freezing foods
Baby foods will stay fresh for up to one month in your freezer, so you might want to try the ice-cube-tray storage method: Pour freshly prepared purées into clean tray compartments, cover with plastic wrap or waxed paper, and freeze. When they are frozen solid, you can dump the squares into larger freezer bags to seal, label, and date, with one type of food per bag. Do not refreeze leftovers.

SERVING YOUR BABY'S FOOD
Your baby's food can be warmed quickly in a microwave oven, which is convenient when you have a hungry baby hollering. But it's always a good idea to spoon out the food you intend to feed the baby and heat it in the plastic serving bowl. You can also warm baby food by standing the glass jar in a pot of hot water on your stove. Always test it before feeding.

With frozen home-cooked baby food, put some cubes into a bowl to thaw in the refrigerator half an hour before a mealtime. After the cubes are thawed,

you can heat the food in a double boiler, oven, or microwave oven.

Always check the temperature before offering food to your baby. Don't heat and reheat the same food under any circumstances.

At the end of the meal, throw away any food that your baby's spoon has been dipped into because when saliva mixes with food, it can spoil it.

FINGER FOODS
When teeth start to appear —as early as six months— and your baby gains control over his thumbs and fore-fingers—about nine months—he's ready for

finger foods. This first important step toward self-feeding calls for food he can chew and grasp. Try bagels, crackers, or unsalted pretzels but save hard-to-bite raw vegetables and fruits for later to avoid worries about choking.

■ WARNING ■
Never give a preschool child whole nuts, particularly peanuts. It's extremely easy for her to inhale a fragment of nut, which could make her choke, and the oil that peanuts contain can severely irritate your child's lungs.

FOODS TO TRY

Pasta Buy tricolored packages and don't oversauce.

Rice Brown rice is good, too, if well-cooked.

Finger foods Try celery and carrot, avocado, peeled apple, peach, and apricot.

Lean ground beef or pork If possible make your own.

Steamed broccoli Offer it cool as a finger food.

Chicken Chop it small so your child can manage it.

Green beans Cook whole as a finger food.

GETTING STARTED ON SOLIDS

PUTTING A LITTLE SPOONFUL of food to the lips of a six-month-old is one of those milestones most parents savor. Your baby's facial expressions alone may amaze you and keep your family smiling at the memory for years afterward. Whether you choose a small glob of pabulum, mashed banana, applesauce, or puréed pear, or take this first taste straight from a jar of strained carrots, keep in mind that what you are doing is introducing the idea of solids. Your child is still receiving all the nourishment she needs from bottle, breast, or perhaps a combination of both. Try "sandwiching" a first taste into the middle of your regular feeding. She won't be as frustrated if she isn't famished, but it might take a while, so be patient.

■ YOU WILL NEED ■
Bib
Small plastic bowl or custard cup
Small spoon
About a tablespoon of applesauce, pear purée, or baby rice cereal
Damp tissue or washcloth

FOLLOW YOUR BABY'S CUES

The American Academy of Pediatrics divides infant feeding into three stages: (1) the nursing period when only formula or human breast milk is given, (2) a transitional period when solids are added, and (3) a modified adult phase during which the bulk of your child's caloric intake comes from the table and less and less from bottle or breast. Most children reach the third stage after their first birthday. Be spontaneous and creative at mealtimes. If your child detests cereal for breakfast and loves sweet potatoes, listen to him. He may not be able to talk but he's speaking his mind loudly and clearly.

FEED HER FIRST

Sit down with your baby's bowl of food within reach. Put a bib on her, then give her half her usual breast- or bottle-feeding—let her empty one breast, for instance, or give her half her bottle. Burp her to bring up any gas. She will need her breast milk or formula for several months to come.

"SANDWICHING" HER FIRST TASTES

1 With her still on your lap, scoop a little food on to the spoon—enough to coat the tip. Put the spoon between your baby's lips so that she can suck the food off. Don't try to push the spoon in—she may gag if she feels food at the back of her tongue. She may be surprised at the taste and sensation at first, so be patient and talk to her encouragingly.

2 She may quickly discover that she enjoys this new experience. If she pushes the food out, scrape it up and put the spoon between her lips again. When she's had about a teaspoonful of purée or rice, wipe her mouth and chin and go back to her normal feeding.

IF SHE REFUSES THE SPOON

Dip the tip of a clean finger into the food and let your baby suck that. If she still protests, she may not like the taste of that food; try another next time.

YOUR BABY'S NUTRITIONAL NEEDS

HOW YOU BALANCE breast- or bottle-feedings with solid foods will depend very much on your baby's temperament and your lifestyle. Don't rush her away from her bottle or your breast. Take one step at a time and let her adjust before taking the next. The chart below is just one way you might approach feeding. Some mothers and fathers feel more comfortable having a schedule to rely upon; others prefer a more laissez-faire approach. This schedule begins at the six-month mark, but you and your pediatrician will know the best time to begin. If you are breast-feeding, keep in mind that your body's production of milk must wind down gradually, so don't drop more than one feeding every three or so days.

A STAGE-BY-STAGE GUIDE TO INFANT FEEDING

Stage/Age	What to do	Drinks	Meals and feedings				
			EARLY AM	BREAK-FAST	LUNCH	DINNER	BED-TIME
Weeks 1 and 2 Age 6 months (ages are guidelines only)	Offer small tastes of baby cereal, fruit, or vegetable purée at lunchtime, halfway through the breast- or bottle-feeding. Give the same food for one week to accustom your baby to it.	If you are bottle-feeding, offer your baby occasional drinks of cool water.	■	■	■■■	■	■
Weeks 3 and 4 Age 6½ months	Introduce solid food at breakfast: baby rice cereal or another single grain iron-fortified baby cereal is ideal. Increase the amount of solid food at lunchtime to 3 to 4 teaspoonfuls.	Offer cool water or diluted fruit juice in a bottle. Don't worry if she doesn't want any.	■	■■■	■■■	■	■
Weeks 5 and 6 Age 7 months	Introduce solid food at dinner, halfway through the feeding. A week later, offer two courses at lunch: follow a vegetable purée with a fruit one, giving 2 to 3 teaspoonfuls of each.	Introduce a training cup, but don't expect her to be able to drink from it yet—it's just a toy to her.		■■■	■■■■	■■■	■
Weeks 7 and 8 Age 7½ months	Offer solid food as the first part of lunch, then give breast or bottle. She can have two courses at dinner now, a vegetable and a piece of banana, for example. At breakfast and dinner, continue breast- or bottle-feeding first. She may eat 5 to 6 teaspoonfuls of solid food at each meal now.	You can start to give your baby drinks in her cup, but hold it for her as she drinks from it.		■■■	■■■	■■■■	■
Weeks 9 and 10 Age 8 months	After lunch solids, offer formula or breast milk from a cup instead of the bottle or your breast. After a few days with no lunchtime bottle, offer solid food as the first part of dinner.	Offer formula in a cup at each meal and cool water or diluted juice at other times.		■■■	■■	■■■	
Weeks 11 and 12 Age 8½ months	Offer your baby a drink of formula in a cup instead of a full feeding after her dinner. You may find that she often refuses the bottle or breast after her breakfast solids now.	As before.		■■	■■	■■	■
Week 13 onward Age 9 months	Offer a drink in a cup before breakfast: now your baby is having solids at three meals a day, plus formula to drink. Some doctors suggest cow's milk after the first birthday.	As before. Your baby may be able to manage her own training cup now.		■	■■	■■	■
		Key ■ feeding ■ solid food					

HOW YOUR BABY LEARNS TO FEED HERSELF

YOUR BABY WILL WANT to feed herself long before she's able to do so efficiently. However messy this is —be prepared for food to go all over her face and clothes, into her hair, and on the floor—and however long-drawn-out it makes mealtimes, encourage her as much as you can, it is her first real step toward independence. Keep a relaxed attitude at meals: if your baby finds them interesting and enjoyable occasions, you are less likely to encounter problems over food and eating in the future.

AT EIGHT MONTHS

Your baby may be making determined efforts to feed herself by this age, but she won't be coordinated enough to get all the food she needs into her mouth. Feed her yourself, but don't stop her from playing with her food. Smearing it over her face may be messy, but it's the first step in learning to feed herself. Have a clean washcloth ready to wipe her when she's finished. Give her plenty of different finger foods, too. They're easy to handle, so she will gain in confidence and dexterity.

1 She will be hungry at the start of the meal. You may want to hold the bowl and spoon-feed her.

2 Once you've satisfied her initial hunger, let her join in but continue feeding her yourself.

Your baby *won't be very skillful yet, but will love the challenge*

3 Your baby may get so absorbed in the pleasure of dabbling her fingers in her bowl and pushing the food into her mouth that she will lose interest in you feeding her with a spoon. If she's still hungry, she may cry and squirm out of frustration because she can't get the food in quickly enough, so offer some more spoonfuls. Otherwise let her practice her feeding skills: feeling "I can do it myself" is important to her. She knows when she's had enough.

TIPS TO HELP

■ If she grabs for your spoon, use two spoons at the same meal. Fill one and put it in her bowl so she can pick it up. Fill the other one and keep it ready for when her spoon turns over on the way to her mouth. When this happens, pop your full spoon in, and fill hers so she can try again.
■ Have clean spoons ready for when she drops hers on the floor.

4 Solid food may make her thirsty, so offer formula and tip the cup for her—she won't be able to hold it herself yet. Don't introduce cow's milk until your doctor suggests it.

QUESTIONS & ANSWERS

"How much food should I offer?"
Let your baby decide how much food she wants at each meal. At six months, start with no more than four teaspoons of food in her bowl, and offer more if she eats it all. With cereal, start with about two tablespoons. Some days she will eat voraciously, others hardly anything. If she is gaining weight normally, there's no need to worry that she's not getting enough.

"My child will eat only strained fruits and no meats. What can I do?"
Food fads are common, and usually don't last more than a couple of weeks. Don't stop offering a variety of foods but don't worry if he won't eat them. He will not suffer if he's getting vital nutrients from other sources. If you are concerned, ask your pediatrician about diet and supplemental vitamins.

"Should I make him eat things he doesn't seem to like?"
Respect your child's opinions. If he doesn't like something, don't mix it with something he does like because he will only end up disliking both. Try varying the form. For instance, if he doesn't like vegetables, he might eat them raw or in soup; or egg custard might be a good alternative to scrambled or hard-boiled eggs, if he always refuses eggs.

FIFTEEN MONTHS
Your child will be making a good attempt to feed himself with a spoon or fork with rounded prongs, so cut his food into bite-sized pieces. He may need your help on some days.

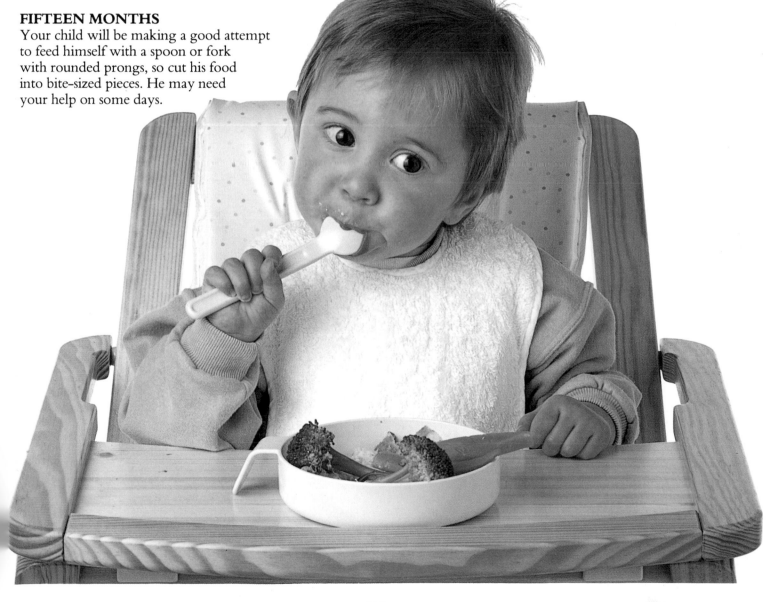

EATING AND YOUR OLDER CHILD

BY THE AGE OF TWO your child will probably be ready to graduate out of his high chair and join you at the table. Mealtimes are important social occasions, and learning how to participate as a member of the family is a vital part of your child's social development. What he eats is important too; it's your job to offer enough good food and it's up to him to eat it. Don't force-feed or hover over him worrying about every bite he does or doesn't take. He won't starve, and he knows best how much food he wants.

A healthy snack
An apple is always a good source of fiber and vitamins. Wash it well first, or peel it.

Avoiding mealtime problems

The secret to avoiding mealtime problems is to keep your own attitude relaxed and friendly. From the beginning, make your child feel that eating is a pleasurable way to satisfy his hunger. It is always a mistake to battle over eating—you will end up more upset than your child, and he may refuse more vehemently next time. Instead, keep the eating issue in perspective for both of you, for it should be an enjoyable experience:
■ Offer your toddler a varied diet, and let him choose what he wants to eat. He will soon make his likes and dislikes clear.
■ Don't punish him for not eating a particular food, and don't reward him for eating something either. "If you finish your carrots, you can ride your tricycle" will make any child think there must be something terrible about carrots if he has to be rewarded for eating them.
■ Don't spend a great deal of time preparing food especially for him: you will only feel doubly resentful if he doesn't eat it.
■ If he dawdles over his food, don't rush him to finish it. He's bound to be slower than you. If you would expect him to stay at the table while you finish your meal, then you must do the same and wait for him to finish when he's slow.
■ Don't force him to eat more than he wants. Let him decide when he has had enough. He won't starve, and if he's growing normally, you know he's eating enough.

The right diet

Variety is the keynote of a good diet: if you offer many different foods throughout the week, you can be reasonably sure that your child is getting the nutrients he needs. His diet will only be unhealthy if for long periods he eats too much of some kinds of food. For instance, a diet based entirely on crackers, cakes, cookies, highly processed snack foods, or hot dogs and take-out hamburgers is a terrible idea.

Snacks and sweets

Your child will often need a snack to give him energy between meals. Rather than cookies or crackers, offer him healthy, nutritious snacks such as a piece of wholegrain bread, an apple, a carrot, or a banana. If he's not very hungry at the next meal, he won't have missed out nutritionally.

Sweets can be a battleground, but it's not fair or realistic to ban them altogether; your child may learn to covet them even more. But sweets provide few nutrients, and they are very bad for your child's teeth.

Control your child's love of anything sweet by keeping sugary and sweetened foods to a minimum:
■ Provide fruit or unsweetened yogurt for dessert at meals. Cheese is excellent too, because it neutralizes the acid that forms in the mouth and attacks tooth enamel.
■ When you do let your child have sweets, offer them at the end of the meal, not in between.
■ Choose sweets that can be eaten quickly, rather than sucked or chewed for a long time.
■ Give pure fruit juices rather than presweetened or carbonated beverages, and provide them only at meals; offer milk or water at other times.
■ Don't use sweets to reward or punish your child: they will become intensely valuable to him, and thus harder to control.
■ Make brushing with a fluoride toothpaste a routine at least after breakfast and before bed (see pages 144–45).

WAYS TO IMPROVE YOUR FAMILY'S DIET

■ Use vegetable margarine and olive oil instead of butter for spreading and cooking.
■ Keep red meat to a minimum: once or twice a week is enough.
■ Cook chicken or fish at least three times a week.
■ Grill or broil rather than fry.
■ Use fresh rather than processed foods—they will contain more nutrients and less salt and sugar.
■ Buy wholegrain bread and avoid presweetened cereals.
■ Serve vegetables raw as often as possible, or cook them only lightly. Any cooking destroys nutrients, but steaming is best.

CRYING AND YOUR BABY

Your baby is bound to cry a great deal throughout his first year. To begin with, it's his only means of communicating his need for food and comfort, but from around three months you will notice a change. Instead of spending much of his waking time crying, he will use that time to learn about the world around him. The crying spells will lessen, and you will become more adept at understanding what he wants. When your baby cries, your instinct will be to pick him up and cuddle him; you don't have to worry that by doing so you are spoiling him, or encouraging him to cry more. Your baby needs to know that he can rely on you. Nevertheless, constant bouts of crying are exhausting for you. If you find that your baby cries so much that you are losing patience, talk to your pediatrician: he may be able to put you in touch with other mothers or voluntary organizations that can help you find ways to cope.

WAYS TO SOOTHE YOUR NEWBORN

THE IMPORTANT THING when your baby cries is to respond quickly, without making a fuss: letting him cry for a long time will agitate him more. See the next page for other possible causes.

SEVEN WAYS TO SOOTHE YOUR CRYING BABY

Feed her In the first months hunger is the most likely reason for your baby crying, and offering a breast or bottle is the most effective way to soothe her—even if that means frequent feedings day and night. If your baby is bottle-fed and sucks hungrily at her bottle with short gaps between bottles, try offering cool water: she may be thirsty.

Cuddle her Very often this will be just the sort of loving contact your baby needs to calm down and stop crying. If she quiets when you hold her upright against your shoulder, or face down in your arms (see page 83), it may have been gas that was making her cry. If she has been passed around for relatives and friends to hold, she may just want a few quiet moments of being cuddled by a familiar parent.

Rock her rhythmically Movement often comforts a cranky baby, and may put her to sleep. Rock her in your arms, and if she doesn't quiet down, try rocking faster—perhaps 60 to 70 rocks per minute. Or just jiggle her up and down by shifting from foot to foot, perhaps with your baby in an infant carrier on your chest (see page 85). Or rock with her in a rocking chair, if you have one. Or put her in her stroller or carriage and push her back and forth; if you can take her around the block, the gentle bumping over the pavement will soothe her.

Swaddle him Wrap him up quite firmly in a baby quilt or receiving blanket, tucking the ends under him to make a neat bundle (see page 123)—it may comfort him to feel safe and secure. Carry him around in your arms still swaddled up until he seems happier, and put him down to sleep on his side without unwrapping him. If your baby is crying because of something you've had to do to him—perhaps he hates being dressed or washed, for example—swaddling may be the best way to reassure and calm him, and stop the crying.

Pat her Rhythmically patting and rubbing her back or stomach will often calm her down, and may help her to bring up gas. The feel of your hand will often comfort her when you first put her down to change her diaper, too.

Give him something to suck Almost all babies are soothed by sucking, and nowadays mothers are often sent home from the hospital with a pacifier for their newborn. Obstetrical nurses have been known to use them, so don't be afraid to try one. You might also offer your cranky baby your own clean little finger. Some newborns suck their own thumbs or fists.

Distract your baby Something to look at may make your baby forget why he was crying, at least for a while. Bright, colorful patterns may fascinate him: he will often gaze intently at postcards, wallpaper, or your clothes. Faces and mirrors are also excellent distractions, and a walk around the house to look at photographs or to peer into a mirror may calm him.

SEVEN REASONS YOUR BABY MIGHT BE CRYING

Often you won't really know why your young baby is crying or why he stopped. There may be times he is crying for no reason at all. If you've tried the simple remedies such as feeding and cuddling, and you've tried the soothing tactics that usually work (see previous page), all without success, there may be another reason. Listed below are other possible causes.

Illness may be making your baby cry, particularly if his crying sounds different from normal. *Always* call your doctor if your baby shows any symptoms that are unusual for him. A blocked nose from a cold may prevent him from feeding or sucking his pacifier or thumb, so he can't comfort himself even though he may not be very ill. Your doctor can prescribe medication to help him breathe easily. (See pages 174–75.)

Diaper rash or a sore bottom may make your baby cry. If he has a sore bottom, take his diaper off, clean him thoroughly, and, if possible, don't put a diaper back on for the rest of the day: just lay him on a towel. Try to stop the rash from getting worse (see page 150).

Colic, often called three-month or evening colic, is characterized by a pattern of regular, intense, inconsolable screaming at a particular time each day, usually the late afternoon or evening. The pattern appears at about three weeks, and continues until 12 or 14 weeks. The crying spell may last as long as three hours. Always ask for medical advice the first time your baby screams inconsolably. Colic isn't harmful, but you might misdiagnose it and miss other, serious symptoms.

Your baby's surroundings may sometimes make him cry. He might be too cold: your baby's room temperature should not be less than 68–70°F (20–21°C), and you can try making this even warmer—up to 80°F (31°C) —if he is very restless. Or he might be too hot: if the back of his neck feels warm and damp, pull down any quilt or blanket covering him and undo some clothes to cool him off. If he is sweating, a towel under the crib sheet may make him more comfortable. Bright lights can make him cry too: make sure an overhead lamp or the sun isn't shining in his eyes.

Activities he hates can't always be avoided, however loudly he voices his dislike. Dressing and undressing, bathing, having eye or nose drops are all common dislikes in a new baby, but all you can do is get them over with as quickly as possible, then cuddle him to calm him down.

Your own mood may be a reason for your baby's distress. Perhaps it's evening and you're tired; perhaps his crankiness is making you irritable. Knowing that your baby is often just reacting to your mood may help you to be calmer with him.

Too much fussing can sometimes make an upset baby cry all the more. Passing him between you, changing a diaper that doesn't need to be changed, offering to feed him again and again, discussing his crying in anxious voices, may all make him even more agitated, so he cries all the harder. If there's no obvious reason for his crying, don't keep trying to find one: he probably just wants to be held.

COPING WITH COLIC

All you can do if your baby has colic is learn to live with it, in the certain knowledge that he isn't ill or abnormal, and that the colic won't last. Don't suffer alone: this will be a difficult three months for you, your partner, and your baby. Try to remember these three points:
■ Do whatever you can to try to soothe your baby. Keeping him in motion, feeding him frequently, rubbing his stomach rhythmically, or just cuddling him, may all soothe him for a short while.
■ Don't resort to medications. You can't cure his colic, so you will be giving your baby large doses of medication for no real purpose.
■ Try to have an occasional evening out. You can leave your partner or a competent, trusted relative to take charge.

YOUR CRYING— OLDER BABY

FROM THE AGE of about three months, you may notice a real change in your baby. She's now much more aware of what goes on around her, she's responsive and interested in everything— more of a person altogether. She'll still cry a lot, and will continue to do so for many months to come, but by now you may have a much better idea of why.

SIX REASONS WHY YOUR OLDER BABY MIGHT BE CRYING

Hunger is still an obvious reason for your baby to cry. As her first year progresses and she becomes mobile and moves on to solid food, she will often get tired and cranky between meals—her life is a busy one. A snack and a drink may restore her energy and cheer her up.

Anxiety will be a new reason for crying from the age of seven or eight months, because by then she's discovered her unshakable attachment to you. You are her "safe base;" she'll be happy to explore the world, provided she can keep you in sight. She may cry if you leave her, or if she loses sight of you. Be patient with her, and let her get used to new people and situations gradually.

Pain, from bumps as she becomes mobile, will be a frequent cause of tears. Often it will be the shock that makes her cry, rather than any injury, so a sympathetic cuddle and a distracting toy will usually help her forget it quickly.

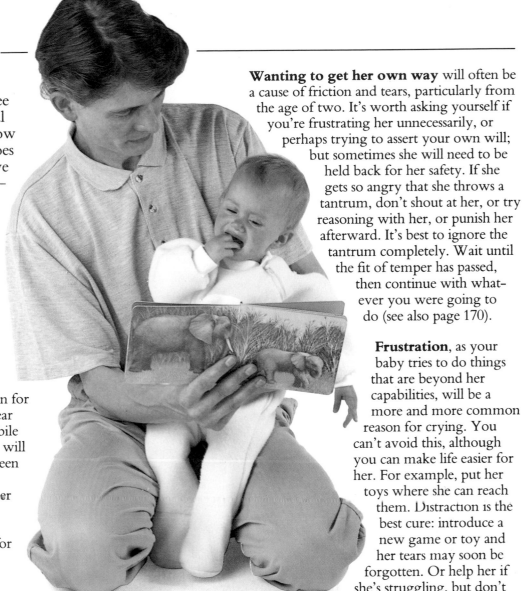

Wanting to get her own way will often be a cause of friction and tears, particularly from the age of two. It's worth asking yourself if you're frustrating her unnecessarily, or perhaps trying to assert your own will; but sometimes she will need to be held back for her safety. If she gets so angry that she throws a tantrum, don't shout at her, or try reasoning with her, or punish her afterward. It's best to ignore the tantrum completely. Wait until the fit of temper has passed, then continue with whatever you were going to do (see also page 170).

Frustration, as your baby tries to do things that are beyond her capabilities, will be a more and more common reason for crying. You can't avoid this, although you can make life easier for her. For example, put her toys where she can reach them. Distraction is the best cure: introduce a new game or toy and her tears may soon be forgotten. Or help her if she's struggling, but don't take over completely.

Overtiredness will show itself in whinincss, irritability, and finally tears. By the end of her first year your child's life is so full of new experiences that she can run out of energy before she's run out of enthusiasm. She needs you to help her relax enough to get the sleep she needs. A quiet time sitting on your lap listening to a story may work, and a calming, enjoyable bedtime routine (see pages 124–25) that you all stick to every evening will help, too.

QUESTION & ANSWER

"Every new tooth my toddler cuts is preceded by days of crying. What can I do to help him?"
The first teeth shouldn't cause any trouble, but the back teeth, cut during the second year, can be painful. Your child will probably dribble a lot and have a red cheek for a couple of days. There are ways you can help him:
■ Rub his gums with your little finger.

■ Give him something firm to chew on: a carrot is ideal, and is even more soothing if you chill it in the refrigerator first.
■ If you use a gel- or water-filled teething ring, put it in the refrigerator, not the freezer: frozen ones can cause frostbite.
■ Check for sharp edges on his smaller toys.
■ Avoid giving repeated doses of medications or teething gels.

SLEEP AND YOUR BABY

Your newborn baby will sleep as much as she needs to; the only trouble is, she may not always sleep when you would like her to. Broken nights and lack of sleep for you will be a fact of life for many weeks until she settles into a routine that coincides more closely with yours. At around nine months, new problems might develop. She may be very reluctant to let you say good night and leave her, or she may settle into a pattern of night waking. Careful handling at bedtime from around the middle of your baby's first year can help to avoid problems later: a relaxing and loving bedtime routine, that takes place in exactly the same way *every* night, will give her the sense of security she needs. Until at least the age of two-and-a-half, and probably much longer, some daytime sleep will be essential. Your toddler's life is an active, exciting one, and she will need a reviving nap during the morning or afternoon to prevent her from becoming overtired and irritable.

EQUIPMENT FOR SLEEP

WHAT YOU BUY for your baby to sleep in will be a significant investment, so shop around and ask friends what worked well for them. If you buy a secondhand crib, make sure any paint is lead-free, and that decorative trim cannot be picked off. You will need plenty of machine-washable bedding. A comforter is light and warm but a restless child might sleep better tucked in securely with a sheet and blankets.

Crib Your baby will be sleeping in this from at least three months to around age three, so it's worth investing in a sturdy, well-made one. Safety is paramount: choose a crib that conforms to Consumer Products Safety Codes.

WHAT TO SLEEP IN

Convertible carriage (see page 156) For your young baby, a carriage that will eventually convert into a stroller is a good-value investment. She can sleep in it day or night, indoors or out, and you have a stroller for later on, too. A bassinet or a cradle that rocks is a good alternative.

Infant seat

For the first few months a seat with carrying handles is very useful. Your baby is portable while she's asleep, and the base is adjustable so that when she's awake she can sit up and even rock.

Watch for *any sharp edges: sand them down if necessary*

A fitted sheet *in 100% cotton is easy to put on and comfortable for your baby*

Carrying handles *mean you won't disturb your sleeping baby when you have to transport her*

The spaces *between the bars should not be less than 1in. (2.5cm.), so she can't get an arm or leg stuck; and not more than 2½in. (6cm.), so she can't slip out feet first*

YOUR BABY'S BEDDING

Mattress Choose a foam type with a fabric cover and air holes at the head end. Vinyl over the rest of the mattress protects it from leaky diaper damage.

Valance or dust ruffle

Air holes *are for added safety*

Fitted sheet and comforter Your baby will find a crib-sized quilt or comforter light: choose a non-allergenic man-made filling, which should be machine washable.

Crib bumper This will cushion and guard against drafts. Make sure any ties are no longer than 7in. (18cm.). Cut them down if necessary.

Lambskin (optional) Buy a treated, machine-washable type only (see page 125).

TOYS FOR THE CRIB

The dropside mechanism *should be one that your baby can't release by herself*

A crib bumper *protects your baby's head if she bumps it against the bars, and keeps drafts out*

If the crib *doesn't come complete with a mattress, follow the instructions on what size to buy. It must fit snugly so your baby can't get her face trapped*

The mattress base *should be at least 2ft. (60cm.) from the top edge of the crib, so your baby cannot climb out. You should be able to lower the base*

Mobile Hanging just out of reach above your baby's crib, a colorful mobile will amuse and interest her.

Board book

Teddy bear

Activity center

She will love to look at **books** propped up; an **activity center** clipped to the crib bars; a **soft toy**; or her reflection in a non-glass mirror.

■ SLEEPTIME SAFETY ■

▲ **Never** let your baby sleep with a pillow until at least two: it could smother her.

▲ Put your baby to sleep on her side, so that if she spits up any formula or milk there is less risk of choking (see page 123).

▲ Remove any plastic packaging from the mattress you buy.

▲ Don't use a plastic sheet for her first two years.

YOUR BABY'S ROOM

■ Keep the room warm: about 68–70°F (20–21°C) is the ideal temperature.

■ Install a dimmer switch or night-light, so you can check on your baby while she's asleep without disturbing her.

■ You may need a smoke alarm installed in your baby's room, unless you live in a small apartment and already have one in a nearby hallway.

■ Never tie a toy to a string, as it could entangle her.

DAYTIME AND NIGHTTIME SLEEP

IN THE EARLY DAYS your baby will sleep in short bursts randomly throughout the day and night. The chart below shows how her sleep pattern might develop: as the months pass, her longest period of sleep coincides more and more with the hours of night, and her wakeful times become longer. However, babies vary. Don't worry if yours takes longer than you expected (or hoped) to sleep through the night.

Emphasizing day and night

Right from the newborn stage, make a clear distinction between how you treat daytime and nighttime sleep, to help your baby learn which time is for play, and which for sleep. During the day put her to sleep in a carriage, cradle, or bassinet: if you're using a crib already, save it for nighttime only. A carriage or stroller can go outside in a shady spot, *always* covered with an insect net and with the brakes on. Indoors, make sure pets can't get into the room where your baby is, but there is no need to keep the house especially quiet for her. When your baby cries, pick her up and make the most of her waking time: help her to associate daylight hours with play and wakefulness.

At night, swaddle your baby firmly so her jerking limbs won't wake her, and put her to sleep in her crib, if you're already using one. Keep the room dark. When she wakes and cries for a feeding, pick her up and feed her quietly, talking as little as possible and only changing her diaper if she's very wet or messy. She will gradually learn that nighttime feedings are business only, not social times, and her sleep pattern will become more like yours as the weeks go by.

Your toddler's naps

From the age of about six months, bedtime will become a more and more important ritual in your baby's day, and she needs to be tired and ready for bed if she is to sleep through the night. She needs some daytime sleep to give her energy for her active life, and will go on needing it throughout toddlerhood, but don't let her nap for too long. Allow two hours for each nap (she may wake earlier), then wake her. She may be grumpy and confused if she was deeply asleep, so give her plenty of time before introducing the next activity.

QUESTION & ANSWER

"My ten-month-old wakes up at 6 am, and won't go to sleep again. Is there anything we can do?"
Early-morning waking probably just means your baby has had enough sleep. Put a few toys in his crib each night to occupy him for a while when he wakes, and, in case he's thirsty, a drink in a training cup with a top that closes tightly. When he tires of his toys and calls for you, changing his diaper and offering some new toys in his crib may gain you an extra hour's sleep.

If early waking is a regular pattern, you could try adjusting his sleep times throughout the day so he has a later bedtime. Put thick curtains up in his bedroom so the sun won't wake him.

HOW MUCH WILL MY BABY SLEEP?

Age of Baby	Daytime (1 am – 8 pm) and Nighttime (9–11)	Key
4 weeks		▪ Nighttime sleep
3 months		□ Daytime sleep
6 months		
12 months		
18 months		
2 years		
3 years		

SWADDLING YOUR NEWBORN BABY

YOUR BABY will probably drift off to sleep much better in his first three months if you wrap him up snugly in a blanket. It makes him feel safe and secure, and stops his limbs from jerking and twitching as he drops off to sleep. Such involuntary movement can startle and wake him. Fold your baby's blanket in half diagonally. If he is crying, don't upset him by putting him down to swaddle him: wrap him up on your lap.

HOW TO SWADDLE YOUR BABY

Folding the second point underneath

Keep your hand *under his head all the time*

1 Hold your baby against your shoulder while you arrange the blanket over your lap, the long edge of the triangle along one thigh, the point hanging down on the other side.

2 Supporting his head, lay your baby across your knees, his neck just level with the edge of the blanket. Bring the far corner up, pulling it taut.

3 Tuck the corner under his bottom, smoothing it out. Bring the other corner up, again pulling it taut, and take it over to tuck under him. Fold the point beyond his feet loosely under his bottom.

PUTTING HIM DOWN TO SLEEP

Once your baby is swaddled and has calmed down, he's ready to be put into his carriage or crib for sleep. Lay him down on his side, smoothing his ear flat under him, and for the first three months put a rolled-up blanket along his back so he can't roll over. He's safest like this: if he sleeps on his back and brings up any milk or formula he might choke, and if he sleeps on his stomach he may accidentally get his mouth and nose buried in the mattress. After three months, he will roll into different positions no matter how you put him down.

A rolled-up *blanket or crib sheet will be sufficient to stop him from rolling over*

SETTLING DOWN TO SLEEP

THE FEELING of a full stomach will often be enough to send your baby contentedly off to sleep; but there will also be many times when she needs you to help her relax. Be confident, calm, and gentle when you're soothing her for sleep. Tickles, giggles, and jerky movements won't help: she needs a quiet period in your arms to make her feel safe, secure, and relaxed.

SOOTHING CONTACT
Rubbing your baby's stomach rhythmically may soothe her enough to put her to sleep. Don't alter the rhythm or you will disturb her; and don't stop until her eyelids have closed.

ROCKING
Rock your baby back and forth in your arms to lull her to sleep. A rocking chair is a wonderful device for a new mother. You may have to rock for some time, but it's still a good method of getting her to sleep.

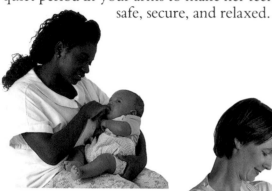

SUCKING
Your baby will be soothed by sucking, and a pacifier is perfectly acceptable. He may suck his own fist or thumb. And on occasion, your own clean little finger will do nicely. Ask your pediatrician for recommendations on pacifier shapes.

Ensure adequate support for his head

AN INFANT CARRIER
If your baby wakes every time you put him down, try using an infant carrier. The motion of your body will keep him asleep (see page 85).

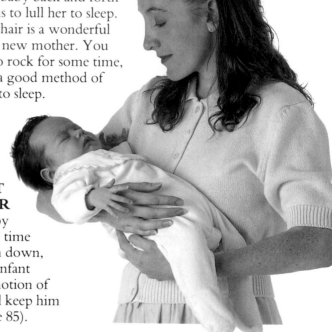

YOUR OLDER BABY'S BEDTIME ROUTINE

FROM ABOUT six months, your baby will settle down to sleep much more happily if the whole process of going to bed takes place in exactly the same way every evening—babies love routine and rituals. From now on she won't be quite so ready to go to sleep in strange surroundings, and her sleep patterns will be easily upset by a change in daily life, such as a vacation, so try to impose the normal routine even if you're away from home. Make getting ready for bed as much fun as you can, so it's a pleasurable but undemanding part of your baby's day.

WHAT TIME IS BEDTIME?
It's up to you and your partner to choose a time that fits in well with your own routine—and one that you can stick to more or less every day. Make sure it's late enough that you're both home, and not so late that the routine takes up all your evening. Any time between 6 pm and 8 pm would be suitable.

THE BEDTIME ROUTINE
1 Start the routine in the same way every evening: a bath is ideal, because it's both fun and relaxing. If she doesn't like being bathed, twenty minutes spent playing a gentle game together might help her unwind.

2 If your baby still has a bedtime feeding, give it to her in her room so she understands this to be a friendly, familiar place, not somewhere she is banished to at night while family life continues elsewhere.

3 Put your baby into her crib with her favorite teddy or soft toys, and her security blanket if she has one.

4 Now perhaps your partner could take over, so you're both involved in the bedtime routine. This last half hour or so needs to be always the same, and as enjoyable as possible for your baby, to mark it clearly as the end of the day.

RHYTHMIC MOVEMENTS

Pushing her back and forth in her carriage will often soothe her to sleep, although she may keep trying to roll over to look at you. When she does drop off, don't lift her out to put her in her crib, even if it's nighttime.

A CAR RIDE

If you get desperate, try putting your baby in his car seat and going for a drive around the block: the motion will probably put him to sleep automatically. When you get home again, leave him undisturbed in his seat and carry both indoors. Cover him with a blanket to keep him warm.

A lambskin *intended for babies' use is machine washable*

The soft fleece *is soothing against your baby's skin*

A LAMBSKIN

Try giving your baby a fleecy lambskin to lie on. The feeling of soft fur on his face and hands will often soothe a baby to sleep, and you can take the fleece with you wherever you go. Buy a lambskin that has been specially treated for babies' use only.

OTHER METHODS

Lullabies, as you rock your baby back and forth, are an age-old method of soothing her to sleep. Your baby won't mind if you can't sing in tune. **Taped music** sometimes helps: gentle music playing softly in her room may calm your baby through a period of light sleep, when she wakes easily. For difficult sleepers, a **soothing tape** of the sounds she would have heard in the womb may work.

5 Read a favorite story with your baby to relax her and help her wind down. Don't give up if you think she isn't paying attention: she will be tired and won't respond to the pictures with her usual lively interest, but that doesn't mean she isn't listening.

6 Position your baby's favorite toy or security blanket next to her and kiss her good night. Turn the light down or switch a night-light on. Don't leave abruptly: spend a moment or two puttering around the room before you go out.

QUESTION & ANSWER

"Is it a good idea to take my baby into bed with me?"

While this practice has always been a little controversial in the United States, night feedings are definitely easier if you take the baby into bed with you. There's little risk of an adult actually rolling onto an infant, so put him in the middle of the bed where he won't be in danger of falling off. Be aware, however, that sleeping with you can become a habit, which may be hard to break later.

OVERCOMING SLEEPING PROBLEMS

■ NIGHT FEEDINGS ■	■ NIGHT WAKING ■	■ UNSETTLED BEDTIME ■
By the time your baby is six months old, she can go until morning without food; but she may well settle into a pattern of waking to be fed. If you want to wean her off these nighttime feedings, start by reducing the feedings gradually, then stop them but go in to see her and offer reassurance for as long as she cries.	The tactics below provide a way of reassuring your older baby when she wakes at night that all is well and you have not abandoned her, while conveying the message that she is only going to get the minimum of attention from you during these hours. If she is not sleeping through within a week, ask your pediatrician's advice.	From the age of about nine months, establish a method of handling bedtime, then stick to it. If your baby gets into a pattern of not settling when you put her to bed, a week of resolutely following the tactics below may break it. She will soon get the message that you *will* always come to her if she cries, but you *won't* pick her up again.

NIGHT FEEDINGS	NIGHT WAKING	UNSETTLED BEDTIME
At her bedtime feeding, try not to let your baby fall asleep with the breast or bottle in her mouth: she needs to learn to fall asleep on her own, not rely on sucking to relax her. As soon as her eyelids droop, take her off the bottle or breast. Tuck her in the crib.	If your baby whimpers at night, wait a few minutes to see if she goes back to sleep again.	Keep to a bedtime routine, making it fun for your baby but relaxing and loving as well. If she cries when you leave her after tucking her in for the night, go back and give her a reassuring kiss, but *don't* pick her up, and *don't* stay more than a moment or two.
↓	↓	↓
For a few nights, feed her when she wakes, but reduce the amount. Put her back in her crib, asleep or not, kiss her, and *leave*.	If she cries loudly, go in to make sure that nothing is wrong. Soothe her and calm her down: rubbing her back may be enough, but you may need to pick her up and cuddle her. When the crying has subsided into sniffles, put her back into her crib, tuck her in so she is snug and warm, and kiss her good night. Then go back to bed yourself.	If she cries again, call out to her reassuringly, but wait five minutes before going in again.
↓		↓
If you are breast-feeding, your partner will have to take over at this point because your baby will smell your milk and want to be nursed. If she continues to cry, wait five minutes, then go back in to give her a pat and rub her back to reassure her. Then go back to bed, even if she's still crying.	↓	When you do go in, make sure that nothing's wrong, such as a wet diaper or something chafing. Pat her back to soothe her, kiss her good night again, and tuck her in. Be cheerful but firm, and then *go*. Don't hesitate—your baby's will is stronger than yours at this point, and you'll be only too easily persuaded to stay.
↓	If the crying continues, or increases in intensity again, call out reassuringly from your own bed if you are near enough to be heard, but wait five minutes before going in to her.	
Continue to go back every five minutes. Pick her up only if she is beside herself with crying; when her sobs subside put her back in her crib and leave her for a few minutes more. You may have a couple of hours of this, but persevere.	↓	↓
	When you do go back, just reassure her by patting and rubbing her back—don't pick her up unless she's really upset—then tuck her in and leave her.	If she keeps on crying, continue going in for a brief look at five-minute intervals. After half an hour, start to increase the intervals between visits, but never let your baby cry for longer than a quarter of an hour.
↓	↓	↓
For the next few nights, stop offering the feeding; instead, adopt the tactics for night waking for as long as it takes to teach your baby to sleep through the night.	Continue going back in this way at five-minute intervals for as long as it takes her to fall back to sleep. After half an hour increase the intervals between visits to ten minutes, but never let her cry for more than 15. A week of gentle firmness on your part should be enough to establish a more sociable sleeping pattern.	Eventually she will realize that the brief reward of you coming in at intervals isn't worth all the effort that she's putting in, and she will drop off to sleep.

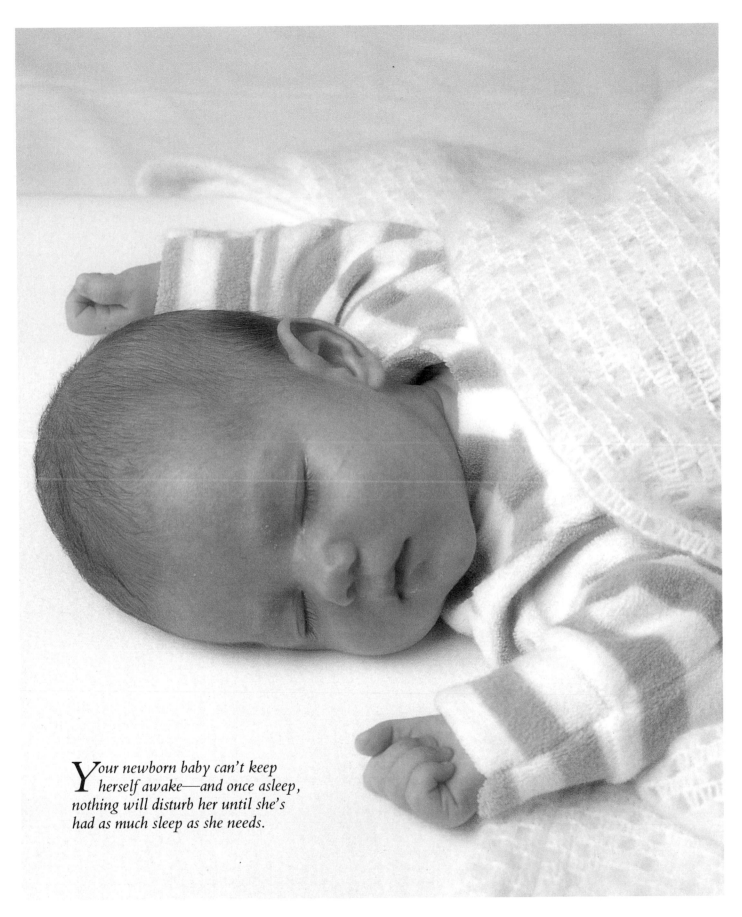

Your newborn baby can't keep herself awake—and once asleep, nothing will disturb her until she's had as much sleep as she needs.

CLOTHES AND DRESSING

In the early weeks you will be dressing and undressing your baby frequently; he may need clean clothes as often as he needs a clean diaper, so you will want to have plenty of newborn sizes on hand. Ask friends and relatives for hand-me-downs. When your child turns into a toddler, start looking for clothes that are as comfortable and unrestricting as possible, but be reassured that you may not need as many outfits then. Don't invest in an extensive "dress-up" wardrobe unless you have very special occasions in mind; fancy clothes are often outgrown long before they are outworn. It's much better to buy a few things at a time, and replace them when they become too small. Choose carefully: easy-to-manage openings and pants with elastic waistlines, for example, will help him as he learns to dress and undress himself. Above all, buy clothes that are easy to care for and machine washable. Staying neat and clean is not number one on a child's list of priorities. In fact, neither of you should need to worry about his clothes.

BUYING CLOTHES FOR YOUR BABY

CLOTHES FOR A YOUNG BABY should be easy to put on, machine washable, and if possible made from natural fibers, which allow your baby to regulate his own temperature as well as he can. Don't use harsh detergents or fabric conditioners to wash baby clothes, because they may irritate his skin. The basic item of clothing now and throughout the first six months is the all-in-one stretchsuit.

Look for suits *with a large cotton content*

Simple cuffs *are best; if your suit has scratch mitts, don't use them*

Envelope neck *stretches wide*

Undershirt

Bodysuit with snap crotch

Underwear
Look for a wide or an envelope neck to help you get it over your baby's head, wide sleeves, and 100% cotton.

Stretchsuit
Look for snaps up the front and around the crotch—this type is the easiest to put on. Avoid scratch mitts— your baby needs to learn about his hands. A tight stretch- suit can cramp and inhibit his movement, so always dress him in one that is baggy all over.

Warm hat

Mittens

Sun hat

On a cold day, your baby needs a **warm hat** that ties under his chin and tie-on **mittens** to stop him from losing heat. In hot weather he needs a **sun hat**.

Sweater
Avoid mohair or fluffy wool, and any knit with large holes that could catch his fingers.

For your newborn, a **nightgown** or stretch-suit is ideal sleepwear. For an older baby, a **sleepsuit** with attached feet will keep him warm, but make sure that there is plenty of room for leg movement.

100% cotton *is best*

Nightgown

Sleepsuit

A drawstring *gives you easy access to your baby's diaper*

BASIC ITEMS FOR YOUR NEW BABY
For a newborn, you'll need lots of changes, or you will be constantly washing. Start with the following, in an infant size. (Sizes are determined by weight.)
- minimum of eight stretchsuits
- six undershirts
- two sweaters
- two nightgowns
- two pairs of socks
- fabric bootees
- tie-on mittens
- sun hat or warm hat
- padded outdoor clothes.

Padded outdoor *clothes keep the wind out and trap a layer of warm air*

Elastic around *the legs should not be too tight*

Snaps *at the crotch make diaper-changing easier*

Cotton suit
A cotton suit with short sleeves and no legs is very cool for your baby during hot weather.

Socks
Should be roomy and soft.

Elasticized fabric bootees
Useful in cold weather before he is walking; they must be very roomy inside.

Outdoor clothes
Put your baby in an extra layer of clothing when you go out, because newborns lose heat easily.

HOW TO DRESS YOUR BABY

DRESSING and undressing your baby is a lovely opportunity to let him learn about his own body by stroking and caressing his soft skin. He may hate being dressed, but you can make it pleasurable with lots of nuzzling, cuddles, kisses, and talk; be especially gentle, too. Gather the clothes you need and undo all the snaps. Lay your baby on a changing pad.

PUTTING ON UNDERWEAR

1 Hold the shirt or bodysuit with the front facing you and gather it into your hands. Put the back edge at his head.

Position the back edge at the top of his head

2 With one swift, gentle movement bring the front edge of the shirt down to your baby's chin. Hold all the fabric gathered together and stretch it as wide as you can, so that none of it drags on his face and upsets him.

3 Gently lift your baby's head and upper body and pull the back of the shirt down so it is around his neck and lying behind his shoulders. Lower him to the pad without jolting or letting his head flop.

4 If your baby's shirt has sleeves, put the fingers of one hand down through the first sleeve and stretch it wide, then with the other hand guide his fist into your fingers.

5 Hold your baby's hand with your first hand, and ease the sleeve over his arm with the other. Pull the shirt down below his arm. Do the same with the other sleeve, pulling the fabric, not your baby.

6 Pull the shirt over his stomach. If it's a one-piece bodysuit, lift his lower body by his ankles and pull the back down. Close the snaps at the crotch.

Lay the stretchsuit out flat

PUTTING ON A STRETCHSUIT

1 Pick your baby up while you lay the clean stretch-suit out flat on the changing pad, the front facing up and all the snaps undone. Lay your baby on top of it, his neck in line with the stretchsuit's.

A shirt *underneath the stretchsuit is essential in anything but the hottest weather*

Pull the suit, *not your baby*

Guide your baby's *fist into the sleeve*

2 Gather the fabric of one stretchsuit leg in your hands, to open up the foot part. Ease your baby's foot in, getting his toes right into the toe of the suit, and pull the leg of the suit up. Do the same with his other foot.

3 Push the thumb and fingers of one hand up through one sleeve from the wrist end, gathering up the fabric of the sleeve over your hand. Stretch the opening as wide as you can. With your other hand, guide your baby's fist into your first hand.

Make sure his *toes are not cramped*

4 Holding your baby's hand between your thumb and fingers, ease the sleeve over your hand and up his arm, drawing it up to his shoulder. This way your baby's fingers and nails can't get caught.

5 If the stretchsuit is on the large side, fold up the cuffs so he can explore with his hands and learn about his body.

6 Close all the snaps, starting with the ones around his thighs and crotch and working up to his neck.

UNDRESSING YOUR BABY

YOUR BABY may be unnerved by the feeling of cold air against his skin as you undress him, so nuzzle his bare body, and make the most of this opportunity for skin-to-skin contact. Have a towel on hand to wrap your baby in when you've undressed him, or dress him again quickly. Lay your baby on his changing mat or table.

TAKING OFF A STRETCHSUIT

1 Undo the stretchsuit snaps. Hold one ankle inside the suit and pull the suit leg off. Do the same with the other.

Hold his ankle *while you pull the leg of the suit off*

2 Undo the snaps on his undershirt, then lift his lower body by his ankles and slide the underwear and stretchsuit up underneath him as far as you can.

Be gentle *as you undress your baby*

Support *your baby's head*

3 Put your hand inside the sleeve and hold his elbow. Grasp the cuff and pull the sleeve off; then repeat on the other arm.

4 Slide your hand underneath your baby's head and neck and lift his upper body so you can remove the stretchsuit.

TAKING OFF A BODYSUIT OR UNDERSHIRT

1 Hold his elbow inside the shirt with one hand and ease all the fabric over his fist. Do the same on the other side.

2 Gather the whole shirt in your hands, so there is no spare fabric that might drag over your baby's face as you take it off.

3 Stretch the opening as wide as you can, then with one movement take it over your baby's face to the top of his head.

4 Slide your hand underneath your baby's head and neck and lift his upper body so you can slide off the underwear.

HOW YOUR CHILD LEARNS TO DRESS HIMSELF

BY ABOUT TWO, your child will probably manage to pull off his own socks or T-shirt, and many children can dress themselves by age three. Encourage this independence by buying clothes that are easy for your child to manage, and by letting him dress and undress as much as he wants, even though you can do it faster.

WAYS TO HELP

■ Allow plenty of time—if you're not in a rush, you won't be irritated by his slowness.
■ Lay out his clothes in the order he needs to put them on.
■ Buy pants or skirts with elasticized waistbands. Avoid pants with zippers for a preschool boy. He may get his penis caught.
■ Look for clothes with large buttons, snaps, or Velcro fastenings.
■ Teach him to start buttoning from the bottom up.
■ Let him choose his "favorite" foot, then mark that shoe so he can get it on the correct foot.
■ Avoid jackets with difficult zippers.
■ When you have to help, make a game of getting dressed, playing "peek-a-boo" as you put garments over his head.
■ Once he's dressed, let him stay dressed—even if he gets dirty.

CHOOSING SHOES

Bare feet are best for babies who are learning to walk. They make it easier to balance, and walking barefoot makes for healthy feet.

Once your child is ready to walk outdoors he will need shoes, but even then, let him go barefoot as much as possible. Shoes are necessary only to protect feet, not to "support" them—the muscles give all the support the foot needs. Buy shoes from a store where children's feet are carefully measured for length *and* width. Have the fit checked every three months.

Buy new socks at the same time as new shoes: too-small socks can be just as constricting as shoes.

What sort of shoes should I buy?

Any leather or canvas shoe is suitable *provided* your child's feet have been properly measured and the shoes fit in length *and* width. Sneakers are fine and come in a wide variety of sizes and designs. Rubber boots aren't always available in half-sizes, but they're still essential for wet weather walks. Buy them on the large side, and use an insole inside.

Avoid all plastic shoes: plastic doesn't mold itself to the shape of your child's foot like leather, so instead his foot will have to mold itself to the shoe—and this could cause permanent damage.

What to look for in your child's shoes

The space between *your child's big toe and the shoe end should be ¼ to ½in. (0.5–1.25cm.)—no more and no less*

Wide toes *are important to give your child's toes room to spread out inside*

T-bar shoes with buckles

The fastening *should hold your child's foot snugly: buckles or Velcro are easiest for your child to manage*

The seams *must be smoothly finished, so nothing can rub your child's skin*

Undressing himself
Your two-year-old will enjoy the challenge of undressing himself, given lots of time.

BATHING AND WASHING YOUR BABY

One day you will look back at your baby's baths as some of the most luxurious moments of parenting. But at first, that's not always the case. You may be nervous, and newborn babies don't always enjoy the sensation of being naked or being in water. Many babies cry that first month. Talk to your pediatrician about when to introduce a full bathtub, but be assured that little babies don't really need daily bathing. In fact, until the belly button is completely healed, you'll probably be advised to stick to sponge bathing. Change diapers often and keep bottoms free of wet or soiled diapers. Get into a habit of washing his face, hands, and diaper area with a soft baby washcloth at the same time every day. This will help inch you both toward a more predictable schedule. Coo, cuddle, and reassure your baby if he is unhappy. He knows your voice already, and soon you will both enjoy those bathing experiences.

EQUIPMENT FOR BATHING AND WASHING

THERE ARE plenty of products available designed to make bathtime easier for you, but you can keep costs down by just buying the things you genuinely need. Some mothers even use the kitchen sink at first. It's the right height and with a bath towel on the bottom for soft cushioning, you'll be all set. Don't use adult shampoos, soaps, or creams. They contain too many additives and chemicals to be safe for a baby.

EQUIPMENT FOR BATHING

Baby bathtub
Until your baby is ready to go into an adult bathtub (some time between three and six months), a baby tub may make bathtime easy for you. Place it at a convenient height on a tabletop, or put it on a towel on the floor and kneel beside it. If you put it on a changing table, make sure it's secure.

Cotton balls

Tissues

Baby wipes

Baby washcloth

You may want to position such essentials near the bathing area and within easy reach.

A rubber bath mat *stops your baby slipping*

Waterproof apron
A cotton fabric with waterproof backing will feel softer to your baby than plastic.

Rubber bath mat
Once your baby moves into the big bathtub, a suctioned rubber bath mat is a must to stop him sliding on the bottom of the tub. The small size will also fit into a baby bathtub to give you more confidence.

BABY TOILETRIES

Bath liquid **Lotion** **Oil** **Moisturizer** **Powder** **Shampoo** **Soap** **Cotton swabs** **Fluoride toothpaste**

Baby bath liquid is an excellent alternative to both soap and shampoo.
Baby lotion is useful for cleaning your baby's diaper area, particularly if his skin is very dry.
Baby oil is a good moisturizer when your baby's skin is dry or scaly.

Baby moisturizer can be used instead of baby oil.
Baby powder will absorb any dampness left on your baby's skin—though it can also cake in the creases and cause irritation if you use too much. Don't put any powder on an area where you will be putting diaper cream.

Baby shampoo may be needed once a week.
Baby soap is very mild so there is no chance of your baby's skin reacting adversely to it. With a young baby, soap him all over on your lap, then rinse the soap off in the bathtub—but remember his body will be slippery.

Cotton swabs are useful for cleaning between your baby's fingers and toes, but never push them into his ears, eyes, nose, or bottom.
Toothpaste can be an adult brand. Try not to let your child eat it—if he does, avoid using it until he's old enough *not* to eat it (see page 144).

HAIR, NAILS, AND TEETH

A **hairbrush** should have soft bristles and be small enough for your child to brush his own hair from about eighteen months. Choose a small **comb** with rounded teeth, and make sure there are no sharp points or edges.
Baby nail scissors have rounded ends and short blades, so there's no danger of accidentally jabbing your baby.

Baby hairbrush and comb

Nail scissors

Toothbrush

Your child's **toothbrush** must have a small head so it can reach into the corners of his mouth, and soft, rounded bristles. Nylon or bristle is equally good. Let your baby play with a baby-size brush, but use a child-size brush to clean his teeth for him. Change his brush regularly, and check with your dentist that it is cleaning adequately.

Towel

Keep a large, very soft towel for your baby's use only. Some baby bath towels have a corner piece that makes a hood.

Natural sponge

Baby washcloth

Keep a new washcloth or sponge for your baby's use, and put the washcloth in the washing machine regularly. Don't let an older baby suck on the sponge.

TIPS FOR WASHING YOUR YOUNG BABY

■ Until your baby's navel has healed, rely on sponge baths. When you do start using a tub or sink, keep the water level to 4in. (10cm.).
■ Only clean the parts you can see—do not try to poke right inside your baby's nose or ears, just wipe away any visible mucus or wax with damp cotton balls. Otherwise you may push the dirt back up into the nose or ear.
■ With a baby girl, never try to separate her vaginal lips to clean inside them. You will hinder the natural flow of mucus that washes bacteria out.

■ With an uncircumcised baby boy, never push back his foreskin to clean under it: you may hurt him, or damage the foreskin.
■ Always wipe from front to back when you are cleaning a baby girl's diaper area. This prevents germs from spreading into the vagina and causing infection.
■ When wiping your baby's eyes and ears, use a fresh cotton ball for each one, or you may spread minor infections.
■ Always clean your baby's bottom last, and use a moistened washcloth, tissues dipped in baby oil, or a diaper wipe, whichever you prefer.

SPONGE BATHING A YOUNG BABY

SPONGE BATHING simply means cleaning only the parts of your baby that really need attention—her hands, face, neck, and diaper area. You don't even need a "sponge." A baby washcloth or cotton balls will do. Sponge bathe as part of your routine. It's an excellent alternative to a bath during the first six weeks, when neither of you will feel very sure about bathing in a bathtub. Make sure the room is warm. Wash your hands. Lay your baby on her changing table or pad on the floor and undress her down to her underwear and diaper. Sponge bathe her in this position or on your lap.

■ YOU WILL NEED ■
Warm tap water
Cotton balls
Tissues
Washcloth
Warm towel
Diaper-changing equipment
Clean clothes

1 Wipe each eye from the nose outward with a cotton ball dipped in water. Use a fresh ball for each wipe, and for each eye. Dry gently with a tissue.

Wipe away *dirt and fluff behind her ears*

5 Uncurl her fingers *gently to wipe her hands*

2 With a fresh moist tissue, cotton ball, or washcloth, wipe each ear. Don't try to wipe inside: just go over and behind it. Dry with the towel.

CLEANING YOUR BABY'S NAVEL
The shriveled up stump of your baby's umbilical cord will probably remain until he is about ten days old. Until it drops off, you must clean it every day. Your pediatrician or the nurse in the hospital can show you how. Careful cleaning prevents infection and helps the cord to separate. Dry the stump with a cotton swab dipped in rubbing alcohol.

Once the stump has dropped off, you will need to clean the navel area every day as part of your routine until it is fully healed.

Consult your pediatrician or midwife as soon as possible if the navel looks red, swollen, inflamed, or starts to ooze fluid of any kind. Keep in mind that a small amount of bleeding is normal.

1 Using a cotton ball or swab moistened with rubbing alcohol, wipe carefully in the skin creases around the navel. (After two weeks you can use clean water.)

2 Dry with a fresh cotton ball. Dust a little baby powder on a piece of cotton and dab it over the navel like a powder puff to absorb any remaining moisture.

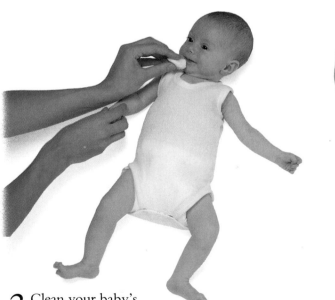

3 Clean your baby's face of formula and dribble by wiping around her mouth and nose, then go over her cheeks and forehead. Dry with the towel.

1 Wipe each eye *with a fresh cotton ball*

3 Remove all traces *of formula and dribble*

2 Never poke *a cotton-tipped swab into your baby's ears*

4 Clean carefully *in the neck creases*

6 Take off her diaper *and pull up her shirt to clean her*

4 Wipe under her chin and in her neck creases with fresh moist cotton balls, tissues, or a washcloth. Sweat can irritate her skin. Dry well.

Wipe over the backs of her hands too

5 Wipe under her arms, gently pulling her arms up to flatten out the creases. Dry well. Uncurl her fists to wash and dry all over her hands and between her fingers.

Always wipe *a girl's genitals from front to back*

6 Now clean your baby's diaper area: undo his or her shirt and diaper and clean in your usual way (see pages 150–51): use tissues dipped in warm water with baby oil added, or moistened with baby lotion. Diaper wipes are also good. Put on barrier cream and a fresh diaper, and dress your baby in clean clothes.

Never pull back *an uncircumcised boy's foreskin*

BATHING YOUR NEW BABY

MOST BABIES eventually love getting a bath; but in the early days you and your baby will probably both have mixed feelings. A new baby often dislikes the feeling of being "unwrapped," and you may feel nervous holding the small, slippery body. In the first weeks you can just sponge bathe your baby to keep her clean; practice with a full bath once a week, and a hair wash every two weeks. Make sure the room is warm. Kneel, sit, or stand to bathe your baby, but don't strain or your back will start to ache.

■ YOU WILL NEED ■
Baby bathtub
Changing mat
Two baby bath towels
Waterproof apron
Cotton balls
Baby soap
Diaper-changing equipment
Baby powder (optional)
Clean clothes

GETTING READY FOR THE BATH

1 Put in cold water, add hot, and mix. Test with your elbow: the water should feel just warm, and be 4in. (10cm.) deep.

2 Lay the bath towel on the changing mat and undress your baby down to her diaper.

3 Wrap her up snugly in a bath towel and wipe her eyes and face with moistened cotton balls.

RINSING YOUR BABY'S HAIR

1 Cradle her head in one hand, her back along your forearm, and tuck her legs under your elbow. Gently pour water from the tub over her head with a cupped hand. Don't splash her face and do keep smiling and chatting.

Avoid splashing *water over her face*

2 Bring your baby back to your lap to pat her head dry gently with the second towel.

QUESTION & ANSWER

"My four-week-old baby has ugly crusty patches on his scalp. What should I do about them?"
This is a harmless form of dandruff called cradle cap. Rub your baby's scalp with baby oil and leave for 24 hours. Comb very gently, then wash the crusts off. If the cradle cap doesn't improve, ask your doctor for a cream.

SOAPING HER

1 Lay your baby on her mat and unwrap the towel. Moisten the soap and make a lather in your hands; then rub your hands all over her upper body. Rinse your hands.

2 Take off her diaper and clean her bottom (see pages 150–51). Then make your hands soapy again and run them over your baby's bottom and legs.

PUTTING YOUR BABY IN THE BATHTUB

One wrist *supports her head, the other her nearest thigh*

Hold *her far shoulder all the time*

1 Unwrap her on your lap, then lift her in: support her head and neck on your forearm, your hand holding her firmly round her far shoulder and upper arm. Put your other hand under her bottom and thighs.

2 Smile and talk to your baby all the time, as you use your free hand to splash water gently over her body. Take it very slowly if she doesn't seem relaxed.

Let her kick *her arms and legs and enjoy the freedom of being naked*

LIFTING HER OUT TO DRY

1 Two or three minutes in the water is enough for a very young baby. Lift her out of the water by sliding your free hand under her bottom: she will be slippery, so hold her firmly.

Support her head *so it can't flop*

2 Wrap her in the towel on your lap and cuddle her dry. Put her on her mat and dry all her skin creases. Put on a clean diaper.

3 If you use powder, sprinkle it on your hands. Run your hands over her, avoiding her diaper area.

BATHING IN THE BIG TUB

YOUR BABY will probably be ready to graduate to the exciting territory of the big tub at the age of three or four months—and some babies are happy in it even earlier. If your baby hasn't yet learned to enjoy bathtime, don't rush the change—give him a few more weeks of being bathed in his own tub, until he really is too big for it, or is more confident.

To bathe your three-month-old, arrange everything you will need beside the tub. Make sure the room is warm. Put the rubber mat on the bottom of the tub and run in cold water, then hot, so that the water is just warm. Put your baby on his changing mat to wash his face, eyes, and ears before you put him in the tub. Take the diaper off and clean his bottom last.

■   YOU WILL NEED   ■
Rubber bath mat
Waterproof apron
Baby soap and baby shampoo (shampoo not needed every time)
Large soft towel
Baby's own sponge or washcloth
Equipment for washing your baby's face
Diaper-changing essentials
Pouring and other toys for an older baby
Toothbrush for an older child
Clean clothes

WASHING YOUR BABY

1 Lay your baby in the tub on a rubber mat. Keep his head and shoulders supported on your arm, his ears clear of the water.

Always kneel *beside the tub so that you can hold your baby securely*

Bathtime *is a time to talk to and enjoy your baby*

The water *should not be deep: 4in. (10cm.) is enough*

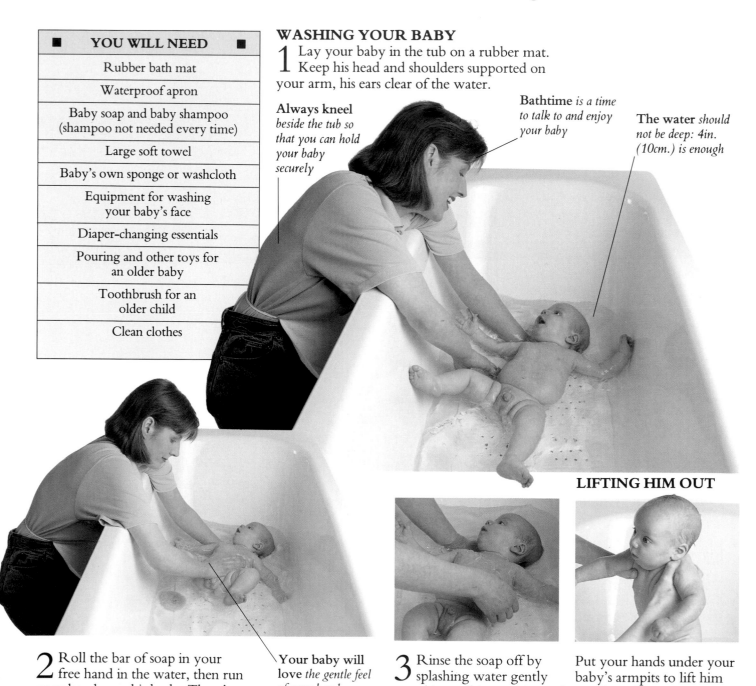

LIFTING HIM OUT

2 Roll the bar of soap in your free hand in the water, then run your hand over his body. There's no need to scrub him—he's unlikely to be that dirty!

Your baby will love *the gentle feel of your hand*

3 Rinse the soap off by splashing water gently over him, talking to him and reassuring him all the time that bathtime is fun time.

Put your hands under your baby's armpits to lift him out: he will be slippery. Wrap him in his towel and cuddle him dry.

WASHING YOUR BABY'S HAIR

1 Wash his hair about once a week. Wet it first. If using shampoo, slide your supporting hand forward and pour a small amount into the palm.

2 Support your baby's head with your free hand and rub shampoo over his hair. Don't worry about hurting the fontanelle, the soft spot on his head.

3 Swap hands again and wipe most of the suds off with a wet, well squeezed out sponge or washcloth.

Take your cue *from him – he might enjoy a teasing game*

■ BATHTIME SAFETY ■

Always follow these few rules:
- ▲ **Never** leave a baby or small child alone in the tub, or move out of easy reach, even for a second. It takes no time for a child to slip and drown, even in very shallow water.
- ▲ **Never** let your child pull himself to standing in the tub even if he can stand steadily and even though you have a rubber mat in the bathtub.
- ▲ Even when your baby can sit steadily, keep a hand ready to support him if he slips.
- ▲ A rubber suction mat in the bottom of the tub is essential.
- ▲ Never add extra hot water while your child is in the water. If any adjustment is necessary, mix hot and cold water in a pitcher so it's just warm, then pour it in.
- ▲ Make sure your water heater thermostat isn't set too high.
- ▲ If the faucet gets hot when you run it, tie a washcloth around it so your child can't be burned.
- ▲ If you bathe with your baby, make the water cooler than you usually have it.

MAKING BATHTIME FUN

Once your baby can sit steadily, bathtime becomes a wonderful playtime—not just a way of getting him clean. Gather together bath toys: things that pour, like plastic beakers and funnels, clean sandcastle buckets with holes, even plastic colanders, will all fascinate him. Floating toys like boats or ducks are ideal too. About once a week use a pouring toy to wash his hair, but don't let water run over his face—he will probably hate it.

Always supervise bathtime, *and never leave your child alone in the bathtub*

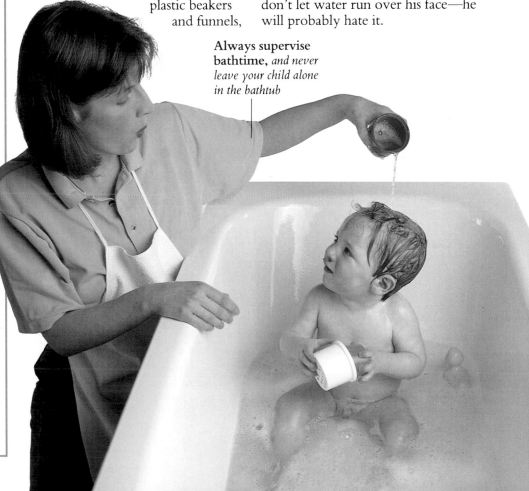

BABIES WHO HATE WATER AND WASHING

BABIES WHO HATE BATHING

Some newborns are frightened by bathtime—and often a baby or toddler may suddenly fight it. Give up baths altogether for a while: light sponge bathing will keep a small baby clean, though a mobile baby may need a thorough sponge bathe on your lap (see below). After two or three weeks, try having a bath with him to help him overcome his fear.

Playing with water
Sit your baby beside a bowl of water on the kitchen floor and let him splash and play. Pouring cups and floating toys can often persuade a child that water can be fun.

BABIES WHO HATE WASHING

Even if your child hates having his hands washed, it's important to do so before and after every meal. Make it more fun by washing his hands between your own wet and soapy ones.

BABIES WHO HATE HAIR WASHING

Babies and young children often particularly dislike having their hair washed, even if they love bathtime—around two and a half to three years is often the most difficult time. If your child doesn't like it, abandon it for a couple of weeks. Help him to be more reasonable about his dislike: for example, go out together in the rain and show him how pleasurable raindrops feel on his face.

Reintroduce hairwashing at bathtime gradually. It may help to give him a washcloth to hold over his eyes and face: often it's the feel of water on their face that children hate most. If your child will wear one, you could try putting a plastic "halo" around his hairline to keep the water off his face.

Sponging her hair
You can keep your child's hair clean by sponging out any bits of food and dirt with a damp washcloth or sponge.

SPONGE BATHING AN OLDER BABY

IF YOUR BABY doesn't like water, there's no need to bathe him: once he can hold his head up, a daily sponge bath on your lap is enough. First, lay your baby on his mat and wipe his eyes, face, and ears with a clean washcloth or cotton balls. Sit him on your lap, with everything you need within reach.

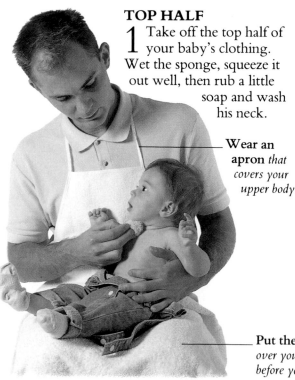

Wear an apron *that covers your upper body*

Put the towel *over your lap before you begin*

■ YOU WILL NEED ■
A sink filled with warm water
Baby soap
Waterproof apron that covers your upper body
Your baby's own sponge or washcloth
Warm towel
Diaper-changing equipment

TOP HALF

1 Take off the top half of your baby's clothing. Wet the sponge, squeeze it out well, then rub a little soap and wash his neck.

2 Wet and soap the sponge again, squeezing it out so it doesn't dribble, then wash all over his chest and stomach. Rinse the soap off as before. Dry him well with the towel.

3 Hold your baby's arms up to wash, rinse, and dry his underarms, where sweat and lint can accumulate. Wash, rinse, and dry his forearms, then let him dip his hands in the water if he wants to. Dry them with the towel.

4 Lean him forward over your arm to wash, rinse, and dry his back and shoulders. He won't like water trickling down his back, so squeeze the sponge out.

LOWER HALF

1 Put on a clean undershirt and take off his pants and socks. Wash his feet and legs next. Rinse, and dry well, particularly between his toes.

Hold your baby's **arms** *up to flatten out his skin creases*

2 Lastly, take off your baby's diaper and clean his stomach, genitals, and bottom in your usual way (see pages 150–51). Lay him on your lap if you feel confident, or put him on his mat. Put on a clean diaper and dress him in a set of clean clothes.

Hold your baby *firmly all the time: he will wriggle*

CARING FOR YOUR CHILD'S TEETH

IT'S NEVER TOO EARLY to start cleaning your child's teeth. Once your baby has two or more, wipe his teeth and gums each evening with a wetted handkerchief. Twelve months is a good age to introduce him to a child's toothbrush: clean his teeth for him (see below) after breakfast and at bedtime, but let him play with a brush himself at bathtime too. Taking care of the first, or "milk," teeth helps to ensure that

when the permanent teeth come in around age six, they will be correctly positioned and in healthy gums—and you will be establishing good, lifelong habits in your child.

At any age, the more of a game teeth cleaning seems, the more your child will be encouraged to co-operate. Playing dentist, cleaning your own teeth with him, and spitting out messily will all help.

CLEANING YOUR BABY'S TEETH

1 Wet a clean handkerchief. Sit your baby on your lap. Wrap the handkerchief around your finger and spread on a pea-sized helping of fluoride toothpaste. There's no need to use toothpaste if your child objects, or wants to eat it, but if you do, use your own brand: children's brands may contain sugar.

2 Rub your finger over your child's gums and teeth. Let her spit into the sink if she wants to copy you.

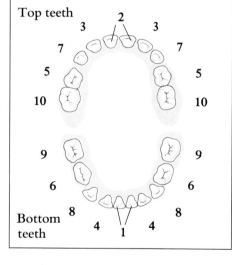

HOW THE TEETH COME IN
Your baby might cut his first tooth at any time during the first year, and he will be teething into his third year. Babies' teeth usually appear in the same order.

Top teeth

Bottom teeth

WHY DO TEETH DECAY?
Teeth decay because bacteria in the mouth react with sugar to form acid, which eats through the hard enamel covering the teeth. Sweets and sugary foods increase the risk of tooth decay, particularly if they're eaten between meals because the teeth are bathed in sugar most of the time. So try to confine sweets to mealtimes, brush your child's teeth afterward, and give him snacks that don't contain a lot of sugar (see page 116).

Fluoride
Children can have their teeth protected with fluoride, a chemical which hardens tooth enamel, and

even heals small breaches in it. Twice-daily brushing with a fluoride toothpaste will help protect your child's teeth from decay, particularly if you let it linger in his mouth. Fluoride is present in some water supplies, or is given in drops or tablets. Your pediatrician can advise you.

Too much fluoride?
You needn't worry if your child swallows a little toothpaste as you brush his teeth, but he might love the taste so much that he wants to eat it from the tube. Don't let him. If he's getting fluoride from water or supplements, the extra in the toothpaste might be excessive.

VISITING THE DENTIST
From the time your child has a complete first set of teeth (at around two and a half) you should arrange regular dental check-ups every six months. Your dentist will have treatments available to prevent tooth decay, and he will be able to advise you about fluoride supplements—so keep up the visits even if you are sure your child's teeth are healthy. If there are any cavities, it's important that they are spotted in good time. Get your child used to the idea of going to the dentist before he has any treatment. If he seems frightened, sit him on your lap in the chair and show him what the equipment does.

CLEANING YOUR CHILD'S TEETH

From the age of 18 months, start cleaning your child's teeth for him with a wetted toothbrush and a pea-sized helping of fluoride toothpaste. Brush them for him for as long as he will let you; he will probably want to brush them himself from the age of about two. Always supervise—he needs to brush correctly. Teach him by standing behind him in front of a mirror, and, holding his hand, showing him the correct movements.

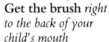

Top teeth: *brush downward, away from the gums*

All biting surfaces: *brush back and forth along the flat tops of the teeth, all around the mouth*

Bottom teeth: *brush upward, away from the gums*

Get the brush *right to the back of your child's mouth*

Brush the gums *with a circular motion, both on the outsides and inside by the tongue*

Making a game of teeth cleaning
Play games at bathtime to encourage your child to copy you; clean his teeth properly afterward.

Cleaning your child's teeth
Stand your child on a step at the sink, with you behind her and to one side. Hold her head back so you can see into her mouth as you brush. Let her rinse and spit out—that's most of the fun.

CUTTING NAILS

YOUR NEWBORN BABY

Keep your baby's fingernails short so that there's no chance of him scratching himself. In the first few months the nails are so soft that the simplest way to trim them is to bite them off gently yourself. If he wriggles, bite them off while he's sleeping.

YOUR OLDER BABY

Sit your baby on your lap, facing forward. Hold one finger at a time and cut her nails with baby scissors, following the shape of her fingertips and checking for sharp points.

CUTTING TOENAILS

Lay a young baby on a mat; sit an older baby on your lap. Hold her foot firmly as she will kick. Cut the nails straight across, otherwise the side edges might grow into the skin.

DIAPERS AND DIAPER CHANGING

The first few weeks of your newborn's life will probably seem like a constant round of diaper changing. Because your baby's bladder is small, she wets often, so at the very least you need to change her after a feeding, after she wakes, before she goes to bed, and in the early weeks often after night feedings too. In fact, change her whenever her diaper is wet or soiled, because a dirty diaper makes it more likely that she will get diaper rash. Changing her isn't always your first priority: when she wakes in the morning she will be hungry, so try taking her wet diaper off, wrapping her in a towel, and feeding her before you change her. You may both get wet but it's not fair to make her wait. Diaper changing need not be a chore: it's a time for games and cuddles, and an important way to show your baby that you love her. Make it easy on yourself by keeping a full set of everything you need in one place; if you live in a two-story house, put a duplicate set downstairs for the first weeks. As the months go by, you'll notice that her diaper needs changing less and less often. By around the age of two your child will start to recognize the feeling of a full bladder, and may be ready for potty training.

THE CONTENTS OF YOUR BABY'S DIAPER

All these are common sights on a baby's diaper:

- **greenish-black, sticky tar (first two or three days only):** this is meconium, which fills the bowels before birth and must be passed before digestion begins
- **greenish-brown or bright green semifluid stools, full of curds (first week only):** "changing stools" show that your baby is adapting to feeding through her digestive system
- **orange-yellow, mustardlike stools, watery with bits of milk curd in them, often very copious:** the settled stools of a breast-fed baby
- **pale brown, solid, formed, and smelly stools:** the settled stools of a bottle-fed baby
- **green, or green streaked, stools:** quite normal, but small green stools over several days may be a sign of under-feeding

Consult your doctor if:
- the stools are very watery and smelly, your baby is vomiting and not eating: diarrhea is life-threatening in a young baby
- you see blood on the diaper
- anything at all worries you.

Disposable diaper

Cloth diaper

TYPES OF DIAPER

Your baby won't mind whether you use disposable or cloth diapers, provided the diaper fits snugly and she's not left in a wet or dirty one. Disposables give your baby a neat, slim-line appearance. Cloth diapers are bulkier, and the clothes you buy your baby may need to be a few sizes larger to accommodate the diaper. Using a diaper service, especially in the newborn stage, is a good idea. Many are as cost-effective as disposables.

A mat with a raised edge *won't stop your baby from rolling off*

CHANGING YOUR BABY'S DIAPER

Since you will be changing your baby's diaper frequently, make your changing area a pleasant place for both of you: a mobile above your baby's head, a teddy bear nearby, bright decals on the walls or furniture alongside will all amuse your baby— and encourage her to lie still for you. A changing mat is cheap and very convenient, and your baby will be safe if you put the mat on a reasonably clean and dry floor. A specially designed changing table may be useful for storing clean diapers and toiletries, but your baby can fall off unless she is buckled on with a restraining belt, and she will soon outgrow it. If you do buy one or use a countertop, chest of drawers, or your bed to change the baby, never turn your back even for a second.

Changing time
Changing your baby's diaper is the perfect opportunity for you or your partner to talk to and play with her: incorporate lots of games and tickles, to make changing time fun.

A game *or two before you put a clean diaper on her will allow air to reach her bottom*

EQUIPMENT FOR CHANGING YOUR BABY'S DIAPER

SUCH AN EXTENSIVE ARRAY OF EQUIPMENT need not seem daunting: the cotton balls, washcloths, and baby wipes, for example, are alternatives. The cotton balls or washclothes can be moistened with water, baby lotion, or baby oil. You may be able to flush used tissues, diaper liners, and wipes down the toilet, but put disposable diapers into a pail lined with a plastic bag. Drop dirty cloth diapers into a special pail, too, so you can launder them separately or send them out with the regular diaper delivery service.

EQUIPMENT FOR CLEANING YOUR BABY'S BOTTOM

Changing mat
A padded, plastic coated mat with raised edges is invaluable. In warm weather put a cloth diaper under your baby's head: the plastic may make her sweaty.

Clean the mat *with a mild solution of disinfectant whenever it gets dirty*

Cotton balls
Pull out a handful of balls before you start the diaper change so you don't have to put a dirty hand into the bag.

Washcloths
Use some wet, some dry, washcloths to clean her bottom.

Tissues
Needed to wipe away feces and to dry your baby's bottom.

Use a little **baby oil** or **lotion** on a cotton ball or washcloth. If your baby gets diaper rash, some lotions can sometimes irritate the skin further.

Baby oil   **Baby lotion**

Baby wipes
Ready-moistened tissues, useful for cleaning your baby's bottom.

Barrier cream
A & D ointments or petroleum jelly form a protective, waterproof layer over the skin. Don't use talcum powder in the same area.

WHAT KIND OF DIAPERS SHOULD YOU USE?
You really have three choices when it comes to diapering your baby: Use disposables, hire a diaper service or buy and wash your own cloth diapers. Cotton cloth diapers that you'll be washing at home really are the cheapest option, but don't forget to consider your time and labor when it comes to cost. You'll also be buying more laundry soap and using more water to run all of the diapers through the washing machine rinse cycle several times to help rid the diaper of soap. When economists compare the costs of diaper services to disposable diapers, they are almost even. A good service provides up to 90 diapers each week, picks up dirty ones and returns a properly washed and dried supply. You still need to purchase rubber pants and diaper pins, however. Disposables, which are the most extensively used, are clearly the most convenient. Initially at least, you may want to use both cloth and disposable diapers. Having some cloth handy for emergencies is always a good idea. You'll need up to 70 disposables weekly so plan shopping trips ahead; big boxes of disposables take up grocery cart space.

DISPOSABLE DIAPERS

Disposable diapers are absorbent paper pads and plastic pants all in one. When you're happy with a brand, buy in large quantities: in the first weeks you may be changing your baby ten or twelve times a day, so 70 diapers will only be one week's supply. A diaper that is too small might be uncomfortable, so buy the next size up if it looks tight. "Ultra" brands are slim and very absorbent; those labeled "standard" are cheaper and bulkier, but you will have to change your baby more often.

You will also need:
Plastic bag or pail with a liner inside: drop the used diaper into this, then when the bag is full, seal it and put it with your garbage. Disposable diapers are guaranteed to stop up your toilet.
A dozen cloth diapers: for general mopping up around your baby.

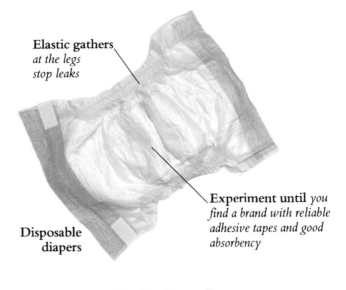

Elastic gathers *at the legs stop leaks*

Disposable diapers

Experiment until *you find a brand with reliable adhesive tapes and good absorbency*

Single-sex diapers
Diapers for baby boys have greater absorbency toward the diaper front than those for girls.

Sticky tape or diaper pins for when the tapes won't stick, or you need to reseal the diaper.

DISPOSING OF THE DIAPERS

Diaper pail Place the used disposable diapers in a pail with a plastic liner inside.

Recycling disposables
Several disposable diaper manufacturers have joined forces to solve the growing problem of trash. Used plastic-covered, disposable diapers are being converted into pulp for wallboard and plastic that can be molded into park benches.

CLOTH DIAPERS AND RUBBER PANTS

When you use **cotton cloth diapers** you will need a pair of rubber pants over the top. Unless you hire a service which provides diapers and launders them weekly, you will have the extra work of washing the diapers. Buy the best quality **100% cotton cloth diapers** you can find; you need 24 to begin with. They are bulkier than disposables, so the smallest sizes of baby clothes may not fit her for long.

Cloth diapers

Always buy *100% cotton cloth diapers*

Diaper liners
These are sometimes used inside a cloth diaper to allow moisture to seep through to the diaper but not back again. The disposable type can be flushed down the toilet with your baby's messes.

Safety diaper pins The hood locks the pin shut. Pin each pin to your clothing as you take it off, and discard any that become blunt.

Pull-on pants
These do prevent leaks, but can also promote diaper rash.

Snap-on pants
When you leave the bottom snaps undone, air circulates inside.

CLEANING A GIRL

CLEAN your baby's bottom thoroughly at every diaper change, otherwise she will soon get red and sore. Wash your hands first. Put your baby on a mat or changing table and undo her clothing and diaper. If she's wearing a cloth diaper, use a clean corner to wipe off most of any mess. With a disposable, wipe off the worst of the mess with tissues and push them down into the diaper. Lift your baby's legs and fold the diaper down under her.

Fold underneath

1 Wipe away feces with tissues, then using a moist baby washcloth, clean all over her stomach up to her navel.

2 With a fresh washcloth clean inside all the creases at the tops of her legs, wiping downward and away from her body.

Dry the skin creases well

3 Lift her legs up with a finger between her ankles and clean her genitals next: always wipe from front to back to prevent germs from the anus entering the vagina. *Do not* try to clean inside the vaginal lips.

4 With a fresh washcloth or baby wipe clean her anus, then her buttocks and thighs, working inward toward the anus. When she's clean remove the disposable diaper, seal the tapes over the front and drop in the pail. Wipe your hands.

5 Dry her diaper area with tissues, then let her kick for a while without a diaper so that her bottom is open to the air.

6 Apply A & D ointment above and around the genitals, on the vaginal lips and anus, and over the buttocks.

DIAPER RASH

All babies get a red or sore bottom from time to time. Consult your doctor if the rash won't clear up.

To avoid diaper rash:
■ change your baby's diaper frequently
■ clean and dry her bottom and skin creases thoroughly
■ let your baby go without a diaper if possible
■ use a diaper rash cream
■ if using cloth diapers, buy snap-on rubber pants, because they allow air to circulate

■ wash and rinse cloth diapers thoroughly.

At the first signs of redness:
■ change diapers more frequently
■ use a healing diaper rash cream
■ let your baby go without a diaper for as much of the day as possible
■ if using cloth diapers, try an absorbent type of liner
■ stop using rubber, vinyl, or plastic pants: they make a rash worse because they help keep urine close to the skin. If you don't like the leaks, switch to disposables for a while.

CLEANING A BOY

YOUR BABY BOY'S urine may go everywhere, so you need to clean his bottom very thoroughly at every diaper change to guard against diaper rash. Wash your hands. Put your baby on a mat or changing table and undo his clothing and diaper. If he's wearing a cloth diaper, wipe off the worst of any mess with a clean corner. With a disposable, undo the tapes, and pause. He may wet then.

1 Your boy baby will often urinate just as you take his diaper off, so pause for a couple of seconds with the diaper held over his penis.

2 Open the diaper out. Wipe off the mess with tissues and drop them into the diaper, then fold it down under him. Moisten cotton balls with water, or use a washcloth or diaper wipe to clean him: wipe his stomach up to his navel.

Clean carefully under his testicles

3 With fresh cotton balls or a diaper wipe clean thoroughly in the creases at the tops of his legs and at the base of his genitals, wiping away from his body. Hold his testicles out of the way while you wipe underneath them.

4 With fresh cotton balls or diaper wipes clean your baby's testicles, including under his penis. There may be traces of urine or feces here. Hold his penis out of the way if necessary, but take care not to drag the skin.

5 Clean his penis, wiping away from the body: do not pull the foreskin of an uncircumcised boy back to clean underneath.

6 Lift your baby's legs to clean his anus and buttocks, keeping a finger between his ankles. Wipe over the backs of his thighs too. When he's clean, remove the diaper.

7 Wipe your hands, and dry his bottom with tissues. Let him kick for a while if he has a rash but keep tissues close at hand just in case he urinates.

Put petroleum jelly or A & D ointment *over his stomach for protection*

8 Apply a barrier cream generously above the penis (but not on it), around the testicles and anus, and over the buttocks.

PUTTING ON A DISPOSABLE DIAPER

IF YOU WANT a disposable diaper to stay on your baby, there are two things to keep in mind: choose the right size for her weight and always wipe your own hands before you open the tabs. When they get greasy, they don't stick.

1 Open out the diaper with the tapes at the top. Lift your baby by her ankles with one finger between them and slide the diaper under her, until the top edge lines up with her waist.

Bring the diaper *straight up: don't twist it to one side*

Spread the diaper *taut over your baby's stomach*

2 Bring the front up, pointing a boy's penis down, where the diaper will be most absorbent.

3 Hold one corner in position and with the other hand unpeel the tape and pull it forward to stick to the front, parallel with the top edge of the diaper.

4 Do the same with the other side, making sure the diaper is snug around your baby's legs, and not twisted around to one side.

QUESTION & ANSWER

"How can I make my 15-month-old son lie still while I change his diaper? He wriggles so much I can't clean him properly or get the diaper on."
No self-respecting toddler will lie quietly while you change him— but you must still get his bottom clean. First of all, make sure to use disposable diapers. They go on very quickly, with no awkward pins to worry about. Remember to make changing time fun, with tickling games and some interesting toys for him to hold. If he's very dirty, it will be easiest to clean him by standing him in the bathtub on a non-slip mat and, if possible, hose his bottom down with warm water from a shower attachment. Dry him well.

Fold the waistband *over. When it is too high, it might irritate your baby's belly button*

5 The diaper should fit snugly around your baby's waist—just room enough for one of your fingers. Check the fit, and if it's too loose reposition the tapes.

PUTTING ON A CLOTH DIAPER

YOU WILL QUICKLY get to know the best way
to put on your baby's diapers. Be creative,
and experiment with the folding until
you get maximum absorbency
right where it's needed.

1 Lift up her lower
body by the ankles
and slide the folded
diaper under her.

**Make sure
A & D cream**
*is applied all over
your baby's bottom*

2 Bring the front edge up
over her stomach.
Draw one front corner of
the diaper over to meet the
back corner above her hip.

FOLDING A CLOTH DIAPER

1 Lay the diaper and
liner out flat. Fold
the side edges in: make
the folds shallow for a
large baby, deep for
smaller one.

3 Keeping the fingers of
one hand between the
diaper pin and her body,
pin the back edge of the
diaper on to the front corner. Make sure the hood
locks the pin shut.

4 Pulling the diaper tight
over her body, pin the
second corner in the same
way as the first.

Extra padding *at
the front is good
for a baby who
likes to sleep on
her stomach*

2 Fold in each end to
give most padding
wherever your baby
seems to get wettest.

**The diaper
should** fit
tightly at first:
it will loosen.

5 Put rubber pants over your
baby's diaper, holding the
leg hole wide as you ease them
up over her foot and knee.
Then pull them over the
diaper, lifting her at the ankles
to pull them up at the back.
Tuck the cloth edges up into
the pants to keep the wetness in.

Tuck the diaper
*edges inside the
pants—but watch for
chafing on your
baby's soft skin*

GIVING UP DIAPERS

Becoming toilet-trained is a big, complicated step in your toddler's life. You can't force him to use a potty chair any more than you can force him to walk. It's all part of his natural development and it may take a day, a week, a month, or half a year. All you need to do is wait until he is ready and then provide encouragement while you help him to understand what's happening. Until your child turns two, he is probably physically incapable of recognizing the signs of a full bladder or bowel or of using his muscles to control them. And if he happens to be one of those children who finds no discomfort in wearing a dirty, wet diaper, there's no reward for him to become potty-trained. Be patient when he has an accident, and remain nonjudgmental. Bowel control usually comes first, during the second year, followed by daytime bladder control, and staying dry at night is last.

Training pants
Extra padding and sometimes a waterproof backing make these more absorbent than ordinary underpants.

TIPS TO HELP
Remember, too much pressure from you can be confusing, as your child struggles to understand and do what you want.
■ Choose a time for potty-training when your child's life is relatively free of new situations, *and* when you can approach it with a relaxed attitude, infinite patience, and a sense of humor.
■ When he's successful, don't be wildly enthusiastic because you want him to accomplish this big step for himself and not just to please you.
■ When he has an accident, be sympathetic, not angry or irritated about it.

Your child and his potty chair
Let him play with it and on it. He will soon understand what it's for.

ACHIEVING DAYTIME CONTROL

1

Wait until your child is ready
Your child can learn to use the potty chair only if he:
■ is two to two and a half (some boys may not be ready to do so until age three)
■ recognizes that he's done something in his diaper, perhaps by pointing and shouting, or by telling you that it's wet
■ is often dry after a nap.

2

Introduce the potty chair
Show him a potty chair and tell him what it's for. Put it in the bathroom for a few days or even months, so he gets used to it. Show him how to sit on it, with or without his diaper on at first.

3

Set aside a suitable time
The ideal arrangement for potty-training is to start in the summer when your child can wear training pants while playing outside in the yard. Accidents won't be as disastrous in the grass and you won't have to worry about outer clothing. Set up his potty where he can see it outside. You might try letting him play in a pail of water or a little wading pool. Don't start when your routines are upset for any reason or when you are away from home.

4

Buy or borrow a pile of training pants
Make sure that you keep a stack of clean training pants in the bathroom so when he has an accident, he can quickly discard one pair for another. Buy or borrow a dozen. Don't put him in overalls with complicated straps, difficult zippers, or buttons. Time is of the essence when he's got to go.

5

Help him to use the potty chair
Be encouraging about sitting on the potty chair, but don't pressure him. Buy him pants he can pull down by himself but help him to sit down on the chair, tucking a boy's penis in. If he's managed to *tell* you he needs it, thank him.

If your child jumps up immediately
Suggest that he sit a little longer and make it easier by distracting him with a toy or a book. If nothing happens, let him get up and keep on playing.

When he does go in the potty
When he does use the potty chair successfully, praise him and tell him what a good boy he is. Wipe off any drips of urine with toilet paper or clean his bottom quickly (wipe a girl from front to back). Hold the potty steady as he stands up. Offer to pull up his pants for him. Don't show disgust at the potty contents, just flush it away, wipe the pot clean, rinse it, and wash your hands.

6

When your child has an accident, don't scold him
You can't expect him to be able to use the potty every time at this stage. When he wets or dirties his pants, don't scold him. Clean him up and be sympathetic. Have a supply of clean training pants handy in the bathroom.

7

Take the diaper off during naps
Once your child is using the potty chair fairly reliably during the daytime, *and* his diaper has been dry after a nap for about a week, you can take his diaper off—he may even ask you to remove it. Suggest that he sit on the potty chair after he wakes from his nap. Napping without diapers will help him stay dry at night.

8

When you go out
Until your child is fairly reliable, put a diaper on him when you go out, but talk to him about it. Try to make sure, without forcing him, that he uses his potty chair beforehand. For car trips, a diaper might be essential unless you will be able to stop easily. Take a potty chair along, spare clothes, and an old towel in case of accidents.

9

Suggest using the toilet
After a few weeks or months of using the potty chair during the day, suggest that he might try using the toilet. Clip a child's seat on it to give him confidence that he won't fall in, and put a step in front so he can climb up. Help him the first few times, until he gets the hang of it. If he just wants to urinate, lift the seat and lid and show him how to aim his penis. Otherwise help him pull his pants down and climb up to sit on the seat; do the same for a girl. Stay nearby until he's finished, wipe his bottom and help him down. Many children aren't able to wipe their own bottoms until at least four. He will probably want to flush the toilet afterward— that's part of the fun. Then wash his and your hands.

Potty chair
This chair converts into a seat that sits on an adult toilet with two steps up.

ACHIEVING NIGHTTIME CONTROL

1

Wait until your child is already dry at night
If you have taken a dry diaper off your child in the morning for at least a week, he can start going without one at night.

2

Don't force the issue of staying dry at night
Your child will stay dry at night. when his bladder is mature enough and you aren't pressuring him. If you make a toddler nervous or anxious about something he has no control over—urinating when he is asleep—achieving nighttime control will only take longer. If you both feel more comfortable wearing the diaper at night, keep it on. If he wants to wear his training pants, let him.

3

If he wets the bed
If your child starts to wet his bed, do not scold, punish, or blame him. Has he suffered some upheaval in his life? There are numerous explanations for why some children never wet their beds and others are unable to stay dry. Because bed-wetting seems to run in families, doctors have looked for physical causes. Is he a deep sleeper, unable to wake when the urge to use the bathroom might be extreme? The size of the bladder is also linked to bed-wetting. Whatever you do, be patient and keep in mind that your child isn't unusual. Put a night-light in his room alongside the potty chair itself. Try waking him to use the toilet at 10 or 11 pm. and protect his mattress with plastic garbage bags under the bottom sheet.

TAKING YOUR BABY OUT

Some form of carriage or stroller and a car seat are essential pieces of equipment for your new baby. Other useful items are an infant carrier (see page 85) or a backpack if your baby is older. A diaper bag with detachable changing mat is convenient for parents on the go: pack it with disposable diapers, changing equipment, spare clothes, plastic bags for used diapers, and whatever feeding equipment you need (but see page 101 for how to transport formula safely). It's a good idea to take a container of diluted juice or water and a bottle or training cup, and don't forget her favorite toy or security blanket. Your older baby will get enormous enjoyment from your adventures. Whether you're going to the zoo to show her the animals, to the park or a friend's house, there's always something to see. Everything is fascinating to her—traffic jams, store windows, other people—so try to look at the world through her eyes, answer her questions, and don't dismiss her when she points excitedly at something that seems trivial or mundane to you.

WHAT KIND OF CARRIAGE?

WHILE IT MAY NOT be quite as difficult as buying a car, deciding on what kind of carriage to purchase for your baby can be almost as troublesome. These checklists should help you sort out the pros and cons of baby carriages and strollers. Before you go shopping, however, consider how many months of the year you'll be using your purchase, how old your baby is, and where you'll be walking. You don't want to succumb to a sale on an old-fashioned baby carriage if you'll be able to use it only for a month, for instance.

CARRIAGE
Use from birth
☑ Gives your young baby good protection in bad weather.
☑ Gives your baby a comfortable ride.
☑ Can be used up to about one year.
☒ Can't easily be used on public transportation.
☒ Needs ample storage space at home.

CONVERTIBLE CARRIAGE-STROLLER
Use from birth as a carriage
Use from three months as a stroller
☑ Your young baby can ride facing you.
☑ When your baby is older you can convert to the stroller position so she can ride looking forward and see around her.
☑ As a carriage, it gives your young baby good protection in bad weather.
☑ Your young baby can sleep in the carriage day and night.
☑ Your young baby can be snug under a baby blanket or comforter.
☑ As a stroller, the rigid seatback gives good support.
☑ In either position the carriage is light, and easy to maneuver.
☑ It can be easily stored when folded flat.
☒ It can be awkward to take on public transportation.

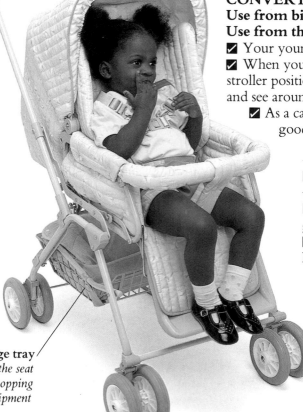

As a carriage
To your newborn baby, the carriage position gives all-round protection and comfort so she can catch her daytime naps in it.

A large tray
underneath the seat is useful for shopping and changing equipment

As a stroller

UMBRELLA-STYLE FOLDING STROLLER

☑ Folds up neatly so it's good on public transportation and if storage space is limited.

☑ The cheapest option; also the lightest.

☒ Soft seatback offers poor support, so not suitable for babies under six months.

☒ Some models don't feature shopping pockets or trays.

YOUR WALKING CHILD

A harness is an ideal way to keep your child from wandering off, and gives her more freedom than holding your hand. Take the stroller with you too.

■ CARRIAGE AND STROLLER SAFETY ■

▲ Check that a stroller is firmly locked into position before you put your baby in.

▲ In a stroller, always strap your child in with the seat belts or stroller harness.

▲ In a carriage, fit and always use a harness when your baby starts to sit up.

▲ Put the brake on as soon as you stop.

▲ Never let your child pull herself up or stand in the carriage: she may tip it over.

▲ Never hang heavy shopping bags on the handles: you may tip the stroller over.

▲ Never let your child play with a folded stroller.

SAFETY IN THE CAR

EACH STATE has different requirements for protecting young children during car travel. You might check with your pediatrician for specific guidelines, but you can be certain of one rule: every child under age four must be securely strapped into an approved safety seat when traveling in a car.

IN-CAR ENTERTAINMENT

Make car trips fun by:
■ bringing along children's cassettes of songs or stories
■ singing songs or reciting nursery rhymes
■ packing a bag full of finger puppets, books, puzzles, teethers, toy cars, and an activity center
■ having portion-sized snacks and drinks handy
■ stopping frequently.

WHAT SEAT FOR WHAT AGE?

Birth to 20lb.: Tub-shaped infant seats are specially constructed and will hold your baby in a semi-reclining position. Designed to face the rear of the car whether in the backseat or front, they can be slipped into and out of a car easily so a sleeping baby need not always be disturbed.

Birth to 40lb.: Convertible seats often feature three positions so a newborn can recline and sit facing backward while an older baby may sit up higher to look out the window.

20–40lb.: Toddler seats are made especially for babies who have outgrown infant seats, can sit up without support, and will want to ride facing forward.

30–60lb.: Booster seats are designed for children who have outgrown other types.

FREE SHOPPING GUIDE

If you are uncertain about what kind of seat would best suit your child and your car, you can obtain a free booklet by writing:
National Highway Traffic Safety Administration, NTS – 13
400 Seventh Street, S.W.
Washington, D.C. 20590.

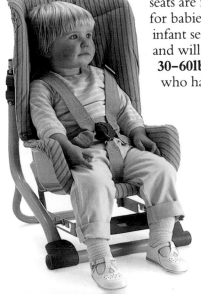

■ TRAVELING TIPS ■

Don't fool yourself into thinking that a baby is safe in an adult's arms when you are in a car. In a crash, no one could hold on. You should **always**:

▲ Select a child safety seat that fits your child and your car, use it correctly and every time.

▲ Face infants toward the **rear**.

▲ Fasten the safety seat with the car's safety belt, properly routing the belt through the safety seat frame, according to the manufacturer's directions.

▲ Fasten the child seat harness snugly over her shoulders.

▲ Buy a new child safety seat if you buy a new car and the old safety seat doesn't fit properly.

▲ Use only child safety seats that meet Department of Transportation requirements and have a stamp of manufacturing after January 1, 1981.

GROWING AND LEARNING

Watching your child grow and learn is a fascinating experience. Physically and emotionally, being a parent is the hardest work you may ever do, but every stage brings something new and rewarding from your baby: at first it's rolling over, using his hands, sitting, crawling, walking. The next thing you know he'll be talking to you. Throughout these preschool years, play is critical. Everything your child knows about the way things behave, colors and shapes, cause and effect, he learns through playing with toys and everyday objects. He needs your stimulation and responsiveness, and he needs some structure to his play time, whether at home, at the child care center, nursery school, or with the babysitter. If you are working away from home and burdened by chores, try to approach them, as well as your baby, like a wonderful game. When you turn on a "let's play" mentality, getting him dressed, unpacking groceries, setting the table can become happy times together. That's what your baby needs from you.

THE FIRST SIX MONTHS

DURING THESE MONTHS you will see your baby develop into a real personality. He'll become someone who is able to reward you with enchanting smiles and gurgles. Although there are toys aimed at this age group, he needs—and loves—people most of all. When he's wakeful, take the time to talk, smile, and respond to the facial expressions. Stimulate him with things to look at, sounds to hear, and textures to explore. You don't really need expensive toys. Position old postcards and photographs near him. Try a child's nonglass mirror so he can smile at himself. Put a rattle in his hand and take him on a tour around your home.

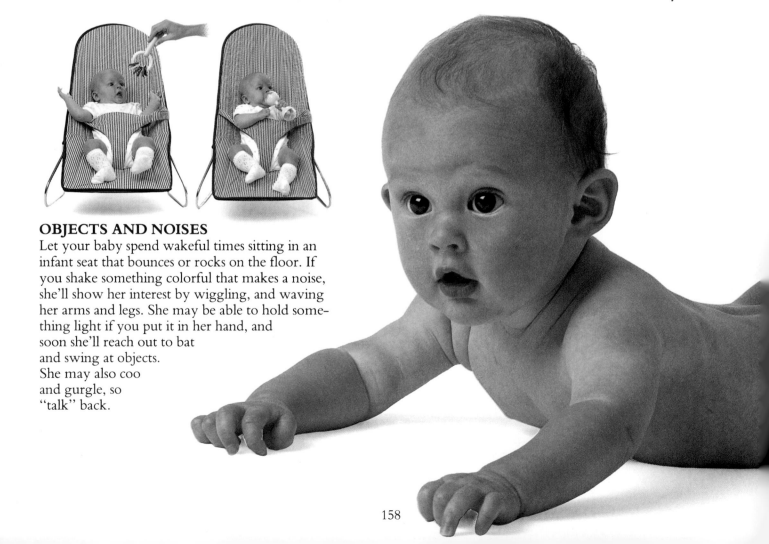

OBJECTS AND NOISES
Let your baby spend wakeful times sitting in an infant seat that bounces or rocks on the floor. If you shake something colorful that makes a noise, she'll show her interest by wiggling, and waving her arms and legs. She may be able to hold something light if you put it in her hand, and soon she'll reach out to bat and swing at objects. She may also coo and gurgle, so "talk" back.

LEARNING ABOUT EACH OTHER

During the first few months of life, your baby focuses best on objects that are 8–12in. (20–30cm.) away. Keep this in mind when you talk to her by exaggerating your expressions and smile. It's this kind of contact that helps your baby become a person, and shows her what a loving relationship is all about.

ROLLING OVER

Sometime during these six months, your baby will learn to roll over, from front to back first, then from back to front. It will give him a great sense of achievement: at last he's beginning to make his body move for him. Remember that even before he's learned to roll he can fall, so never leave him unattended on a high surface, not even the center of a bed.

SITTING

As your baby gains more control over his body, help him learn to sit by surrounding him with pillows. They will let him balance, and protect him if he falls over.

PREMATURE BABIES

Your premature baby will probably reach all his developmental milestones later than other babies. Remember that in reality he has two "birthdays:" one is the day he was born, but the more important one for the first few months is the date on which he was *expected* to be born. If you take those missing weeks in the womb into account, you may find that his progress is not slow at all. Your pediatrician will be monitoring him each month, and he should catch up with other children born at the same time by the age of two.

USING HER BODY

Give your baby the chance to explore what she can do with her limbs and body. Lying on her stomach, she will push up on her arms and kick her legs out behind her; she may even balance on her stomach. She will probably enjoy your massaging her gently with baby oil too.

THE SECOND SIX MONTHS

YOUR BABY will cram a great deal into these months. He will sit up unsupported, he may crawl, stand, and even walk by his first birthday. It won't be steady progress, and not every child goes through each stage. Some children never crawl, for example, but this doesn't hinder walking development. This is the age when he learns to explore every new thing by putting it in his mouth—so finger foods are ideal. From now until around two, make sure he can't grab anything sharp or toxic or small enough to swallow.

EXPLORING BOXES
Don't be surprised if your baby finds the boxes her toys arrive in just as fascinating as the toys. Be sure to remove any staples.

MAKING NOISES
A wooden spoon and a saucepan make a perfect drum—your baby will love banging away and listening to the noise.

SITTING UP
Your baby will lean forward and spread her legs out wide and straight when she first learns to balance sitting up. (Put a pillow behind her until she's really steady.) Now she has both hands free to explore. A board book is easy to handle, and even more fun if you look at it with her and point out the action, objects, and characters.

CRAWLING
Moving around on all fours is a great achievement. She may not use each leg in the same way: a lopsided shuffle with one knee and the other foot is quite normal.

"PAT-A-CAKE"
Teach your baby to clap his hands together and play pat-a-cake. Sing the rhyme and use toys, too.

WATER PLAY
Fill a plastic kitchen bucket or tub half full and let your baby splash, scoop, pour, and feel the wonder of water.

BOXES AND OBJECTS
Offer your baby a box of small plastic toys, blocks, or shapes. She may play this "fill and dump" game over and over again.

INTRODUCING A BALL
At seven months, your baby may be fascinated to see a ball rolling around, but surprised when she accidentally makes it move. By a year, she may be able to pick it up, throw it, and roll it—she's learned how a ball behaves.

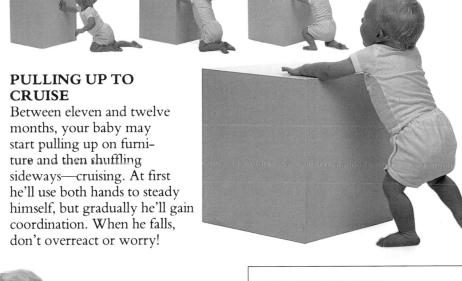

PULLING UP TO CRUISE
Between eleven and twelve months, your baby may start pulling up on furniture and then shuffling sideways—cruising. At first he'll use both hands to steady himself, but gradually he'll gain coordination. When he falls, don't overreact or worry!

GOING UP AND DOWN
As soon as your child shows interest in stairs, start teaching him how to go up and come down safely. Make a game of it and get down on all fours with him, facing into the stairs. Invest in security gates for doors and stairways.

PLAYPENS AND BABY WALKERS
Though it has fallen out of favor, a **playpen** can be one of the safest spots for an active baby when you have to temporarily leave him alone. A playpen can serve as a great storage spot for toys, too. The key to a successful playpen is not overusing it.

A **baby walker** is a seat on wheels. It will give your baby mobility before he can actually walk because he propels it around using his feet. **Never** leave him unattended: some models tip easily, and if allowed to wander in a walker he could get hurt.

GREAT GAMES TO PLAY WITH YOUR BABY

THERE ARE A FEW favorite games that most parents find themselves playing with their child, and that all young children seem to love. Peek-a-boo, catch, hide-and-seek, clapping games: once you start, your child probably won't let you stop. These games have an educational value, as well as being fun to play.

PLAYING CATCH

Sit down on the floor with your baby directly opposite you and try a game of simple catch. Roll a soft ball or toy car to him. He may pick it up and want to return it. Or he may not want to release it to you at all. He may puzzle you by holding out a toy for you to take and then pulling it back. This is common, and he isn't trying to frustrate you. He may not be very good at physically releasing something from his grasp yet, or he could simply be showing you what a wonderful toy he has. Don't try to pull it away from him. Just tell him what a nice toy it is and keep chatting.

HIDE-AND-SEEK

Start by putting one of his favorite toys under his blanket or a towel right in front of him. Then ask him to find it. Or simply close your hand around a small toy and, making two similar fists, ask your toddler which hand holds the toy. Step up the excitement by using three towels to hide the toy. "Where did the toy go?" you wonder aloud. Search-and-find games can be fascinating to a toddler. They require him to follow rudimentary instructions and remember clues. For instance, he has to recall under which towel his toy has gone.

PLAYING PEEK-A-BOO

"Peek-a-boo, I see you!" is an immensely popular game with babies of all ages. The surprise of seeing your face dip out of sight and then come back into view can send a little one squealing with pleasure. Try playing it with your baby in a "bouncer;" as he twirls around, you'll disappear, then he'll shout delightedly as he bounces around to face you again.

And even if your baby loved it when he was only six months old, he will still enjoy variations on this search-and-find game later on. As he grows older, he'll imitate you and may "hide" from you behind his hands or under a diaper or hand towel. He'll pass through a stage where he thinks you can't see him simply because he can't see you. This is normal and can be fun when you turn it into a game. Some experts believe that playing peek-a-boo with your baby will help him handle any potential separation anxiety easier. By realizing that you will always "come back" and that he can be "missing" from you and then "return," he learns that his world is a safe, reassuring place in which to live.

Attach the "bouncer" *to a door frame or to a hook secured in a beam. Set the height so that your baby's feet just touch the ground*

WHEN YOU HAVE TO LEAVE YOUR CHILD

ONE OF THE MOST DIFFICULT things you may have to do as a first-time parent is to leave your baby—crying, smiling, or (heaven forbid) ignoring you—with a sitter or at a child care center. No matter how much outside advice you hear or read, saying good-bye for the first time is rarely simple. Some women even experience a real physical ache, along with the emotional pain. Others feel guilty because they are so happy to be suddenly free of the baby care. You may be on your way back to a full-time job, having an afternoon "off duty," or going out for an evening of relaxation with your mate. Whatever the reason, you need a babysitter you trust, and an ability to look at the situation from your child's point of view.

BABYSITTERS

Unless you begin working with a regular babysitter when your child is extremely young, your baby is bound to experience some degree of upset and anxiety about separating from you and being with a "stranger." There are several ways to approach the sitter situation to make it easier on everyone concerned.

■ Talk about what is going to happen beforehand. Even babies who are too young to know exactly what's up will understand a calm voice.

■ Don't try to begin what might be a stressful encounter when your baby is tired, hungry, or sick. To introduce any new babysitting arrangement or caretaker, pick a time of day when you think he'll be at his most alert and happiest.

■ Make your baby see that this "stranger" is going to be a loving friend. If you are suspicious and upset, he will be, too.

■ Don't rush. Sit quietly even if your baby is crying and pulling at you. Hold him lovingly and keep talking so he can have time to survey the situation and size up this new person in his life.

■ Have some favorite toys handy to begin a real exchange. Hand the sitter a toy, for instance, talk about it, and begin to play a little game of give and take. Invite your child to join.

Arranging for child care is rarely easy on a new parent, emotionally or physically. By establishing a routine, having confidence in your sitter or child care center, and learning how to unwind when you and your baby are together, you can make even the busiest lives much happier.

SEPARATION ANXIETY: WHAT IS IT?

If your mild-mannered baby suddenly starts to cling to you when you try to put him down or cries inconsolably when you leave him with a sitter, then he's suffering from a bout of separation anxiety. Don't worry. It actually indicates a step forward for him developmentally because it means that he recognizes you as separate from him and he knows he's dependent upon you for so much in his life. Some children show signs of separation anxiety as early as seven months, while others start becoming terribly anxious when parents leave only after they are toddling around on two feet. Be patient. Take it seriously because his fears are very real. Reassure him when you have to be away and tell him where you are going as well as when you will return; don't sneak out.

FAVORITE TOYS AND SECURITY BLANKETS

By eight or nine months, most children form a strong attachment to a favorite soft toy, a blanket, or a special object. This powerful need for something cuddly will only grow stronger after the first birthday. Experts say it's a wonderful way for a toddler to cope with the fears and frustrations of growing up, so don't worry about it or try to persuade your baby to give it up. Keep it handy. Tell babysitters about it, and be assured that having a security blanket will help her as she separates from you. If she adopts a blanket, cut it in half or buy a duplicate one, so that you have a spare should she lose the original or when it needs to be washed.

Most boys and girls *enjoy playing mothers and fathers using dolls as their babies*

YOUR ONE-YEAR-OLD

THERE IS NOTHING SWEETER for parents than to light that single candle on a child's first birthday cake. After a long, exhausting, yet exhilarating twelve months, your baby is about to turn some pretty significant corners. In fact, he's stepping into toddlerhood. If he hasn't already, during his second year he'll walk, talk, take great delight in little friends, and pull away from you as he becomes more independent. Physical growth slows down now. He may gain only 6–8lb. (3–4kg.) in the coming year. But watch for the marvelous emotional and intellectual spurts.

First steps will be unsteady

USING STAIRS
Toward the end of this year, your child may grow confident and skillful enough to go up and down stairs upright and facing forward.

LEARNING TO WALK
Once your child has taken her first hesitant steps unsupported, it will only be a few days before she's toddling about enthusiastically, if unsteadily. She may keep her feet wide apart and her arms out for balance. Let her go barefoot as often as possible: she needs shoes only for walking outdoors.

BUILDING A TOWER
From about 18 months, your child will be able to build a tower of four or even five blocks.

WALKING SKILLS
A pull toy will help her sense of balance.

IMITATING YOU
Copying you is how your child learns—and "helping" is always a favorite game. Toy tools make it easy for him to join in.

GREATER MOBILITY
At around 18 months, a simple, stable, ride-on toy will improve coordination and confidence, and provide a new challenge.

USING CRAYONS
Introduce nontoxic crayons during the second half of this year. She may scribble now; soon she'll make up and down strokes.

WHAT KIND OF SHAPE SORTER?
Pick a shape sorter with some secondary play value, too, such as a bucket for water, or a dump truck.

PRACTICING SPEECH
A telephone is an invaluable toy for practicing the art of communication by copying what you and your partner do and say.

THE NAME GAME
You can help your child learn the parts of his body by playing the name game. Ask him to point to his nose, for instance. Then tell him that a nose is for smelling. Use a mirror. Page through a magazine and point out faces. Work your way down and around his body, laughing.

LEARNING TO TALK
Your child's first word, probably "Dada" or "Mama," will appear sometime around his first birthday, and from then on he may acquire roughly two or three new words a month. By the age of two he may be able to string two words together—"me go," say—and will know about 200 words in all. Help him learn and improve:
- Talk to him.
- Use picture books and rhymes when you play together.
- Listen to him, be interested in what he's saying.
- Don't interrupt to make him repeat words "properly."
- Use adult language when you talk to him, but don't try to be his "language teacher." Talk normally.
- Be clear and direct: "Put the block on the top" is less confusing than a string of explanations or commands such as, "Let's see if we can get this nice red block on top of the other one."

YOUR TWO-YEAR-OLD

THIS YEAR, your child may surprise you with his imagination, which can be wildly creative, and the strength of his will, which may be fiercely insistent. If you make sure he has little friends to play with and free time to spend, he can make an absorbing game of anything. Don't waste money on expensive toys that may actually stifle creativity. A big cardboard box can become a house, a car, a boat, or a spaceship. A sheet draped over two chairs is a marvelous hiding place, a tent, or a house. Try not to interfere except when tempers flare, and watch how he plays with his peers, developing social skills and devising games. You may want to begin looking into nursery schools for him now.

DRESSING UP
The perfect "let's pretend" game at any age. Your old clothes, shoes, handbags, and hats are all ideal items for a dressing-up box, and much more fun to play with than the special store-bought outfits in toy departments.

PUZZLES
Jigsaw puzzles demand concentration, dexterity, and visual understanding. If he gives up quickly, hand him a simpler one.

COLOR AND PAINT
Painting is a good way to learn about color and texture. Provide thick brushes, nonspill pots, and lots of paper. Protect his clothes.

IMAGINARY FRIENDS
Dolls and teddy bears will become friends to your girl *or* boy. Watch how she models her play on real-life situations.

JUMPING AND RUNNING
Learning to jump, run, and balance are physical challenges. Jump with him to show him how to bend his knees as he lands.

USING HIS HANDS
Help your child refine his hand movements. He can screw and unscrew small objects and may enjoy using cookie cutters to make shapes out of play or even real edible dough.

PLAYING TOGETHER

A sandbox is always fun. Show your child how to use buckets and shovels, and step in when she tries to throw sand. She will soon find her own level of creativity. Cover the box when not in use to stop animals from getting into it.

SHARING AND PLAYING

Taking turns and sharing toys are difficult lessons for toddlers. Sometime around the age of two and a half to three, your child will start to play *with* other children more often, sharing his toys amicably and joining in a common project. This is the ideal age to introduce him to a play group if he's not already enrolled in a day care center or preschool. The more your child is with others his own age, the quicker and easier he will learn to join in—and to fit in. You can provide plenty of good play opportunities yourself: a sandbox, a wading pool, interlocking plastic blocks, dressing up, making holiday decorations —are all excellent ways for children to learn to play with peers constructively. Adult supervision is important, though, to keep everyone safe or to step in when tempers get out of hand.

BECOMING A PERSON

You will quickly become familiar with your baby's own particular temperament. She may be placid and "easy," she may cry a lot and be hard to comfort, or she may have a somewhat suspicious attitude toward anything new. Those characteristics will tend to persist as your child gets older, but her personality is also shaped by what happens to her, and the way other people behave toward her—particularly you and your partner. You can help her to be secure, confident, and outgoing by showing her, right from the beginning, how special she is to you. Treating her as an individual with her own wishes and opinions will give her confidence in herself. There will be times during toddlerhood when her enthusiasm outstrips her limited abilities, and you will need all your tact to help her succeed without letting her think you're taking over. But if you can put yourself in her position, and see why life is sometimes frustrating for her, the preschool years should be a time of enjoyment and discovery for both of you.

GETTING ALONG TOGETHER

LEARNING TO GET ALONG well together in the preschool years is a process of adjustment for both of you. Your child has to learn the boundaries of acceptable behavior, while you may have to adapt your own natural style as a parent. It's not always easy to remain tolerant, consistent, and fair. Yet your child needs you to show her, not just tell her, how to behave well. Kindness, gentleness, politeness, thoughtfulness—all this she will learn only by copying you when you show the same behavior toward her.

How to handle your child
Your child will almost certainly respond to you best and do as you say willingly if you can be both affectionate and firm. It isn't always easy to get the balance right.
■ Be consistent in what you say and do. If you spank your child when she acts up, she will hit other children when she's angry with them, even if you tell her not to.
■ "Do's" work better than "Don'ts." "Hang your coat up so no one will step on it" elicits a more positive response than "Don't drop your coat on the floor."
■ Say please—and thank you—when you ask her to do something.
■ Agree with your partner on rules and behavior limitations, and back each other up.
■ Try to persuade rather than coerce. If she's in the middle of some absorbing activity, say, "Let's just finish this and then it'll be time to go to bed," rather than "Put away those toys now—it's bedtime."
■ Don't be too restrictive. Try listening to the way you talk to your child. Are you always issuing orders—"Stop that. Do as you're told. Don't touch"?

■ If you were unreasonable over something, say so, and apologize.
■ Don't assert your authority unnecessarily—avoid a clash of wills.
■ Always explain *why* she shouldn't do something as well as *what* it is she shouldn't do, even if she's still too young to understand fully.

Watch your rules!
Until your child has reached at least two and a half, you can't expect her to understand reasons for not doing things, or to remember what she shouldn't do. It's your responsibility to make sure her curiosity won't lead her into danger, and that the important rules are enforced.

For example, "Don't ever go out of the yard on your own" is an abstract rule that your toddler cannot comprehend, much less remember when she's busy playing. It's up to you to keep an eye on her, and *make sure*—with a secure lock or fence around your yard—that she doesn't wander out.

Childproof your home to minimize dangers and to avoid repeatedly reprimanding her—otherwise her curiosity will lead the two of you into conflict

(see pages 226–28). For instance, move stereos out of reach, don't let cords from electrical appliances or lamps hang loose, put child-resistant locks on drawers, cabinets, and the refrigerator, and childproof electrical sockets with guards. Sometimes keeping her away from danger is the only answer, so gate doorways to the kitchen when you can't watch her.

Loving and spoiling
You may worry that the normal affection you give your child will spoil her. It won't. She needs your love, combined with plenty of attention. But you *can* spoil her by being overly lenient when confronted with obnoxious behavior. Letting her get her own way through tears and tantrums will not help her develop social skills to deal with peers and adults.

If you are working outside your home, you may find yourself feeling guilty about not being with her. Don't lavish toys or treats on her to make up for your being away. Toys can't take your place and you are giving her unrealistic expectations about life. Instead, when you *are* home, give her lots of affection.

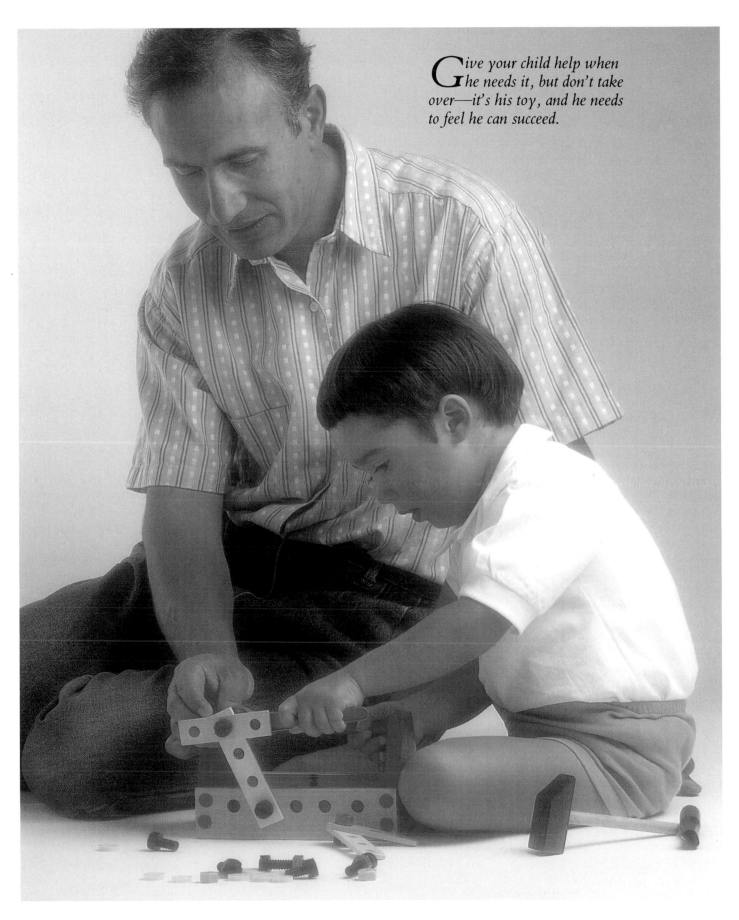

Give your child help when he needs it, but don't take over—it's his toy, and he needs to feel he can succeed.

GOOD AND BAD BEHAVIOR

WHEN THEY ARE HEALTHY and happy, most children usually behave beautifully. But every child has off days, and every child wants to test her limits—and yours—by seeing how far she can go. Bad behavior is often an effective way of gaining your attention, too. The time of greatest conflict will probably come at some stage during the "terrible twos:" tears and tantrums often go hand in hand with being age two.

Dealing with bad behavior
A golden rule is: Act quickly. Step in right away, and remove the source of the trouble—take away the food that's being thrown, or the toy that's being fought over, or pick your child up and remove her with a firm "NO." At the same time distract her attention with some other activity or toy. You don't have to be angry or upset, just consistent, so your child gets the clear message that she's *never* allowed to behave in that way.

Some types of bad behavior—whining, for example—are best simply ignored. If your child never manages to elicit a response from you, and is *never* allowed to win any arguments by such behavior, she will soon stop.

Even tantrums are best ignored. You may be able to divert her attention if you recognize one brewing, but once she's throwing herself to the floor in a rage, just be calm, businesslike and go on as if nothing is wrong. If necessary, put her outside the room until she calms down.

Rewards for good behavior
To your preschool child, the best reward you can give is your time, attention, and love. Praise, a cuddle, a story on your lap, admiring words—all these make your child feel good.

It's very easy to give your child more attention when she behaves badly than when she is good. You're bound to react when you see her pulling the cans off the shelves in the supermarket but you don't always notice or comment on her good behavior when you are busy.

Rewarding her with praise and affection when she behaves well is very effective: "What a good girl you are to wait here so patiently," for example. You will encourage the behavior you want, and teach her a useful lesson—that being nice works much better than being nasty in life.

Punishments
Whatever punishment you decide upon, it has to be *immediate* if it is to have any effect on your toddler. Threats of future action, perhaps the withdrawal of treats and privileges, are useless and unfair for young children. Your child won't be able to understand why she is having a delayed punishment.

When you are confronted by constant bad behavior that you can't ignore, or when a situation has gotten out of hand, an immediate punishment that your child *will* understand is to be isolated for a short while to cool off. Fifteen minutes spent somewhere safe but alone will be long enough for her to forget whatever it was she wanted to do, and give you time to compose yourself.

Should I spank my child?
Spanking is often a sign that you have reached the end of your patience, and it's not a good way to deal with bad behavior. It doesn't deter your child from doing the same thing again, and next time you will probably hit her harder. What's more, you are teaching her that physical force is an acceptable way to make people do what you want.

QUESTIONS & ANSWERS

"My child seems very shy and fearful. What should I do?"
Always respect your child's fears. A little wariness will help keep him safe in some situations—being afraid of dogs or strangers, for example, is reasonable and normal. If he seems very anxious and fearful, discuss his fears with him and take them seriously. Something simple like a night-light to dispel his fear of the dark may make him feel more secure. Fear is contagious: if you have a phobia yourself, make an effort to control it in front of your child.

"Should I try to stop my two-year-old from playing with his penis when I change his diaper?"
Baby boys—and girls—are just as interested in their genitals as they are in every other part of their bodies, and they soon discover that touching them feels nice. Their actions are quite normal. If necessary, you can tell your child that touching his penis is something people do in private. If he seems to masturbate a lot during the day, discuss the habit with your pediatrician.

"Why has my two-year-old suddenly become so difficult to manage?"
The third year of your child's life is a crucial phase in growing up. She is becoming an independent person, wanting to take charge of her own life, yet she is hampered and frustrated by her limited language and abilities. Often she isn't able to make you understand what she wants. Give her as much independence as you can, and be firm in handling this frustrating and troublesome stage. She will eventually grow out of it.

How to avoid running out of patience

No matter how creative you become at managing your child, there will be days when her behavior seems completely unbearable and you know you are close to losing control.

When this happens, take your child out. Whatever the weather, a trip to the park, the stores or to an understanding friend will distract both of you from your respective moods and help you recover your sanity and sense of humor.

Dealing with aggressive children

All small children fight occasionally, especially when they are bored or tired, and boys are often more aggressive than girls. When fights get out of hand, step in quickly:
- separate the fighting children
- divert them by introducing some other game or change of scene
- don't take sides—it's nearly always impossible to work out the rights and wrongs of any situation.

If your child bites another child:
- give all your attention and concern to the bitten child
- remove the biter right away and put her somewhere else, safe but alone, for a quarter of an hour.

Your child is bound to pull and grab when she first starts to play with other children, but with help from you she will soon learn to share, and be kinder to others. A few children continue to be very rough and aggressive, and their behavior will eventually make them unpopular. So for your child's sake, help her to be gentle with others:
- Be a good model for her by always trying to be gentle, patient, and loving toward her.
- Make it clear through the way you act that it's your child's *behavior* you dislike, not her.
- Always step in and stop your child immediately if she starts to hit another child. Be firm, but don't shout or be aggressive yourself.
- Try not to let her get her own way by behaving aggressively or unpleasantly. If it works the first time, she's bound to do it again.

DEVELOPING A SENSE OF IDENTITY

AT AROUND EIGHTEEN MONTHS, your child may declare his independence. It's not always a declaration of war, although some toddlers make it seem that way. Stay calm, and be proud because his defiance and "I'll do it myself!" behavior simply indicates that he knows he's a separate person from you. He shows you his self-determination now by knowing his name as well as words like "me" and "no!"

Encouraging independence

- Make things easy. Organize his possessions so that he can do as much as possible for himself. Buy clothes that are easy to manage, so he can dress and undress himself; put a stool by the bathroom sink so he can wash his hands without your help; and put some hooks in your coat closet within his reach so he can hang up his coat.
- Encourage him to help you. "Helping" is a game at the moment, not a chore. Simple jobs, such as unpacking the grocery bags, setting the table, or sweeping the kitchen floor, make your child feel he's achieved something, and show him that helping is part of family life.
- Let him make decisions. The opportunity to make simple decisions gives your child the feeling that he has some control over his own life. So let him choose which T-shirt he wants to wear, or how his room is arranged, or where he'd like to go for a walk.

Helping your child to feel special

Your child, just like every child, needs to feel that he's special—that you love him and that he is worth loving. It's this message that helps to make him emotionally strong and able to cope away from the security of home. There are plenty of little ways you can show how special he is to you:
- Don't forget to *say* you love him, or be too busy to give a hug or a cuddle when he wants one.
- Respect his feelings and respond to his needs. When he's miserable, he needs to cry and be comforted. Saying "Don't be a crybaby" denies him the right to feel sad.
- Praise him and be enthusiastic about each new achievement.
- Listen and show interest when he talks to you.

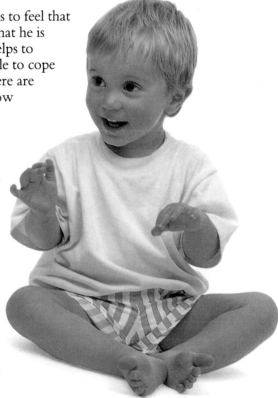

Becoming a person
Appreciate your child for the fascinating, lively, independent individual he has become.

3

HEALTH
CARE

■ ■ ■ ■ ■ ■

*Everything you need to know to recognize
and treat common childhood
illnesses, plus a guide to first aid.*

THE FIRST THREE MONTHS

It is always difficult to be sure whether or not a baby is truly sick, especially when you are a first-time parent. Everything about your infant is new in those early months, including the way he'll let you know when he isn't feeling well. But babies can become seriously ill quickly and any infection may be dangerous, so don't take chances: be cautious and call your doctor right away if you think your baby might be sick. If you notice anything about his behavior that frightens you, look at the symptoms listed on these two pages. These are the most common health risks for babies under three months old. The guide will direct you to the relevant section on pages 176–79, but is not intended as a definite medical diagnosis—only a doctor can offer you that. If you can't find your baby's symptoms here, look at the guide on pages 180–81, which covers illnesses for babies and children of all ages. Babies are born with a natural immunity to many infections, since antibodies (which destroy germs) are passed to them from their mother's blood. Breast-fed babies also receive antibodies from their mother's milk. This immunity lasts for about six months, so before this age your baby is very unlikely to catch any of the infectious illnesses that are common in childhood.

■ EMERGENCY SIGNS ■

Call for emergency help immediately if your baby:
▲ throws up green vomit
▲ has a temperature over 102.2°F (39°C) for more than half an hour
▲ vomits AND cries uncontrollably as if in great pain
▲ is breathing very noisily or rapidly

Fontanelle

▲ has a taut, bulging fontanelle when he isn't crying

▲ screams as if in pain and turns pale when he screams
▲ has BM's containing blood and mucus, which resemble red currant jelly.

■ CALL THE DOCTOR ■

Call your doctor now if your baby:
▲ cries more than usual, or his crying sounds unusual or abnormal for more than an hour
▲ seems abnormally quiet, drowsy, or listless
▲ refuses two successive feedings, or does not demand to be fed for six hours
▲ seems particularly irritable or restless.

PREMATURE BABIES

Babies who were very small at birth, or who were born a month or more before their due date, are very vulnerable to infections during their first weeks. Until your baby is older and has put on weight, keep him away from anyone who has a cough or cold, and don't take him into public places where he might pick up an infection.

Cold hands and feet, *see Chilling (page 178)*

Areas of dry, flaking skin *mean that your baby's skin needs moisturizing, so rub a little baby oil or baby moisturizer gently into the dry areas.*

Crying

If none of your usual soothing methods calms your baby after an hour or so, or if his crying sounds unusual, **call your doctor now**. If your baby cries inconsolably for two or three hours at about the same time each day, but shows no other signs of illness, he might have colic (see page 118). This may continue for several weeks, but there is no treatment for it.

Loss of appetite

If your baby does not want to be fed, but seems generally healthy and contented, there is no need to worry. If he refuses two feedings in succession, or does not demand a feeding for six hours, **call your doctor now**.

Slow weight gain

If your baby does not seem to be gaining weight at the normal rate (see charts on pages 246–49), consult your pediatrician. Occasionally an underlying illness can make a baby grow more slowly than normal.

Brown, scaly patches
on the head, *see
Cradle cap (page 177)*

Vomiting,
see page 179

Hot, flushed, damp skin,
*especially on the neck or chest,
see Overheating (page 178)*

Tears from
one or both
eyes *even when
your baby isn't
crying: this
happens when
the tear duct has not opened completely, so her tears can't drain
away. It is quite common, and
usually corrects itself by the time the
baby is a year old. Consult your
doctor if it continues beyond this age.*

Pus *in the inner corner
of the eye, or* eyelashes
gummed together *after
sleep, see Sticky eye (page 177)*

Hiccups, *particularly
after feeding: these are nothing to worry about, and will
go away without any treatment.*

Tiny white
spots, *usually
on the nose or
cheeks: these are
called milk spots
or milia. Many
babies develop them during the first
few weeks of life. They need no
treatment, though they may last for
several weeks.*

Red blotches each with
a tiny red center,
*see Spots and rashes
(page 176)*

Diarrhea,
see page 179

Painless bulge
around the
navel *that
increases in size
when your baby
coughs, sneezes,
or cries: this is a hernia and is
caused by a weakness in the
abdominal wall. It will probably
disappear without any treatment
within a year.*

Redness *or* rash
*around the genitals,
see Diaper rash (page 176)*

SPOTS AND RASHES

What are they?

Many newborn babies go through what might be called a spotty stage, so don't worry if your baby develops a few spots—they don't mean that he is sick; it's just that his skin is delicate. One of the most common rashes is newborn urticaria; it usually appears during the first week of life.

What can I do?

If your baby has newborn urticaria (see symptoms box), the spots will disappear on their own within about two or three days, so don't put any lotions or creams on them. Don't alter your baby's feedings—the spots are not due to formula disagreeing with him.

■ SYMPTOMS ■

▲ Red blotches, each with a tiny red center, which come and go on different parts of the baby's body, and last only a few hours.

■ CALL THE DOCTOR ■

Call your doctor now if the spots are flat and dark red or purplish (a petechial rash—a sign of bleeding under the skin). Consult your doctor as soon as possible if:
▲ a spot has developed a pus-filled center
▲ you think a spot has become infected.

DIAPER RASH

What is it?

Diaper rash is an inflammation of the skin on a baby's bottom. It may occur if your baby has been left in a dirty diaper for too long, because as urine and feces are broken down, ammonia is released, which burns and irritates the skin. It can also be due to an allergy to laundry detergent or fabric conditioner used to wash cloth diapers. A similar-looking rash may be caused by thrush, which normally starts in the mouth (see page 206), but can spread through the body and affect the skin around the anus.

■ SYMPTOMS ■

▲ Red, spotty, sore-looking skin in the diaper area
▲ smell of ammonia from your baby's diaper.

What can I do?

1 Buy a diaper rash cream (available at most drugstores) and apply it when you change her diaper, to soothe and heal the skin.

2 Change your baby's diaper frequently, and clean and dry her bottom thoroughly at each change (see pages 150–51). Inside cloth diapers use an extra-absorbent type of liner or switch to disposable diapers.

3 Whenever possible, let your baby lie on a diaper with her bottom exposed to the air. Don't use rubber pants over cloth diapers until the rash subsides.

Spread the cream
evenly all over your baby's diaper area

4 Don't use harsh detergents or fabric conditioner to wash cloth diapers because they can trigger an allergy. Rinse her diapers thoroughly.

5 Look for white patches inside your baby's mouth. If you see any, she may have thrush (see page 206).

■ CALL THE DOCTOR ■

Consult your doctor as soon as possible if:
▲ the rash lasts longer than two days
▲ you think your baby has thrush.

What the doctor might do

The doctor may prescribe an antibiotic cream if the rash has become infected, or an antifungal cream if your baby has thrush.

CRADLE CAP

What is it?
Brown, crusty patches on a baby's head are known as cradle cap. Sometimes it may spread to the baby's face, body, or diaper area, producing a red scaly rash. Although it looks as if it might be irritating, cradle cap doesn't seem to distress the baby.

SYMPTOMS ■

▲ Brown, scaly patches on the scalp.

CALL THE DOCTOR ■

Consult your doctor as soon as possible if the rash spreads and:
▲ seems to irritate the baby
▲ looks infected or begins to ooze
▲ does not clear up after five days.

What can I do?
1 Rub the scales on your baby's head with baby oil to soften them. Leave the oil on for 12 to 24 hours, then comb his hair gently to loosen the scales. Finally, wash his hair—most of the scales should simply wash away.

2 If the rash spreads, keep the affected areas clean and dry. Don't use soap, baby lotion, or baby bath liquid—ask your pharmacist to recommend a mild cleansing product.

What the doctor might do
If the condition proves obstinate, or if the rash looks infected or starts to ooze, your doctor may prescribe a cream to be rubbed gently on the area.

STICKY EYE

What is it?
This is a very common mild eye infection caused by blood or fluid getting into your baby's eye during birth. If your baby develops any of these symptoms after she is two days old, she probably has conjunctivitis (see page 202).

SYMPTOMS ■

▲ Eyelashes gummed together after sleep
▲ pus in the inner corner of the eye.

CALL THE DOCTOR ■

Call your doctor now if your baby has a bad discharge of yellow pus. Consult your doctor as soon as possible if:
▲ your baby develops symptoms of sticky eye after the first two days of life
▲ sticky eye does not clear up after three days.

What can I do?
Clean your baby's eyes twice a day with a cotton ball dipped in warm boiled water. Wipe outward from the inner corner of her eye, and use a fresh cotton ball for cleaning each eye.

What the doctor might do
If the doctor thinks your baby has conjunctivitis, he will probably prescribe antibiotic eye drops.

To give the eye drops, swaddle your baby in a blanket and hold her eyes open very gently, then squeeze in the drops. If necessary, ask another adult to hold her head still.

CHILLING

Why are babies at risk?
For the first few weeks, your baby cannot regulate his body temperature very efficiently. If he gets cold, his body temperature will drop and he may become dangerously chilled quickly. Premature babies are particularly vulnerable to this.

What can I do?

Warm your baby up by picking him up and feeding him. Once he has become chilled, it doesn't help just to pile on extra clothes or blankets.

> ### ■ SYMPTOMS ■
> ▲ Crying and restless behavior
> ▲ cold hands and feet.
>
> ### As the baby gets colder
> ▲ Quiet, listless behavior
> ▲ cool skin on the chest and stomach
> ▲ pink, flushed face, hands, and feet.

How can I prevent chilling?
Keep the room your baby sleeps in at about 68°F (20°C). When you undress and bathe him, the room should be even warmer. Be sensible about taking him out in cold weather—wrap him up well and don't stay out for too long. Never let him sleep outside in his carriage on a cold day.

Put on a hat *under the hood to keep his head warm*

In cold weather, dress your baby in a one-piece outdoor suit, or wrap a blanket over his other clothes and use mittens and bootees.

OVERHEATING

Why are babies at risk?
Since young babies can't control their body temperature very well (see Chilling, above), they can become overheated just as easily as they become chilled.

What can I do?
1 Take your baby to a cooler place and remove a layer of clothing.

2 Take your baby's temperature (see page 187) and, if it is raised, try to reduce it by sponging her with cool water (see page 188).

3 When she seems comfortable, dress your baby in light clothes.

> ### ■ SYMPTOMS ■
> ▲ Restless behavior
> ▲ hot, sweaty skin
> ▲ raised temperature.

> ### ■ CALL THE DOCTOR ■
> Call your doctor now if your baby has a temperature over 100.4°F (38°C).

How can I prevent overheating?
Dress your baby according to the weather—on very hot days, she can sleep in just a diaper and a shirt, but always remember the danger of chilling (see above). Never allow her to sleep directly in the sun, because her skin will burn easily. Provide shade and check her often as the sun moves around.

VOMITING

Why do babies vomit?

All babies spit up a small amount of milk during or just after a feeding. This is perfectly normal, and does not mean that your baby is ill, but until you are used to it, you may think that she is vomiting. If your baby truly has indigestion or nausea, she will vomit most of her feeding. This is unlikely in a breast-fed baby.

Frequent vomiting in a bottle-fed baby, especially if she also has diarrhea, may be caused by gastroenteritis (see page 214). This is very serious because of dehydration.

FORCEFUL VOMITING

Sometimes a baby throws up with great force, so that the vomit shoots across the room. If your baby does this at two successive feedings, **consult your doctor as soon as possible.**

The most likely reason is that she has thrown up part of her feeding with a large burp of gas behind it. However, if it happens after every feeding, especially if your baby seems hungry all the time, she may have a condition called pyloric stenosis, in which the outlet from the stomach becomes blocked. This condition runs in families, and usually develops when the baby is about two to eight weeks old. If your baby has this, she will need a simple operation.

What can I do?

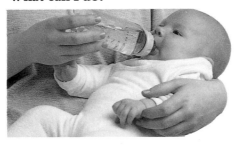

1 Stop bottle-feeding for 24 hours. Give your baby frequent drinks of cool water or a sugar solution (dissolve three level teaspoons of sugar in 7fl. oz. (200ml.) cooled boiled water, or ask your pharmacist to recommend a commercial solution for babies). She needs at least 1 pint ($\frac{1}{2}$ liter) a day.

2 Give your baby diluted feedings for the next three days, made up as described below. To make sure that she has enough to drink, offer her a small amount every hour.
Day 1 Use a quarter of the usual amount of powder or concentrated liquid formula to the normal amount of water.
Day 2 Use half the normal amount of concentrated formula.
Day 3 Use three-quarters the normal amount of concentrated formula.
Day 4 Make up the bottles to the normal strength again.

■ EMERGENCY SIGNS ■

Call for emergency help immediately if your baby:
▲ vomits all feedings in an eight-hour period
▲ has a dry mouth
▲ has sunken eyes
▲ has a sunken fontanelle
▲ has a dry diaper for more than six hours.

■ CALL THE DOCTOR ■

Call your doctor now if:
▲ your baby vomits and shows any other signs of illness
▲ your baby vomits all of two successive feedings.

What the doctor might do

The doctor may prescribe a commercial product for rehydrating babies. However, if your baby has lost a lot of body fluid, the doctor might send her to the hospital, where she may be given fluid intravenously.

How can I prevent an upset stomach?

Breast-fed babies rarely have upset stomachs. If you are bottle-feeding your baby, sterilize all feeding equipment and throw away any unfinished bottles. When you make up bottles, cool them quickly under cold water and store in the refrigerator. Never keep a bottle warm for a long period.

DIARRHEA

What is it?

Until babies start eating solid food, they may have fairly runny bowel movements a few times a day. If your baby's BM's are very watery, greenish, and frequent, he has diarrhea. This is serious in a young baby, since it may dehydrate him quickly.

What can I do?

Make sure that your baby has plenty to drink so that he doesn't become dehydrated. If you are breast-feeding, offer your baby cooled boiled water between feedings. If you are bottle-feeding, dilute the formula in the bottles for a few days.

■ CALL THE DOCTOR ■

Call for emergency help immediately if your baby has any of the emergency signs listed for vomiting. Call the doctor now if your baby has had diarrhea for six hours.

DIAGNOSIS GUIDE

When your child seems sick, one of the most important steps you can take is identifying the symptoms. Relax. This isn't always easy to do. Even when they can talk, children aren't always good at verbalizing exactly where they hurt or precisely what is bothering them. You can end up playing a dangerous guessing game as you look for a specific diagnosis. That's why a guide like the one below can be invaluable for a worried mother or father. If your child is suffering from more than one symptom, focus on the one that appears to be the most severe. Keep in mind that not all children will develop every symptom of an illness and that only your doctor can offer a truly accurate diagnosis. What this guide will do is provide you with *possible* causes and refer you to a more detailed section. For special health risks in young babies, turn to pages 174–75.

Fever
A raised temperature, or fever, may mean that your child has an infection, so look for other signs of illness. However, sometimes healthy children run a slight fever during energetic play or in very hot weather, so check your child's temperature again after she has rested for half an hour. If it is still over 100.4°F (38°C), she may have an infection.

Changed behavior
If your child is less energetic than usual, more irritable, whiny, or simply unhappy, she may be sick.

Unusual paleness
If your child looks white-faced or pale she may be sick.

Hot, flushed face
This may be a sign of a fever.

Loss of appetite
Although a child's appetite varies, a sudden loss of appetite may be a sign of illness. If your baby is under six months old and has refused two successive feedings, or has not demanded to be fed for more than eight hours, **call your doctor immediately**. If your child stops eating for more than 24 hours, look for other signs of illness (see page 183).

Eyes looking in different directions, *see Squint (page 203)*

Red, sore, or sticky eyes or eyelids, *see Eye problems (pages 202–3); if combined with a* **rash and fever,** *see Measles (page 198)*

Itchy eyes, *especially if accompanied by* **runny nose or sneezing,** *see Colds and flu (pages 194–95). Could also be hay fever, particularly if it occurs in summer—consult your doctor*

Aversion to bright light, *especially if accompanied by* **fever, headache, and stiff neck,** *see Meningitis and encephalitis (page 225)*

Runny or blocked nose, sneezing, *see Colds and flu (pages 194–95)*

Sore mouth, *see page 206*

Momentary lapses of attention, *see Absence attacks (page 225)*

Loss of consciousness, *see Fainting (page 225); if combined with* **stiffness and twitching movements,** *see Convulsions (page 225)*

Itchy head or tiny white grains in the hair, *see Lice and nits (page 224)*

Earache, partial deafness, discharge from ears, itchy ears, *see Ear problems (pages 204–5)*

Puffy face, swollen glands *at the angle of the jawbone and on the sides of the neck, see Mumps (page 200);* **swollen glands** *accompanied by* **sore throat,** *see Tonsillitis (page 207) and German measles (page 197)*

Stiff neck, *if accompanied by* **fever and headache,** *see Meningitis and encephalitis (page 225)*

Red lump, perhaps with pus-filled center *anywhere on the body, see Spots and boils (page 218)*

Red, raw skin, *see Chapped skin (page 221)*

Sore throat, *see Throat infections (page 207); if accompanied by* fever and general illness, *see Colds and flu (pages 194–95); if also accompanied by a* rash, *see German measles (page 197); if accompanied by* puffy face, *see Mumps (page 200)*

Spots or rash *anywhere on the body, if accompanied by* sore throat *or* fever, *see Infectious illnesses (pages 197–99); if without other symptoms, see Skin disorders (pages 218–23) and Insect stings (page 244)*

Stomach pain, *see page 212; if accompanied by nausea, vomiting, or diarrhea, see Gastroenteritis (page 214)*

Abnormal-looking feces, *see page 215*

Diarrhea, *see page 215*

Constipation, *see page 213*

Intense itching around the anus, *see Pinworms (page 224)*

Pain when urinating, odd-colored urine, frequent urination, *see Urinary tract infections (page 216)*

Sore tip of penis, *see Genital problems in boys (page 217)*

Painless bulge in the groin or scrotum, *see Genital problems in boys (page 217)*

Vomiting with great force *in babies, see Forceful vomiting (page 179)*

Vomiting or nausea, *see page 214*

Sores around the mouth, *see Cold sores (page 222) and Impetigo (page 223)*

Faint red rash over the face or in skin creases, *see Heat rash (page 219)*

Cough, *see Coughs and chest infections (pages 208–11) and Whooping cough (page 201); if accompanied by a* rash, *see Measles (page 198)*

Breathing difficulty, wheezing, rapid breathing, *see Chest infections (pages 208–11)*

Areas of very itchy, dry, red, scaly skin *anywhere on the body, see Eczema (page 220)*

Red, tender skin *anywhere on the body, see Sunburn (page 221) or Burns and scalds (page 237)*

Dry, painless lump *anywhere on the body, see Warts (page 222)*

Soreness, itching or redness around the vagina, vaginal discharge, *see Genital problems in girls (page 217)*

Intense itching around the vagina, *see Pinworms (page 224)*

White or brown lump on sole of foot, *see Warts (page 222)*

FIRST SIGNS OF ILLNESS

Even if your child has no definite symptoms, often you can tell he is getting sick by his whiny, clingy behavior. Children may become pale, lose their appetite, and drive their parents crazy with irritable temper tantrums. With a teething baby, there's always a tendency to dismiss the change in behavior to new teeth on the way. That can be dangerous, though, so don't do it. Take symptoms seriously because no studies have yet confirmed the connection between illness and teething. Try to isolate the origin of all symptoms by using the guide here. Follow the directions for diagnosing and above all stay calm. Sick children can be very frustrating, testing even the most patient parents. If your child is under a year, watch especially carefully, because babies can become very ill very quickly.

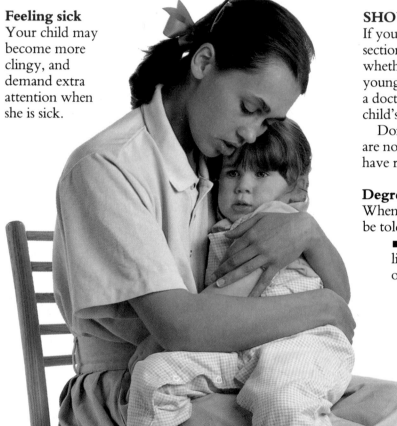

Feeling sick
Your child may become more clingy, and demand extra attention when she is sick.

SHOULD I CALL THE DOCTOR?

If you think you know what is wrong, read the relevant section about complaints on pages 194–225 to determine whether you need to call the doctor. As a general rule, the younger the child, the more quickly he should be seen by a doctor. When you phone your doctor, describe your child's symptoms and remind him of his age.

Don't ever hesitate to call your pediatrician, even if you are not absolutely certain that something is wrong. Some have regular morning calling hours.

Degree of urgency
Whenever you are instructed to call the doctor, you will be told how quickly your child needs medical help.
- **Call for emergency help immediately:** this is a life-threatening emergency, so call for an ambulance, or go to the nearest hospital emergency room.
- **Call your doctor now:** your child needs medical help now, so contact your doctor immediately, even if it is the middle of the night. If you can't reach him, call for emergency help immediately.
- **Consult your doctor as soon as possible:** your child needs to be seen by a doctor within the next 24 hours.
- **Consult your doctor:** your child should be seen by a doctor within the next few days.

■ SYMPTOMS ■

The most common early symptoms of illness in children are:
- ▲ raised temperature—100.4°F (38°C) or more
- ▲ crying and irritability
- ▲ vomiting or diarrhea
- ▲ refusal to eat or drink
- ▲ sore or red throat
- ▲ rash
- ▲ swollen glands in the neck or behind the jaw.

■ EMERGENCY SIGNS ■

Call for emergency help immediately if your child:
- ▲ is breathing very noisily, rapidly, or with difficulty
- ▲ has a convulsion
- ▲ loses consciousness after a fall
- ▲ is in severe, persistent pain
- ▲ has a fever and is unusually irritable or drowsy
- ▲ has a rash of flat dark red or purplish blood spots (a petechial rash—a sign of bleeding under the skin).

CHECKING FOR SYMPTOMS

What can I do?

1 If you think your child is feeling sick, or if he looks as though he has a fever, take his temperature (see page 187). A fever of 100.4°F (38°C) or above can be a symptom of illness.

Tuck the bulb *of the thermometer into your child's armpit*

2 Check your child's throat to see if it's inflamed or infected, but don't try to examine the throat of a baby under a year old. Ask your child to face a bright light and open his mouth. If he is old enough to understand, tell him to say "Aah" to open the back of his throat. If his throat looks red or you can see creamy spots, he has a sore throat (see Throat infections, page 207).

3 Feel gently along your child's jawbone and down either side of the back of his neck. If you can feel tiny lumps under the skin, or if any of these areas seem swollen or tender, your child has swollen glands, which are a common sign of illness.

4 Check your child for a rash, particularly on his chest and behind his ears—the most common areas for one to start. If he has a rash and a fever, he may have one of the common childhood infectious illnesses (see pages 197–99).

QUESTION & ANSWER

"Is my child in pain?"

If your baby is in pain, his crying may sound different from normal. When a baby or small child cries or complains of pain, it can be difficult to discover where the pain is, let alone how bad it is.

Serious pain will affect your child's behavior, so watch him to find out how severe his pain is. Does it make him cry or stop him from sleeping, eating, or playing? Does his face look drawn or has his color changed? Would you know he had a pain even if he didn't tell you? If not, his pain is not severe.

Call your pediatrician and describe your child's symptoms before offering pain medication.

THE DOCTOR'S EXAMINATION

Even though you may have a great relationship with your pediatrician, that initial visit to his office with your sick child can be troubling. His examination may differ from an ordinary checkup and you'll be asked to describe the symptoms in detail. It may help to make notes about your child's illness before you leave home.

1 The doctor may feel the glands that lie along your child's jawbone, down the back of his neck, and in his armpits and groin. These often swell during an infectious illness.

2 He will take your child's pulse to see if his heart is beating faster than usual. This is often a sign of a fever. The doctor may also check your child's temperature.

3 By listening to your child's chest and back with a stethoscope, and asking your child to breathe deeply, the doctor will check the condition of his heart and lungs.

4 If your child has a sore or inflamed throat, the doctor will examine his throat using a small light, pressing his tongue down with a tongue depressor.

QUESTIONS TO ASK THE DOCTOR
Don't hesitate to question your doctor about anything. If it worries you, then ask:
■ how long your child may be sick, and what to expect
■ whether he is infectious, and needs to be isolated particularly from small babies and pregnant women
■ how you can make your child more comfortable while he is sick.

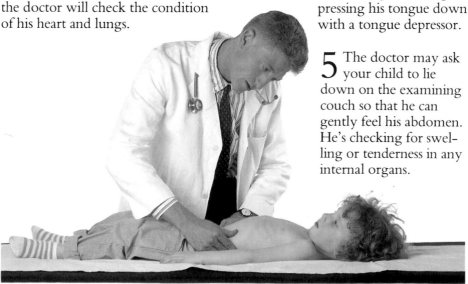

5 The doctor may ask your child to lie down on the examining couch so that he can gently feel his abdomen. He's checking for swelling or tenderness in any internal organs.

GOING INTO THE HOSPITAL

Going into the hospital is stressful for anyone. For a child who is too young to understand why he is there or, indeed, whether he will ever come out, it can be terrifying, especially if it also means that he is separated from his parents. While it helps to explain to your child what is happening, you can't do much to prepare him if he is under two—all he really needs at this age is your presence. If your child is over two, using a favorite toy to explain why he is going to the hospital can help. Tell him, for instance, that even Teddy bears go to the hospital to get better, not as a punishment. Assure him that you will stay with him or visit often, and then do what you promise. Keep explanations simple but truthful; your child will be upset or angry if you tell him something won't hurt, and then it does.

VISITING YOUR CHILD

Hospital personnel know how important it is for a parent to be with a child to comfort and reassure him, and should make it easy for you to visit him at any time. Some even provide accommodations so that you can stay with your child—find out about this before his admission. He won't find the hospital so frightening if you continue to care for him as you would at home, so ask the nurses whether you can still dress, bathe and feed him as normal.

If you can't stay in the hospital with your child, visit him as often as you can, and arrange to bring brothers and sisters to see him if possible. Visiting policies have become more lenient in recent years. Make a special effort to be with him around the clock for the first day or two, and to be there when he has any unpleasant procedures such as injections, or stitches removed.

WHAT TO PACK

Your child may need the following things while she is in the hospital. Call the admissions office to ask for specific guidelines, for instance, on diapers. Label everything clearly.

Bathrobe

Three pairs of pajamas or three nightgowns

Slippers

Favorite toys

Bib and feeding equipment

Washing equipment

Consider packing soap, washcloth, toothbrush and toothpaste, brush, comb, and a favorite bath towel.

HAVING AN OPERATION

If your child is old enough to understand, explain what will happen on the day of his operation. Ask the doctor how the anesthesia will be administered (it may be injected or inhaled through a mask), and find out whether you will be allowed to stay with your child while he is given the anesthesia. Try to be with him when he wakes up after surgery since he may be frightened.

1 Warn your child that he may not be allowed to eat or drink anything on the day of his operation.

2 Tell your child that he will be dressed up for the operation in a hospital gown, and will wear a bracelet with his name on it.

3 While he is still in his room, your child may be given an injection to make him sleepy.

4 Warn your child that he may feel sick when he wakes up.

5 Your child may be wheeled in his bed to the operating room, where the anesthesia is administered. He should fall asleep quickly.

6 If your child has stitches, discourage him from scratching them. If they must be removed, it will hurt only momentarily.

THE CHILD WITH A FEVER

In children, normal body temperature is between 96.8° and 99.5°F (36° and 37.5°C), depending on the time of day. Body temperature is usually lowest in the middle of the night and highest in the afternoon. A temperature above 100.4°F (38°C) may be a sign of illness. A child's temperature can shoot up alarmingly quickly when she is sick, but a slightly raised temperature is not a reliable guide to your child's health. Babies and children can be ill with a normal, or below-normal, temperature, and some children can have a slight fever without being sick. So if your child *seems* ill, she might be, even if her temperature is normal. Her temperature may rise temporarily if she has been playing energetically, particularly in hot weather. If it is still above 100.4°F (38°C) after she has rested for about half an hour, she may be ill, so check for any other signs of illness (see pages 182–83).

READING A THERMOMETER

Normal temperature range

Your child has a fever, *so take her temperature again after 20 minutes. If it is still raised, try to reduce it (see page 188)*

Feel your child's forehead with your cheek if you think he has a fever—don't use your hand because, if it is cold, your child's skin will feel warm by comparison. If his forehead feels hot, take his temperature.

■ SIGNS OF A FEVER ■

Your child may have a fever if:
▲ she complains of feeling sick
▲ she looks pale and feels cold and shivery
▲ she looks flushed and her forehead feels hot.

■ CALL THE DOCTOR ■

Consult the doctor if your child:
▲ has a fever over 103°F (39.4°C) —over 101°F (38.3°C) if she is under a year old—and you can't bring it down
▲ has a fever for 24 hours.

CHOOSING A THERMOMETER

The best thermometers for babies and young children are the easy-to-read mercury thermometer, the digital thermometer, and the temperature indicator strip. The easy-to-read thermometer contains mercury which, as it warms, expands up the tube alongside a temperature scale.

Safe and easy to use, the digital thermometer offers a quick and accurate reading. Although it is more expensive than other thermometers, it is ideal for young children. Always keep spare batteries.

Heat-sensitive panels on the temperature indicator strip glow in sequence and stop when they reach your child's temperature.

Bulb of mercury

Column of mercury

Arrow *indicating normal temperature*

Temperature reading

Easy-to-read thermometer

Digital thermometer

Window *with temperature reading*

Panels *marked with a temperature*

Temperature reading

Temperature indicator strip

—— TAKING YOUR CHILD'S TEMPERATURE ——

When your child is sick, take her temperature at least twice a day, morning and evening. The best method is to place the thermometer under her arm, which gives a reading 1°F (0.6°C) lower than her true temperature. Never put a mercury thermometer into a young child's mouth, since it can break easily. The digital thermometer is not breakable, so it is safe to put it into a young child's mouth, but if she can't hold it correctly under her tongue, place it in her armpit, just like a mercury thermometer. The temperature indicator strip is the easiest way of taking a young child's temperature, but the reading is less accurate than that of a thermometer.

USING A MERCURY THERMOMETER

2 Bring your child's arm down and fold it over her chest. Leave the thermometer in place for the recommended time—usually about three minutes.

Hold the thermometer
firmly in place

3 Remove the thermometer and turn it until you can see the column of mercury next to the scale. Anything over 98.6°F (37°C) is a fever. (Taken under the arm, this figure is slightly different from below.)

1 Hold the thermometer firmly and shake it sharply several times, with a downward flick of your wrist, to shake the mercury back into the bulb. Then sit your child on your knee and lift her arm. Tuck the bulb end of the thermometer into her armpit.

The number
aligning with the top of the mercury column is your child's temperature

USING A DIGITAL THERMOMETER

The number
in the window is your child's temperature

1 Switch the thermometer on and ask your child to open her mouth. Place the thermometer under her tongue and ask her to close her mouth. Wait for about three minutes.

2 Remove the thermometer and read your child's temperature. Anything over 99.5°F (37.5°C) is a fever. Switch the thermometer off, then wash it in cool water and dry it.

USING A TEMPERATURE INDICATOR STRIP

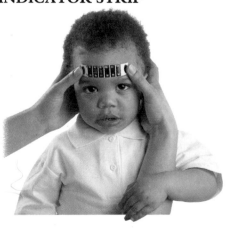

Hold the strip on your child's forehead for about 15 seconds. The highest panel that glows indicates your child's temperature. Anything over 99.5°F (37.5°C) is a fever.

BRINGING DOWN A FEVER

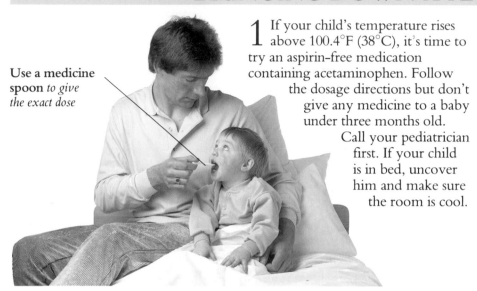

Use a medicine spoon *to give the exact dose*

1 If your child's temperature rises above 100.4°F (38°C), it's time to try an aspirin-free medication containing acetaminophen. Follow the dosage directions but don't give any medicine to a baby under three months old. Call your pediatrician first. If your child is in bed, uncover him and make sure the room is cool.

2 Your child may sweat profusely as his temperature falls, so give him plenty to drink, to replace the lost fluid. Change his sheets and pajamas when his temperature is normal again, to make him comfortable.

SPONGING
If your child's temperature rises above 103°F (39.4°C) and medication doesn't seem to be bringing it down, try sponging her with lukewarm water. In fact, if your baby is under three months, sponging should be among your first steps to reduce fever.

1 Take off your child's blankets and remove her pajama top. Put towels under her so that the bed does not get damp, then fill a bowl with lukewarm water and wring out a sponge in it.

2 Gently wipe your child's face, neck, and arms. Remove her pajama bottoms and sponge her legs. Let her skin dry naturally. Continue for about half an hour, then take her temperature. If it is still above 103°F (39.4°C), **call your doctor now**.

FEVERISH CONVULSIONS
A rapid rise in temperature can cause convulsions in some children. They'll lose consciousness and go rigid for a few seconds, then twitch uncontrollably.

What can I do?
Put your child on the floor and stay with her, but do not try to restrain her. Call your doctor as soon as the convulsion stops.

How can I prevent feverish convulsions?
If a tendency to have feverish convulsions runs in your family, keep your child's temperature as low as you can when she is ill. Follow the cooling methods shown above, and try not to let her temperature rise above 102.2°F (39°C). Your doctor may instruct you to give her children's medicine with acetaminophen at the first signs of illness, to prevent a fever.

DELIRIOUS CHILDREN
Some children become delirious when they have a high fever. A delirious child is very agitated, and may hallucinate and seem very frightened. This state is alarming, but it isn't dangerous. Stay with her to comfort and calm her. When her temperature drops, she will probably fall asleep and be back to normal when she wakes up after a good rest.

ALL ABOUT MEDICINES

Most minor illnesses get better on their own, with or without treatment. Even if you have to consult your doctor, he may not prescribe a medicine. However, if one is necessary, the doctor will tell you how often, and for how long, your child should take it. It is important to follow the directions carefully. Always shake the bottle before pouring out liquid medicine, and measure doses exactly. You can buy child-sized medicine spoons, droppers, and tubes for giving medication to babies at most drugstores. Never mix medicine into your baby's food or bottle or a child's drink, since he may not finish it, or somebody else may, unwittingly, drink it themselves. If your baby or child struggles when you give him medicine or put drops into his nose, ears, or eyes, ask another adult to hold him still while you administer it. You can prevent a baby from wiggling by swaddling or wrapping him firmly in a receiving blanket. If the doctor prescribes antibiotics, your child must take the full course, even if he seems better before the medicine is finished; otherwise the infection may recur. However, antibiotics aren't effective against all illnesses: infectious diseases are caused by either viruses or bacteria, and antibiotics destroy bacteria, but don't affect viruses. This means that there is no real cure for viral illnesses such as colds, measles, mumps, and chicken pox. They simply have to run their course. Many other diseases, such as chest and urinary tract infections, are caused by bacteria, and can be treated successfully with antibiotics.

GIVING MEDICINE TO BABIES

When you give medicine to your baby, put a bib on him in case of a spill, and keep some tissues handy. Sterilize all the equipment in boiling water before giving medicine to a baby under six months. If your baby cannot sit up yet, hold him as if you were going to feed him. If he can sit up, hold him on your lap and tuck one of his arms behind your back. Keep your hand firmly on his other arm to prevent him from struggling.

Using two spoons
Measure the exact dose and pour half into a sterile teaspoon, so it won't spill easily.

MEDICINE SPOON

Measure your baby's dose and pour half into another spoon (see above). Keep both spoons nearby, then pick up your baby. Hold him so that he can't wiggle, then pick up one spoon and rest it on his lower lip. Let him suck the medicine off, then repeat with the rest of the dose.

MEDICINE DROPPER

Measure the dose in a medicine spoon, then squeeze the end of the dropper and suck some of it up into the tube. Put the dropper into your baby's mouth and squirt the medicine in. Repeat until your baby has taken an accurate dose. Don't use a glass dropper if your baby has teeth.

MEDICINE TUBE

Measure the correct dose and pour it into the medicine tube, then pick up your baby and rest the mouthpiece of the tube on his lower lip. Tilt the tube slightly so that the medicine runs into your baby's mouth, but don't tilt it too much, or the medicine will run out too quickly.

FINGERTIP

When all else fails, try letting her suck medicine off your finger. Measure the dose in a medicine spoon, then pick up your baby, keeping the spoon nearby. Dip your finger into it and let her suck the medicine off. It may take time, but continue until she has taken the whole dose.

GIVING MEDICINES TO CHILDREN

Most medicines for children are sweetened or pleasantly flavored, but if your child dislikes the taste, these tips may help to make it more acceptable.

■ Have a favorite drink poured and ready to take away the taste of the medicine.

■ Try bribery—a small treat or reward may help.

■ Tell your child to hold her nose so that she can't taste the medicine, but never do this forcibly for her.

■ If your child is old enough to understand, explain why she has to take the medicine. If she knows that it will make her feel better, she may be more inclined to take it.

■ If you really find it impossible to get the medicine into your child, ask your doctor if he can prescribe it with a different flavor or in another form.

A taste tip
If your child dislikes the taste of the medicine, pour it on to the back of her tongue. It won't taste so strong, because her taste buds are at the front.

> ## ■ MEDICINE AND SAFETY ■
>
> Make sure that your child can't help herself to any medicines in your home.
> ▲ Keep all medications out of her reach, preferably in a locked cabinet.
> ▲ Buy medicines with childproof lids or packaging.
> ▲ Don't disguise medicine by letting your child think she is having a normal soft drink.

Medicine and tooth decay
Clean your child's teeth after giving her medicine, because many medications for children contain sugar. If your child must take medicine for any prolonged period of time, ask your doctor whether a sugar-free alternative is available.

> ## ■ WARNING ■
>
> **Never give aspirin to your child when she is sick.** Use any child's medication with acetaminophen instead. A few children who were given aspirin for a mild illness such as the flu have developed a rare but very serious disease called Reye's syndrome. If your child suddenly vomits and develops a high fever, **call for emergency help immediately.**

NOSE DROPS

CHILDREN

1 Place a small pillow or cushion on a bed and help your child lie on her back with the pillow beneath her shoulders and her head dropped back. If your child is likely to wiggle as you give her the drops, ask another adult to help you by holding her head.

2 Put the tip of the dropper just above your child's nostril and squeeze out the prescribed number of drops. If the dropper touches her nose, wash it before using it again. Keep your child prone and still for about a minute.

BABIES
Swaddle your baby in a blanket, then lay her on her back across your knees, so that her head falls back over your left thigh. Put your left hand beneath her head to support it, then administer the drops as instructed for a child.

EAR DROPS

CHILDREN

1 Most children find ear drops too cold as they go into their ears, so ask your doctor whether you can warm up the medication (some spoil when they are warmed). Place the bottle in a bowl of warm, not hot, water for a few minutes, then check the temperature on the inside of your wrist: it should not be too hot.

2 Ask your child to lie on his side with the affected ear facing up, then place the dropper close to his ear and squeeze the prescribed number of drops into the ear canal. Keep your child prone for about a minute and place a cotton ball very lightly in his ear to prevent excess liquid from running out.

BABIES
Swaddle your baby and lay her on her side across your lap with the affected ear facing up. Support her head with one hand, then administer the ear drops as instructed for a child.

EYE DROPS

CHILDREN

Hold your child's head *steady and pull her lower eyelid down gently with your thumb*

1 Bathe your child's affected eye with a cotton ball dipped in warm boiled water, then ask your child to lie on her back across your knee or with her head in your lap. Put one arm around your child's head with your palm against her cheek, then tilt her head so that the affected eye is slightly lower than the other. Draw her lower eyelid gently down with your thumb.

2 Hold the dropper over the gap between the lower lid and the eye, angling it so that it is out of your child's sight. If necessary, ask someone to hold her head steady. Squeeze out the prescribed number of drops, being careful not to touch the eye or the lid. Even if she cries, enough of the medicine is likely to stay in her eye.

BABIES
Choose a time when your baby is relaxed, then swaddle her and lay her on a firm surface or across your knees. Follow the directions for a child.

EYE OINTMENT
If an eye ointment has been prescribed, squeeze a tiny amount into the outer corner of her eye.

CARING FOR A SICK CHILD

While your child is feeling sick, she will probably demand a great deal of attention, and may be irritable or easily bored. Most children become more babyish when they are sick, and both babies and children need a lot of extra cuddling and reassurance. Try to be very patient and avoid letting your child know you are anxious. Keep your baby with you during the day—let her sleep in her carriage or infant seat, so that you can check on her frequently. Let your child lie down in the living room, or somewhere near you. At night, sleep in the same room as your child if she is very sick. If possible, try to alternate with your partner, so that you have some nights of uninterrupted sleep. Many children vomit when they are ill, so keep a bowl nearby. Vomiting isn't always serious, and can be brought on by emotional upset or excitement. However, frequent vomiting can be a sign of a serious condition, and may lead to dehydration. See page 214 for advice about calling your pediatrician and preventing dehydration.

EATING AND DRINKING

Your child will probably have a smaller appetite than usual while she is ill. Because she is not running around as much, she will use less energy, so don't worry if she doesn't want to eat much for a few days—it won't do her any harm. Allow her to choose favorite foods, and offer small helpings. Let her eat as much or as little as she wants: when she is feeling better, her appetite will return. Babies may demand to be fed more frequently than usual, but take very little each time. Be patient if your baby behaves like this—she needs the comfort and reassurance of feeling close to you as she sucks.

Drinking is much more important than eating when your child is ill. Make sure that she has plenty to drink—about 3 pints (1½ liters) a day, especially if she has a fever, or has been vomiting or had diarrhea—to make sure that she doesn't become dehydrated.

Giving your child a drink
Let your child choose her favorite drink. It doesn't matter whether this is soda, fruit juice, milk, or water.

ENCOURAGING YOUR CHILD TO DRINK
If it is difficult to persuade your child to drink enough, make her choices more appetizing by trying some of the ideas suggested below.

Small container
Offer frequent small drinks from a doll's cup or an egg cup, rather than forcing large amounts.

Straws
Make drinks look appetizing and more fun by letting your child use a straw.

Training cup
Offer drinks in a training cup or bottle. If she has outgrown either, it might be fun to use them again.

Ice cubes
For a child over a year old, freeze diluted fruit juice into cubes, then let her suck the cubes.

Ice popsicle
Your child may prefer an ice pop—the "drink on a stick." Try to avoid ones with artificial coloring.

NAUSEA AND VOMITING

1 Hold your baby or child while she is vomiting to reassure her. Put a big plastic container nearby for her to be sick into. Support her head with one hand on her forehead, and put your other hand over her stomach, just below her rib cage.

2 After she has finished vomiting, reassure your child, then sponge her face and wipe around her mouth. Give her a few sips of water, let her rinse her mouth out, or help her to clean her teeth to take away the unpleasant taste.

3 Let your child rest quietly after vomiting; she may want to lie down and sleep for a while. Wash the container and put it near her, in case she vomits again. If your child vomits frequently, she may have gastroenteritis (see page 214).

COMFORT AND ENTERTAINMENT

STAYING IN BED

There is no need to insist that your child stay in bed. If he is feeling very ill, he'll probably want to remain there. If he wants to get up, make sure he keeps warm and that the room he is playing in isn't drafty. However, your child may want to lie down and go to sleep during the day, even if it isn't his usual naptime. If he doesn't want to be alone, let him snuggle with a pillow and a blanket on the sofa in the living room, or make up a bed for him wherever you are. Your child still wants to feel like part of the family even though he's sick.

ENTERTAINING YOUR CHILD

Try to keep your child occupied so that he doesn't get bored, but remember that he may act younger than his age while he is ill. He won't be able to concentrate for very long, and won't want to do anything too demanding. Bring out an old favorite toy he hasn't played with in a while. If you give him small presents to keep him entertained, don't be tempted to buy toys that are advanced for his age. Babies will enjoy a new mobile or a rattle that makes a new sound. Quiet activities such as interlocking building bricks, felt pictures, simple jigsaws, crayons or felt-tip pens, a kaleidoscope, play dough, or Plasticine are ideal for sick toddlers and children. Protect the bedding with a towel if your child wants to play with something messy while he is in bed.

Playing in bed
If your child feels like staying in bed, but wants to sit up, prop him up with pillows. Make a tray-table by resting a large tray or board on piles of books.

COLDS AND FLU

All children get occasional colds and bouts of flu. As soon as your child comes into contact with other children, he may get one cold after another—some children under six have up to seven a year. Don't worry. As a child grows older, he develops resistance to many of the viruses that cause colds and flu.

EMERGENCY SIGNS

Call for emergency help immediately if your child develops a rash of flat dark red or purplish blood spots. Doctors refer to this as a petechial rash.

Wiping your child's nose

When a child has a non-stop runny nose, it's nearly impossible to prevent the tender skin beneath the nostrils from becoming sore. Use extra-soft tissues, dab gently, and coat the area with cream when he is asleep.

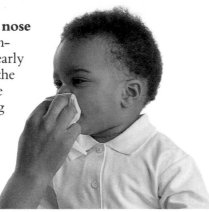

CALL THE DOCTOR

If your child has been feeling absolutely miserable, and especially if he is not yet one year old, consult your doctor as soon as possible if he has:
▲ a temperature over 102.2°F (39°C)
▲ wheezy, fast, or labored breathing
▲ earache
▲ a throat so sore that swallowing is painful
▲ a severe cough
▲ no improvement after three days.

COLDS

What are they?

Perhaps the most common of all illnesses, a cold is a viral infection that irritates the nose and throat, so children don't catch a cold simply by being cold, by going out without wearing a coat, or by getting their feet wet. While it is not a severe illness, a cold should be taken more seriously in babies and children than in adults, because of the risk of a chest or ear infection developing. If your child develops a rash in addition to the symptoms of a normal cold, she might very well have contracted German measles or measles (see pages 197–98).

SYMPTOMS

▲ Runny or blocked nose and sneezing
▲ slightly raised temperature
▲ sore throat
▲ cough.

What the doctor might do

If your baby has trouble sucking because her nose is blocked, your doctor may prescribe nose drops to be given just before a feeding.

Nose drops and decongestants

Use these only if your doctor has prescribed them, and never use them for more than three days. When over-used, they can increase mucus production, which will make your child's nose even more blocked.

What can I do?

1 Take your child's temperature (see page 187), and give her aspirin-free children's medication to bring it down if necessary. Make sure that she has plenty to drink, but don't force her to eat if she's not hungry. A drink before bedtime may help to keep her nose clear at night.

SINUSITIS

The sinuses are air-filled cavities in the bones of the face. The lining of the nose extends into them, so they can easily become infected after a cold. This infection, sinusitis, causes facial pain, but the sinuses that are most likely to become infected don't develop until the age of three or four. For younger children, sinusitis isn't a problem.

FLU

What is it?

Flu (also known as influenza) is a very infectious illness caused by hundreds of different viruses. It tends to occur in epidemics every two or three years, when a new strain of the virus appears to which people have not yet developed immunity. If your child has caught the flu, he will develop symptoms a day or two later, and will probably be sick for about three or four days. He may be sick enough to want to stay in bed and could feel weak for several days after his temperature goes down. A few children develop a chest infection such as bronchitis or pneumonia (see pages 210–11) after having the flu.

■ SYMPTOMS ■

▲ Raised temperature
▲ headache
▲ aching all over the body
▲ shivery feeling
▲ runny nose
▲ cough
▲ sore throat.

What can I do?

Take your child's temperature (see page 187) and give him aspirin-free medicine with acetaminophen to reduce his fever if necessary. Make sure that he has plenty to drink. Offer your baby cooled water.

QUESTION & ANSWER

"Should I have my child vaccinated against flu?"
If your child has a high risk of developing a chest infection after an attack of the flu, a vaccination may be a good idea, so discuss it with your doctor. It will protect him from the illness for about a year. However, since new strains of the virus develop every two or three years, the vaccine (which can only be made from existing forms of the virus) does not give lifelong protection.

2 Spread a barrier cream, such as petroleum jelly, under your child's nose and around her nostrils if the area has become red and sore from a constantly runny nose or frequent wiping.

3 If your child is more than a year old, rub a mentholated rub on her chest before she goes to bed.

4 Dab a little of the mentholated rub or oil on your child's nightclothes or a handkerchief. Tuck the handkerchief next to the mattress at the top of the crib or bed.

5 If your baby has a cold, she will be able to breathe more easily if you raise the head of the crib mattress slightly. Put a small pillow or a folded towel underneath it, then lay your baby in her crib so that her head and chest are slightly raised.

Make sure *that there are no gaps between the mattress and the head of the crib*

6 Keep your child's room warm, but make sure that the air isn't too dry. Breathing very dry air can be uncomfortable. Use a humidifier or hang a wet towel near the heating vents or radiator in your child's room, to add moisture to the air.

HAVING YOUR CHILD IMMUNIZED

At the two-month pediatric checkup, your baby will probably receive her first in a series of vaccination shots designed to protect her from severe infectious diseases. A vaccine is nothing more than a small harmless dose of the germ that causes the disease. It's too weak to cause dangerous problems in your baby but it will make her body produce special cells called antibodies that will immunize her from the disease in the future. Unfortunately, some babies become fussy or run slight fevers after certain immunizations like the DPT (diphtheria, pertussis, and tetanus) shot.

Why should my baby be immunized?

In recent years, some parents have complained that some immunization shots are not necessary, and at times even dangerous. They argue that the risk of catching certain infectious illnesses on the vaccination schedule are slim. Unfortunately, if the number of children being immunized against a particular disease drops dramatically, epidemics are much more likely to occur. By having your child immunized, not only do you protect her but you also help to eradicate the disease altogether.

What are the risks?

Immunization is safe, although it may make your baby mildly sick for a short time. However, if your baby has had a convulsion, or has a close relative with epilepsy, she has an increased risk of a serious reaction to the whooping cough (pertussis) vaccine, so tell your doctor. Do not take her to be immunized if she has a cold, is sick, or has recently had antibiotics.

What are the aftereffects?

Immunization may induce a slight fever, so watch her temperature for 24 hours; if it rises, give her the recommended dose of acetaminophen.

Your baby may develop a small, hard lump at the injection site. This will disappear in a few weeks. The measles vaccine may give her a rash and a fever up to ten days later, and the mumps vaccine might make her face swell slightly three weeks later. If her crying sounds unusual, her temperature rises above 100.4°F (38°C), or she develops any other symptoms, **call your doctor immediately.**

Where is it given?

The doctor may inject her in the top of her arm, in her bottom, or in her thigh. Hold your baby firmly while she has the injection.

When are the shots given?

Childhood immunization means protection against eight major diseases: polio, measles, mumps, rubella (German measles), whooping cough (pertussis), diphtheria, tetanus, and Hemophilus (Hib) infections. Check the table and ask your pediatrician if your child is up to date on vaccines.

All these major diseases are preventable. In order to be protected against diphtheria, tetanus and pertussis, your child needs a shot of the diphtheria-tetanus-pertussis (DTP) vaccine at 2, 4, 6, and 18 months and a booster prior to school entry.

At 15 months your child should have a shot for measles, mumps, and rubella (MMR). A booster should be given to children 10 years or older who have not had measles. **Should a local measles outbreak occur, this MMR booster may be given earlier.**

Children should be tested for tuberculosis in the first year of life. Hib conjugate vaccine is due at 18 months. At 14 to 16 years a tetanus-diphtheria booster should be given.

If you don't have a pediatrician or family physician, call your local public health department. It usually has supplies of vaccine and may give shots free.

YOUR CHILD'S IMMUNIZATION PROGRAM (Recommended by The American Academy of Pediatrics)								
Age	**DTP**	**Polio**	**TB Test**	**Measles**	**Mumps**	**Rubella**	**Hib Conjugate**	**Tetanus-Diphtheria**
2 months	■	■						
4 months	■	■						
6 months	■							
1 year			■					
15 months				■	■	■		
18 months	■	■					■	
4–6 years	■	■						
5–21 years				■	■	■		
14–16 years								■

INFECTIOUS ILLNESSES

Because most children are immunized, many of the ailments in this section are uncommon. If your child is unlucky enough to catch one, he will become immune to that illness for the rest of his life. Infectious diseases are caused by viruses, so medicines can't cure them (see page 189), but recovery is ordinarily quick and uneventful. In years past, a bout with an infectious illness sent someone into quarantine, but today, unless it's German measles (see below), that step isn't even routinely recommended. Warning the parents of your child's playmates is a helpful gesture, however.

■ WARNING ■

If your child has a raised temperature while he is ill with one of these diseases, **DO NOT** give him aspirin to bring the fever down, since it can cause a serious disease called Reye's syndrome (see page 190). Give him an aspirin-free medication with acetaminophen.

■ EMERGENCY SIGNS ■

Call for emergency help immediately if your child has an infectious disease and develops any of these signs:
▲ unusual and increasing drowsiness
▲ headache or stiff neck
▲ convulsions
▲ rash of flat dark red or purplish blood spots.

GERMAN MEASLES

What is it?
German measles is a very mild illness, so your child may feel perfectly well and may not want to stay in bed. She will develop symptoms two to three weeks after she has been infected.

What can I do?
1 Take your child's temperature at least twice a day (see page 187), and if necessary give her acetaminophen to reduce her fever.

2 Make sure that your child has plenty to drink, especially if she has a fever.

■ SYMPTOMS ■

Days 1 and 2
▲ Symptoms of a mild cold
▲ slightly sore throat
▲ swollen glands behind the ears, on the sides of the neck, and on the nape of the neck.

Day 2 or 3
▲ Blotchy rash of flat, pink spots appearing first on the face, then spreading down the body
▲ slightly raised temperature.

Day 4 or 5
▲ Fading rash and general improvement.

Day 6
▲ Your child is back to normal.

Day 9 or 10
▲ Your child is no longer infectious.

■ CALL THE DOCTOR ■

Call for emergency help immediately if your child develops any of the emergency signs above. Consult your doctor as soon as possible if you think your child has German measles, but check with him before taking your child to his office, to avoid the possibility of her coming into contact with a pregnant woman.

What the doctor might do
Your doctor will confirm that your child has German measles, but there is no treatment for it.

German measles and pregnancy
While your child is infectious, prevent her from coming into contact with pregnant women. Although German measles is a mild disease, it can cause defects in a fetus if a pregnant woman catches it.

MEASLES

What is it?

Measles is a very infectious illness that causes a rash, fever, and cough. Symptoms appear one or two weeks after your child has been infected.

Children usually feel uncomfortably ill with measles, and your child will probably want to stay in bed while her temperature is high. A few children develop complications such as an earache.

■ SYMPTOMS ■

Days 1 and 2
▲ Runny nose
▲ dry cough
▲ red, sore, watering eyes
▲ fever that gets steadily higher.

Day 3
▲ Slight fall in temperature
▲ continuing cough
▲ tiny white spots, like grains of salt, in the mouth.

Days 4 and 5
▲ Rising temperature—it may reach 104°F (40°C)
▲ dull red rash of slightly raised spots appears, first on the forehead and behind the ears, gradually spreading to the rest of the face and trunk.

Days 6 and 7
▲ Fading rash and disappearance of other symptoms.

Day 9
▲ Your child is no longer infectious.

■ CALL THE DOCTOR ■

Call for emergency help immediately if your child develops any of the signs listed on page 197. Consult your doctor as soon as possible if you think your child has measles. Call him again if:
▲ your child is no better three days after the rash develops
▲ your child's temperature rises suddenly
▲ your child's condition worsens after she seemed to be getting better
▲ your child has an earache
▲ your child's breathing is noisy or difficult.

What can I do?

1 Check your child's temperature (see page 187) at least twice a day, and every five to six hours when her fever is high on days four and five. Stay with her if she is feeling very miserable while her temperature is high.

2 Make your child comfortable. Try to bring her temperature down with an aspirin-free medicine with acetaminophen and, if necessary, by sponging (see page 188).

3 Make sure that your child has plenty to drink, especially when her temperature is high.

4 If your child's eyes are sore, bathe them with cotton balls dipped in cool water. Although bright light won't damage her eyes, keep her room dark if this makes her more comfortable.

What the doctor might do

There is no medical treatment for measles, but your doctor will confirm the diagnosis and may want to check your child and have you watch her closely until she has recovered. He will treat any complications as they develop.

CHICKEN POX

What is it?

This very infectious illness produces a rash of itchy spots. Your child may not feel very ill, but if she has a lot of spots, she may itch all over. Symptoms appear two to three weeks after your child has been infected.

The chicken pox virus causes shingles in adults, particularly the elderly, so keep your child away from older people while she is infectious.

SYMPTOMS

Days 1 to 6

▲ Groups of small, red, very itchy spots with fluid-filled centers, appearing in batches first on the child's chest, abdomen, and back, later elsewhere on the body
▲ fluid within the spots becomes white and cloudy
▲ slight temperature.

Days 5 to 9

▲ The spots burst, leaving small craters
▲ scabs form over the spots and drop off after a few days.

Day 10

▲ Your child is back to normal.

Day 11 or 12

▲ Your child is no longer infectious.

CALL THE DOCTOR

Call for emergency help immediately if your child develops any of the signs listed on page 197. Consult your doctor as soon as possible if you think your child has chicken pox, and call him again if your child has any of these symptoms:
▲ very severe itching
▲ redness or swelling around any spots, or pus oozing from the spots – this means they have become infected.

What can I do?

1 Take your child's temperature (see page 187), and, if raised, give her the recommended dose of a children's medicine containing acetaminophen to bring it down, and plenty to drink.

2 Try to discourage your child from scratching the spots, because they can become infected and cause scarring when they heal. Cut your child's fingernails short and keep them clean so that the spots are less likely to become infected if she does scratch them.

3 Try to relieve your child's itchiness. Dab the spots gently with cotton balls dipped in calamine lotion.

4 Give your child regular warm baths, each with a handful of baking soda dissolved in the water to help reduce the itching.

5 If your child is very itchy, she will probably find loose cotton clothes the most comfortable.

What the doctor might do

Your doctor will confirm the diagnosis and may prescribe an antihistamine cream or medicine to relieve your child's itching if it is very severe. If any of the spots have become infected, he may prescribe an antibiotic cream.

MUMPS

What is it?

Mumps is an infection that causes swollen glands. It specifically affects the glands in front of the ears, making your child's cheeks look puffy. Your child will develop symptoms two to four weeks after he has been infected.

Occasionally, mumps causes inflammation of the testicles, but this is very rare in a boy before puberty.

■ SYMPTOMS ■

Day 1
▲ Pain when chewing, or facial pain that your child can't locate
▲ raised temperature.

Day 2
▲ Swelling and tenderness on one side of the face

Area of swelling

▲ pain when opening the mouth
▲ fever
▲ sore throat, and pain when swallowing
▲ dry mouth.

Day 3
▲ Increased facial swelling, usually on both sides.

Days 4 to 6
▲ Gradual reduction of swelling and improvement in other symptoms.

Day 13
▲ No longer infectious.

What can I do?

1 Very gently feel your child's glands (see page 183) if he complains of facial pain, or if his face looks swollen.

2 Check his temperature (see page 187) and give him children's medication with acetaminophen to bring his temperature down if it is raised.

3 Encourage your child to drink liquids, but avoid acidic fruit juices. Let him drink through a straw if it hurts him to open his mouth. Be patient when feeding your baby, since he may find sucking painful.

4 If it hurts your child to swallow, give him liquid or semi-liquid foods such as ice cream and soup.

■ CALL THE DOCTOR ■

Call for emergency help if your child develops any of the signs on page 197. Consult your doctor as soon as possible if you think your child has the mumps, and call him again if he develops stomach pain or a red testicle.

5 Fill a hot water bottle with warm water and wrap it in a towel, then let your child rest his cheek against it to soothe the swelling. Don't give a hot water bottle to a baby who may be too young to push it away if it is too hot: heat a soft cloth and hold it gently against his face instead.

What the doctor might do

There is no cure for the mumps, but your pediatrician can offer suggestions for making your child as comfortable as possible.

WHOOPING COUGH

What is it?
One of the most serious childhood diseases, whooping cough is a severe and persistent cough. It is highly infectious, so keep your child away from babies and children who have not been immunized. Even immunized children can get a mild form of the illness. A few children with whooping cough develop a secondary infection, such as bronchitis or pneumonia (see pages 210–11).

■ SYMPTOMS ■

Week 1
▲ Symptoms of a normal cough and cold
▲ slight temperature.

Week 2
▲ Worsening cough, with frequent coughing fits lasting up to a minute, after which your child has to fight for breath
▲ if your child is over 18 months, he may learn to hold his coughs in with a "whooping" sound
▲ vomiting after a coughing fit.

Weeks 3 to 10
▲ Cough improves, but may worsen if your child gets a cold
▲ your child is unlikely to be infectious after the third week.

What can I do?
1 Stay with your child during coughing fits, since he may be very distressed. Sit him on your lap and hold him leaning slightly forward. Keep a bowl or plastic container nearby so that he can spit out any phlegm he coughs up, and in case he vomits afterward. Clean the bowl thoroughly with boiling water, to make sure that the infection doesn't spread.

2 If your child often coughs and vomits after meals, offer him small meals at frequent intervals, if possible just after a coughing fit.

3 Keep your child entertained—he will have fewer coughing fits if his attention is distracted, but don't let him get too excited or overtired since this may bring on a coughing fit.

■ EMERGENCY SIGNS ■
Call for emergency help immediately if your child turns blue during a coughing fit.

■ CALL THE DOCTOR ■
Consult your doctor as soon as possible if you suspect that your child has whooping cough.

4 Sleep in the same room as your child, so that you can be with him if he has a coughing fit at night.

5 Don't let anyone smoke near your child, and don't give him any cough medicines.

What the doctor might do
The doctor may prescribe a cough suppressant and an antibiotic. Although the antibiotic won't cure your child's cough, it may reduce its severity and make your child less infectious. This is particularly important if you have a baby who is at risk of catching whooping cough from an older brother or sister who already has the disease. However, the antibiotic is only really effective if it is given right at the beginning of the infection.

CARING FOR A BABY
Whooping cough is dangerous in babies because they may not be able to draw breath properly after coughing. Your baby will need careful nursing and may be admitted to the hospital. She may find sucking difficult if she vomits frequently, so abandon your regular feeding schedule, and feed her as soon as she has calmed down after coughing or vomiting.

Place a cushion *under the crib mattress*

Coughing fits
When your baby has a coughing fit, lay her in her crib on her stomach with the foot of her crib mattress slightly raised, or face down across your lap. Stay with her until she has stopped coughing and is breathing normally again. Cuddle her to comfort her after a bout of coughing or vomiting.

EYE PROBLEMS

Although most eye disorders clear up quickly when they are treated, all problems affecting the eye should be taken seriously. Eye infections spread easily to other people, so give your child her own washcloth and towel, and change them frequently. Dry her eyes with tissues, using a clean one for each eye. Keep your child's hands clean and try to stop her from rubbing her eyes. These steps will help prevent an infection, and stop one from spreading.

BLEPHARITIS

What is it?
Blepharitis is an inflammation of the edges of the eyelids, which usually affects both eyes. Children with dandruff often develop blepharitis.

■ SYMPTOMS ■
▲ Red and scaly eyelids.

What can I do?
1 Dissolve a teaspoon of salt or baking soda in a glass of warm boiled water, and use this to bathe your child's eyelids. Wash your hands before and afterward, and use fresh cotton balls for each eye. Do this twice a day, making a fresh solution each time.

2 If your child has dandruff, wash her hair with an antidandruff shampoo. Use an anticradle cap shampoo for a baby.

■ CALL THE DOCTOR ■
Consult your doctor as soon as possible if:
▲ your child's eyes are sticky
▲ there is no improvement after about a week of home treatment.

What the doctor might do
The doctor might prescribe a cream to soothe your child's eyelids, or an antibiotic ointment.

CONJUNCTIVITIS

What is it?
Also known as "pink eye," because the white of the eye may turn pink, conjunctivitis is an inflammation of the lining of the eye and eyelids. It can be caused by a virus or by bacteria. It's milder when caused by a virus. If your child's eyelids are gummed together with pus when she wakes up, she probably has bacterial, rather than viral, conjunctivitis. If your baby develops any of these symptoms in the first day or two of life, see Sticky eye, page 177.

What can I do?
1 Try to find out whether your child's symptoms might be caused by something other than conjunctivitis. She might have an allergy such as hay fever, or she may have a speck of dust or an eyelash in her eye. If she has an allergy, her eyes may be itchy and watering as well as red and sore.

2 If you think she has conjunctivitis, dissolve a teaspoon of salt in a glass of warm boiled water, and dip a cotton ball in this. Bathe both of her eyes, using fresh cotton balls for each one. Start with the uninfected one, and wipe from the outside corner to the inside. Wash your hands before and after this procedure.

■ SYMPTOMS ■
▲ Bloodshot eye
▲ gritty, sore eye
▲ discharge of pus
▲ eyelids gummed together after sleep.

■ CALL THE DOCTOR ■
Consult your doctor as soon as possible if you think your child has conjunctivitis or if her eyes are bloodshot and sore.

What the doctor might do
The doctor may prescribe antibiotic drops or ointment for a bacterial infection, which will cure it quickly. Viral conjunctivitis needs no treatment, but may last for a few weeks.

STYE

What is it?
A stye is a painful, pus-filled swelling on the upper or lower eyelid, caused by infection at the base of an eyelash. Some styes simply dry up, but most come to a head and burst within a week, relieving the pain. Styes are not serious and you can treat them at home.

SYMPTOMS
▲ Red, painful swelling on the eyelid
▲ pus-filled center appearing in the swelling.

CALL THE DOCTOR
Consult your doctor as soon as possible if:
▲ the stye does not improve after a week
▲ your child's whole eyelid is swollen
▲ the skin all around your child's eye turns red
▲ your child also has blepharitis.

What can I do?

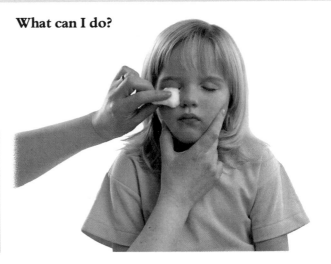

1 Dip a cotton ball in hot water, squeeze it, and press it gently on to your child's stye, to help bring the stye to a head more quickly. Repeat this for two or three minutes three times a day until the stye bursts.

2 When the stye bursts, the pain is relieved. Wash the pus away very gently using a fresh cotton ball dipped in warm boiled water for each wipe.

SQUINT

What is it?
Normally, both eyes look in the same direction at the same time, but in a child with a squint, one eye focuses on an object, while the other does not follow it properly.

A newborn baby's eyes do not always work together correctly, so intermittent squinting is common. This is nothing to worry about—your baby is simply learning to use his eyes. But if your baby's eyes don't move together after he is about three months old, he may have a squint.

Squinting may be constant, but in some children it comes and goes. However, children do not grow out of a squint, so it is essential to have it treated. The younger the child, the more successful the treatment.

SYMPTOMS
▲ Eyes looking in different directions.

CALL THE DOCTOR
Consult your doctor if you think your child has a squint.

How can I check for a squint?
When your baby is about three months old, hold a toy 8in. (20cm.) from his face and move it slowly from side to side. Check that his eyes work together to follow the moving object.

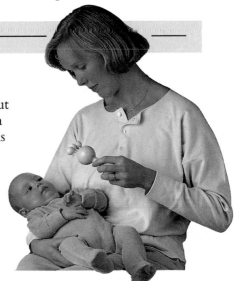

What the doctor might do
The doctor will check your child's vision and may give him a patch to wear over his stronger eye for several hours each day. This forces him to use his weak eye. A toddler may need to wear glasses. If your child is under two, this treatment will probably cure his squint in a few months. If your child has a severe squint caused by muscle weakness, he may need to have surgery to correct the problem.

EAR PROBLEMS

Most ear problems in small children come from an infection of the outer or middle ear, or because the tube connecting the ear and throat becomes blocked. Ear infections should be taken seriously, but they are dangerous only if they are not treated promptly: there is a risk that pus may build up behind the eardrum, and eventually burst it, or that infection may spread into a bone behind the ear (mastoiditis).

Anatomy of the ear

Each ear consists of three parts. From the outer ear (the only visible part) a slightly curved canal leads to the eardrum. The middle ear lies just behind the eardrum and is a cavity housing three small bones that transmit sound vibrations. The inner ear contains the delicate structures that actually allow you to hear and to balance yourself.

Canal

Outer ear

Eardrum *vibrates in response to sound waves*

Middle ear cavity *contains three tiny bones that transmit sound signals to the inner ear*

Inner ear *contains the mechanisms for hearing and balance*

Auditory nerve *takes sound signals to the brain*

Eustachian tube *leads to the back of the throat. It is much shorter in children than in adults, so infection can spread easily*

OUTER EAR INFECTION

What is it?

The skin lining the outer ear canal becomes inflamed when your child has an outer ear infection. This may happen if he swims a lot in chlorinated water, or because he has poked or scratched his ear and it has become infected. Children with eczema are especially prone to such infections if they get water in their ears.

What can I do?

1 Give your child the recommended dose of children's medication containing acetaminophen.

2 Make sure that water doesn't get into the affected ear at bathtime, and just sponge his hair clean. Don't let your child go swimming until the infection clears up.

What the doctor might do

Your doctor will probably prescribe antibiotic or anti-inflammatory ear drops to treat the infection.

■ SYMPTOMS ■

▲ Pain in the ear that is worse when the child touches his ear or lies on it
▲ redness in the ear canal
▲ discharge from the ear
▲ itchiness inside the ear.

■ CALL THE DOCTOR ■

Consult your doctor as soon as possible if you think your child has an outer ear infection.

WAX IN THE EAR

Wax sometimes accumulates in the ear, giving a feeling of fullness or partial deafness. If your child has a lot of ear wax, very gently wipe away any visible wax with a cotton ball, but don't poke anything into the ear. If this doesn't help, consult your doctor.

To administer ear drops, ask your child to lie still on his side while you squeeze drops into the affected ear. It may be difficult, but try to keep him in this position for about a minute afterward.

MIDDLE EAR INFECTION

What is it?

If your child has a middle ear infection, the cavity behind his eardrum becomes inflamed, usually because an infection has spread from the throat. The tube that runs from the throat to the ear is very short and narrow in a child, allowing infection to spread extremely easily. Generally only one ear is infected. Once your child has had a middle ear infection, especially if this happens during his first two years, he is likely to have one in the same ear whenever he has a cold or throat infection.

SYMPTOMS

▲ Very painful ear, which may stop your child from sleeping
▲ crying and rubbing or tugging at the ear, if your child can't talk yet or easily explain that his ear aches
▲ crying, loss of appetite, and general signs of illness in young babies, especially following a cold
▲ fever
▲ partial deafness.

What can I do?

1 Try to relieve your child's earache. Fill a hot water bottle with warm, not hot, water and wrap it in a towel, then let him rest his ear against it. Don't give a hot water bottle to a baby who is too young to push it away if it is too hot. Heat a soft cloth and hold it against his ear instead.

2 If your child's ear is very painful, give him the recommended dose of aspirin-free pain medication.

3 If you notice a discharge, don't clear it away or probe into his ear—just put a clean handkerchief over his ear. Encourage him to rest his head on the affected side, so that any discharge can drain away.

How can I prevent ear infection?

In cold weather, keep your child's ears warm. Use menthol drops or a menthol rub whenever he has a cold (see page 195). These help to clear your child's nasal passages, which reduces the chances of infection spreading to the ear.

CALL THE DOCTOR

Consult your doctor as soon as possible if your child's ear is infected or has a discharge.

What the doctor might do

The doctor may prescribe an antibiotic to clear the infection. If pus has built up behind the eardrum, the doctor may prescribe a drug to help it drain away. If this is not effective, your child may need the minor surgery described below.

GLUE EAR

What is it?

Repeated middle ear infections can lead to glue ear, an accumulation of sticky fluid in the middle ear.

SYMPTOMS

▲ Partial deafness after repeated middle ear infections.

CALL THE DOCTOR

Consult your doctor as soon as possible if you think your child has glue ear.

What can I do?

Make an appointment to see your doctor if your child's hearing seems to be impaired after an ear infection.

What the doctor might do

Your doctor may prescribe a decongestant, but a simple operation may be necessary. Under anesthesia, a hole is made in the eardrum and a tiny tube is inserted. The tube is not uncomfortable, and will not affect your child's hearing, but he can't go swimming while it is in place. After several months it will fall out, the hole will heal, and his hearing will be back to normal.

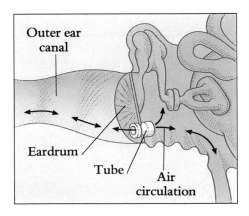

The tube is implanted in the eardrum, to equalize air pressure on either side of the eardrum and to allow the ear to dry out.

MOUTH INFECTIONS

When a baby or young child has a mouth infection, two of life's simple yet satisfying pleasures—sucking and eating—become very painful. Thrush is the most common mouth affliction in babies, while older children may be prone to cold sores (see page 222).

Helping the child with a sore mouth

If your child's mouth is sore, try to make eating and drinking as painless as you can. Allow warm meals to cool before giving them to your child, since hot food generally hurts more than cold, and offer her plenty of very cold drinks. If she is reluctant to eat or drink, try some of the suggestions given here.

Let your child drink through a straw or

use a training cup, since this may be less painful than drinking from a glass.

Soup This is nourishing, easy to eat, and can be served cold. Mix or chop solid food into very small bites.

Cold drinks Serve drinks very cold; avoid fruit juice, since it is too acidic.

Ice cream Your child may find cold food such as ice cream easy to eat.

Water

Cheese Encourage your child to finish meals with cheese and a drink of water to help keep her teeth clean without brushing.

THRUSH

What is it?

Thrush is an infection caused by a yeast that lives in the mouth and intestines. The yeast is normally kept under control by bacteria, but sometimes it multiplies wildly producing a sore, irritating rash. Occasionally, it spreads through the intestines and causes a rash around the anus. It is not a serious infection and, although it does not ordinarily respond to home remedies, it usually clears up quickly under a doctor's care.

■ SYMPTOMS ■

- ▲ Reluctance to eat due to a sore mouth
- ▲ creamy yellow, slightly raised patches on the inside of the cheeks, tongue, or the roof of the mouth, which do not come away easily if you try to wipe them off
- ▲ in babies, a rash around the anus that looks like diaper rash.

■ CALL THE DOCTOR ■

Consult your doctor as soon as possible if you think your baby or child has thrush.

What can I do?

1 Wipe the patches in your child's mouth very gently with a clean handkerchief. If they don't come off easily, she probably has thrush. Don't rub them hard, because if you scrape them off there will be sore, bleeding patches underneath.

2 Give your child food that is easy to eat (see above). If you are bottle-feeding, buy a special soft nipple and clean it carefully, then sterilize it after each feeding.

3 If you are breast-feeding, continue to nurse normally, but take extra care with nipple hygiene to prevent your nipples from becoming infected. Wash them in water only, not soap, after each feeding, and don't wear breast pads. If they are sore or develop white spots, consult your doctor.

What the doctor might do

Your doctor may prescribe a medicine to be dropped into your baby's mouth just before a feeding, or, for a child over two, lozenges to suck. If you are breast-feeding, the doctor may check your nipples for signs of infection.

THROAT INFECTIONS

Sore throats are common in children of all ages, and often accompany a cold or the flu. Most of the time they are caused by viruses and clear up quickly. Call your doctor because it's important to rule out more severe throat ailments, which might require a prescription medication or signal a bacterial infection of the tonsils.

— SORE THROAT —

What is it?
A sore throat is an infection of the throat that makes the area painful and red. It may be part of a cold or flu (see pages 194–95), or one of the first signs of German measles or mumps (see pages 197 and 200). Children are prone to earache when they have a throat infection (see pages 204–5).

■ SYMPTOMS ■

▲ Reluctance to eat, because it hurts to swallow
▲ red, raw-looking throat
▲ earache (see pages 204–5)
▲ slightly raised temperature
▲ swollen glands
▲ stomach ache in young children.

What can I do?
1 Ask your child to face a bright light and open his mouth. Examine the back of his throat carefully (see page 183). If it is sore, it will look red and raw and you may be able to see creamy spots.

2 Gently feel down each side of your child's neck and just below the angle of his jawbone, checking for tiny lumps under the skin, indicating swollen glands (see page 183).

3 Give your child plenty of cold drinks, and mash solid foods if it hurts him to swallow. Very cold food such as ice cream is less painful to eat than warm food.

4 Take your child's temperature (see page 187), and if it is above normal, give him pain medication containing acetaminophen to bring his fever down.

What the doctor might do
Most mild sore throats need no treatment, but if the doctor suspects that the infection is caused by bacteria, he may prescribe an antibiotic.

— TONSILLITIS —

■ SYMPTOMS ■

▲ Very sore throat
▲ red and enlarged tonsils, possibly covered with creamy spots
▲ temperature over 100.4°F (38°C)
▲ swollen glands on the neck.

What is it?
Tonsillitis is an inflammation of the tonsils, causing a very sore throat and other symptoms of illness. The tonsils are glands at the back of the throat, one on either side, which trap infection and prevent it from spreading.

What can I do?
1 Examine your child's tonsils and feel his glands (see page 183). If infected, his tonsils will be large and red, and may have creamy spots.

2 Take his temperature (see page 187), and give him aspirin-free pain medication to bring it down.

3 Encourage your child to have plenty to drink, especially if he has a fever. Offer him cold drinks and liquid or semi-liquid foods.

What the doctor might do
Your doctor will examine your child's throat, and may take a throat culture by wiping a sterile swab across it. He may prescribe an antibiotic to clear the infection up quickly.

If your child has recurring bouts of severe tonsillitis your doctor may recommend that he has his tonsils removed. However, this operation is rarely done in a child under four years of age.

COUGHS AND CHEST INFECTIONS

Most coughs in small children are a symptom of a cold or the flu (see pages 194–95), which produces a dry, ticklish cough. A cough may also be a symptom of a chest infection (see pages 209–11) or an early sign of the measles (see page 198). A severe, persistent cough might be whooping cough (see page 201).

Your child may get a chest infection after having a cold or the flu, if the infection spreads down toward his lungs. If he has a chest infection, he will have other symptoms as well as a cough: he may find breathing difficult, and might cough up some mucus. However, slightly wheezy breathing is normal for a small child with a cold or the flu, because his airways are very narrow and become even narrower if they are swollen when he is ill, so this symptom on its own may not be a sign of an infection. Occasionally, a chest infection develops as a complication of the measles or whooping cough.

> ### ■ EMERGENCY SIGNS ■
> Call for emergency help immediately if your child:
> ▲ has a bluish tinge around his face, mouth, and tongue
> ▲ is breathing very rapidly
> ▲ is breathing so noisily that it can be heard across the room
> ▲ seems to be fighting for breath
> ▲ deteriorates suddenly when he has a cold or the flu
> ▲ is abnormally drowsy
> ▲ is unable to speak or make sounds as usual.

FREQUENT CHEST INFECTIONS
Babies under a year old and children with a longterm chest disorder such as asthma (see page 210) are prone to chest infections. If you smoke, your children are much more likely to develop chest infections than the children of nonsmoking parents.

If your child has frequent chest infections, your doctor may arrange for tests to find the cause.

Breathing
When your child breathes in, air is sucked down his windpipe and bronchi (the airways) into his lungs, where oxygen is absorbed into his bloodstream. His blood then carries the oxygen throughout his body.

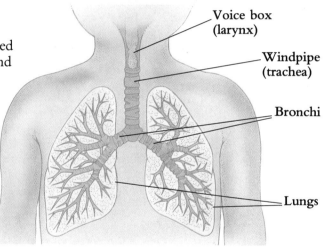

Voice box (larynx)

Windpipe (trachea)

Bronchi

Lungs

——— CROUP ———

What is it?
Croup is an inflammation of the larynx or voice box, which makes it swell, so that your child finds it difficult to breathe. Attacks of croup tend to occur at night, and usually last about two hours.

> ### ■ SYMPTOMS ■
> ▲ Breathing difficulty
> ▲ loud, crowing sound as breath is drawn in
> ▲ barking cough.

What can I do?
1 Keep calm, and reassure your child. He may be very frightened, but if he panics, it will be even harder for him to breathe.

2 Create a steamy atmosphere by taking your child into the bathroom and turning on the hot water full blast. Moist air will help him to breathe more easily. Meanwhile put a cold-mist humidifier in his room to moisten the air there, too.

3 Prop your child up on pillows, or sit him on your lap—he will then be able to breathe more easily.

> ### ■ CALL THE DOCTOR ■
> Call your doctor now if your child has difficulty breathing, or if you think he has croup.

What the doctor might do
The doctor will reassure you and tell you what to do if your child's croup recurs. He might prescribe an antibiotic, and, in case of another attack, may also give some medication to ease your child's breathing. If your child seems very ill, the doctor might recommend going to the hospital.

COUGH

What is it?

A cough can be either a reaction to irritation in the throat or windpipe, or the result of a chest infection. A dry, ticklish cough is rarely serious. It probably means that your child's throat or windpipe is irritated, which may be a byproduct of a cold, because mucus dribbles down the throat and irritates it. Her throat might also be irritated by smoke, if she is with adults who smoke. An ear infection can also cause a dry cough.

If your child's cough sounds moist, particularly if she spits up mucus, she probably has a chest infection. While most coughs like this are not serious, they can be a symptom of bronchitis or pneumonia (see pages 210–11).

■ CALL THE DOCTOR ■

Call your doctor now if, over a period of about half an hour, your child is breathing faster than usual, or if his breathing is labored or very noisy. Consult your doctor as soon as possible if:

▲ your baby is under six months old and has a cough
▲ your child's cough prevents him from sleeping
▲ the cough does not improve in three days
▲ your child has a recurrent cough.

What the doctor might do

The doctor will listen to your child's breathing. If he has a dry cough, the doctor may prescribe a cough suppressant medication to soothe his throat. If the cough is deep, the doctor may carry out some diagnostic tests. He may prescribe antibiotics and perhaps a cough medication to make the mucus easier to cough up.

What can I do?

1 If your child has a sudden attack of coughing, make sure she hasn't inhaled a small object such as a piece of candy or a button. If she has, try to remove it (see Choking, page 234), but don't put your fingers down her throat to pull it out.

2 If your child has a deep cough, try to help her clear the mucus from her chest when she is coughing. Lay her on her stomach across your lap, then pat her back rhythmically but not too hard. Have a bucket or bowl nearby and encourage her to spit out any mucus that she has coughed up.

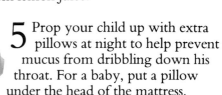

Keep your child's head
slightly tipped down

3 Make sure that your child doesn't get cold while she has a deep cough, otherwise the infection may spread further down into her chest, causing bronchitis.

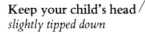

4 If your child has a dry cough, give her a warm drink at bedtime. For a child over 18 months, make this soothing drink by dissolving a teaspoon of honey in a glass of warm water and adding a few drops of fresh lemon juice.

5 Prop your child up with extra pillows at night to help prevent mucus from dribbling down his throat. For a baby, put a pillow under the head of the mattress.

6 If your child's cough is worse in a smoky atmosphere, don't let anyone smoke near him and keep him away from smoky areas.

7 Don't give a cough medication unless your doctor prescribes one.

BRONCHITIS

What is it?
Bronchitis is an inflammation of the lining of the main air passages leading to the lungs. It may follow a cold, the flu or a sore throat because the infection has spread downward.

Your child probably won't feel particularly ill, but he may have difficulty sleeping if his cough tends to be worse at night.

■ SYMPTOMS ■
- ▲ Rattly cough
- ▲ slight wheeziness
- ▲ slight temperature
- ▲ runny nose.

What can I do?
1 Help relieve wheezy breathing and clear your child's lungs during a coughing fit. Lay him across your lap on his stomach and pat his back (see page 209).

2 Take your child's temperature and, if it is raised, give him aspirin-free medication with acetaminophen, and plenty to drink.

3 Put a pillow under the head of your baby's mattress. When your older child goes to bed, prop him up with extra pillows (see page 209).

4 Until your child is better, keep him indoors in a warm, but not too hot or stuffy, room.

■ CALL THE DOCTOR ■
Call for emergency help immediately if your child shows any of the emergency signs on page 208. Consult your doctor as soon as possible if you think your child has bronchitis, and call him again if he:
- ▲ is not better after two days
- ▲ coughs up greenish-yellow mucus.

What the doctor might do
Your doctor might prescribe a cough suppressant to help your child sleep. If he thinks your child has a secondary infection, he might also prescribe an antibiotic to eliminate it.

ASTHMA

What is it?
Asthma is recurrent episodes of narrowing of the tiny airways leading to the lungs. Breathing, especially exhaling is difficult. It may be caused by an allergy, and if other people in your family have asthma, eczema, or hay fever, your baby is susceptible too. Mild asthma is common, and your child may outgrow it.

■ SYMPTOMS ■
- ▲ Coughing, particularly at night or after exercise
- ▲ slight wheeziness and breathlessness, especially during a cold
- ▲ attacks of severe breathlessness, when breathing is shallow and difficult
- ▲ feeling of suffocation during an asthma attack
- ▲ pale, sweaty skin during an attack
- ▲ bluish tinge round the lips during a severe attack.

What can I do?
1 Keep calm and reassure your child. If he has had previous attacks, give him whatever medication the doctor has prescribed. If this has no effect, **call for emergency help**.

2 Sit your child on your lap and help him to lean slightly forward—this makes it easier for him to breathe. Don't hold him tightly; let him settle into the most comfortable position.

Put a small cushion *on his lap for him to lean on*

3 If your child prefers to sit on his own, give him something to rest his arms on—a table top or pile of pillows, for example—so that he leans forward.

PNEUMONIA

What is it?

Pneumonia is an inflammation of the lungs, which causes breathing difficulty. In young children it is nearly always due to the spread of an infection such as a cold or the flu, and is usually caused by a virus, not bacteria. Occasionally pneumonia is the result of a tiny amount of food being inhaled into the lungs and causing a small patch of inflammation and infection to occur.

Pneumonia is a serious disease, but most healthy babies—even those under a year old—recover completely in about a week.

■ SYMPTOMS ■

▲ Deterioration in a sick child
▲ raised temperature
▲ dry cough
▲ rapid breathing
▲ difficult or noisy breathing.

What can I do?

1 Prop your child up with extra pillows in bed, so that he can breathe more easily. For a baby, put a pillow under the head of the mattress.

2 Take your child's temperature and, if it is raised, try to reduce it by giving an aspirin-free medication with acetaminophen or by sponging him (see page 188).

■ CALL THE DOCTOR ■

Call for emergency help immediately if your child develops any of the emergency signs on page 208. Call your doctor now if you think your child has pneumonia.

3 Make sure that your child has plenty to drink, especially if his temperature is raised. Offer your baby cool water.

What the doctor might do

The doctor will advise you how to nurse your child, and, if the infection is bacterial, he may prescribe an antibiotic. If your child is very ill, he might need to be treated in a hospital.

PREVENTING ASTHMA ATTACKS

Try to find out what causes your child's asthma attacks by keeping a record of when they occur. Vigorous exercise and overexcitement can bring on an attack. Some other common triggers are shown here.

Dust
Reduce dust in your house by vacuuming and damp-mopping, rather than sweeping and dusting. Cover your child's mattress with a plastic sheet.

Animal fur If you have a pet, let it stay somewhere else for a while, and note whether your child has fewer attacks.

Feather-filled cushions or pillows
Change these for ones with synthetic filling.

Pollen, especially from grass and trees
Discourage your child from playing in tall grass, and keep him inside when the pollen count is high.

Cigarette smoke
Don't let people smoke near your child.

■ EMERGENCY SIGNS ■

Call for emergency help immediately if your child:
▲ has a bluish tinge on his tongue or around his lips
▲ is severely breathless
▲ does not start to breathe more easily ten minutes after taking his medication
▲ becomes abnormally drowsy.

■ CALL THE DOCTOR ■

Call your doctor now if this is your child's first asthma attack. Consult your doctor as soon as possible if you think your child may have asthma.

What the doctor might do

The doctor may prescribe a drug to be given at the beginning of an attack, or before any activity that causes one. During a severe attack, he may send your child to the hospital.

STOMACH PAIN

Pain between the bottom of the ribs and the groin, or "stomach pain," can be a symptom of many disorders, including gastroenteritis (see page 214) and urinary tract infections (see page 216). It may also be caused by vomiting, and can accompany illnesses such as tonsillitis and the measles. Your child may complain of a stomach ache if he feels generally sick, knows he is about to be sick, or if he has a pain somewhere else, but can't easily describe its exact location.

DEALING WITH A STOMACH ACHE

What causes stomach pain?

Many children have recurrent bouts of stomach pain when something makes them feel anxious or insecure. Provided that your child's pain is not severe and lasts for only an hour or two, you needn't worry; try to find out what is bothering him, and reassure him.

However, if your child is in severe pain for a few hours, you should take it seriously. He might have appendicitis—inflammation of the appendix, a small, blind-ended tube attached to the intestines—though this is extremely rare in children who are under the age of three.

Waves of severe stomach pain at intervals of about 15 to 20 minutes in a baby or toddler may mean that his bowel has become blocked.

What can I do?

1 Take your child's temperature. If it is slightly raised, he may have appendicitis, especially if the stomach pain is severe or seems to be located around his navel. Don't give him medication to ease it, or anything to reduce his temperature.

2 If you think your child may have appendicitis, don't give him anything to eat or drink. If you've ruled out the appendix, give him water if he is thirsty, but don't let him eat.

3 Comfort your child by giving him cuddles and extra attention.

4 If you don't suspect appendicitis, fill a hot water bottle with warm, not hot, water and wrap it in a towel. Let your child lie down with this held against his stomach.

Wrap the hot water bottle *securely in a towel*

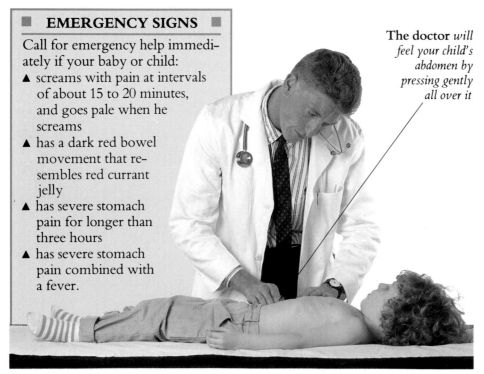

The doctor *will feel your child's abdomen by pressing gently all over it*

◼ EMERGENCY SIGNS ◼

Call for emergency help immediately if your baby or child:

▲ screams with pain at intervals of about 15 to 20 minutes, and goes pale when he screams
▲ has a dark red bowel movement that resembles red currant jelly
▲ has severe stomach pain for longer than three hours
▲ has severe stomach pain combined with a fever.

◼ CALL THE DOCTOR ◼

Call your doctor now if your child:

▲ develops any other symptoms
▲ has stomach pain for longer than three hours.

Consult your doctor if your child frequently has stomach pain.

What the doctor might do

The doctor will examine your child to try to find the cause of his stomach pain. The treatment will depend on his diagnosis, but most of the time, stomach pain disappears on its own. If the doctor suspects appendicitis or a blocked bowel, he will arrange for your child to go to the hospital for emergency surgery.

CONSTIPATION, VOMITING, AND DIARRHEA

A minor change in diet can cause temporary constipation or diarrhea. Vomiting or diarrhea may accompany almost any illness, and can also be caused by excitement or anxiety. If your child vomits or has mild diarrhea, check for other signs of illness (see pages 182–83). Frequent vomiting or severe diarrhea can quickly make a baby or young child dehydrated. This is a serious condition and must be treated promptly (see page 214), before the body loses too much fluid.

CONSTIPATION

What is it?

If your child has constipation, she has bowel movements less frequently than usual, and they are harder than normal. Children's toilet habits vary greatly: some children have a bowel movement twice a day, others go only once every two or three days. Whatever your child's regular pattern, it is quite normal—don't tamper with it. Babies often become slightly constipated when they learn to sit up or crawl, and before they can walk.

> ### ■ CALL THE DOCTOR ■
>
> Consult your doctor as soon as possible if your child:
> - ▲ cries or complains of pain when moving her bowels
> - ▲ has streaks of blood in her bowel movement, on her diaper, or underpants
> - ▲ has constipation for more than three days.

What can I do?

1 Don't worry if your child is temporarily constipated; it won't do her any harm. Don't give her a laxative, since this will upset the normal action of her bowels, and don't add sugar to her bottle.

2 Give your child plenty to drink, especially if the weather is hot, to soften her stool. Fruit juice helps to ease her constipation.

3 Don't hurry your child when she is on the toilet, but don't let her remain there for too long. If she seems constipated, smear petroleum jelly on her bottom before sitting her on the toilet, to make her bowel movement easier.

4 Try to include more fiber in your child's diet (see below). This provides the bulk that helps the bowel to grip and move its contents along.

What the doctor might do

The doctor may prescribe a mild laxative and give you some advice on your child's diet. If your child has streaks of blood in her stool, she could have a small tear in the lining of her anus, so the doctor may lubricate the area very gently.

GOOD SOURCES OF FIBER

Some examples of foods rich in fiber are shown here. Fresh foods are always best. Wash vegetables and fruit thoroughly, remove pits and strings, and peel for a child under one year. Purée the food for a baby under eight months (see pages 110–11).

Fresh fruit Offer your child a variety of fruit such as slices of peeled pear, peach, and banana.

Wholegrain bread

Wholegrain breakfast cereal

Dried fruit Prunes and apricots are ideal for young children.

Fresh vegetables Mashed potatoes and lightly cooked broccoli are high in fiber. Celery and carrots can be served raw.

VOMITING

What is it?
When your child vomits, she may throw up most of the contents of her stomach. Babies under about six months old often regurgitate a small amount of their feedings. This is perfectly normal, so don't worry.

■ CALL THE DOCTOR ■

Call your doctor now if your child:
▲ vomits and seems abnormally drowsy
▲ throws up green-yellow vomit
▲ has vomited repeatedly for more than six hours
▲ shows any signs of dehydration.

IDENTIFYING AND TREATING DEHYDRATION

Your child may be dehydrated if she shows one or more of these symptoms:
▲ dry mouth and lips
▲ dark, concentrated urine
▲ no urine passed for six hours
▲ sunken eyes
▲ sunken fontanelle
▲ abnormal drowsiness or lethargy.

If your child is dehydrated, or is in danger of becoming so, speak to your doctor. There are commercial oral rehydration products available at your drugstore to replace salt and sugar.

What can I do?
1 Hold your child over a bowl and comfort her while she is vomiting (see page 193). Wipe her face afterward and give her some sips of water.

2 Make sure that your child has plenty to drink —she needs more than the usual amount of fluid to make up for her losses (see Dehydration). If your baby won't take a bottle, try using a teaspoon or a medicine dropper (see page 189) to feed it to her.

What the doctor might do
The doctor will examine your child to find out what is making her vomit, and will then treat her according to the diagnosis.

If she shows signs of dehydration, the doctor may prescribe a commercial rehydration solution for her to drink. If she is very dehydrated, the doctor might arrange for her to be admitted to the hospital, where she can be given fluid intravenously.

GASTROENTERITIS

What is it?
Gastroenteritis is an inflammation in the stomach and intestines that can be caused by contaminated food. It is serious in babies, since it can dehydrate them very quickly, but it is rare in breast-fed babies. A mild attack in a child over two is not serious.

■ SYMPTOMS ■

▲ Vomiting and nausea
▲ diarrhea
▲ stomach cramps
▲ loss of appetite
▲ fever.

What can I do?
1 Make sure that your child drinks about 2–3 pints (1 to 1½ liters) a day. A special drink, made as described above, is best.

2 Don't give your child anything to eat until he stops vomiting, then introduce bland foods. Give your baby diluted formula (see page 179).

3 If your child has a fever, give him an aspirin-free medication with acetaminophen.

4 Let your child wear a diaper again if he has just outgrown them.

5 Make sure that your child washes his hands after going to the bathroom and before eating. Wash your own hands after changing his diaper and before preparing his food.

DIARRHEA

What is it?

If your child has diarrhea, her bowel movements will be watery and more frequent than normal. This may be the result of eating food that is too rich for her or that contains more fiber than she is used to.

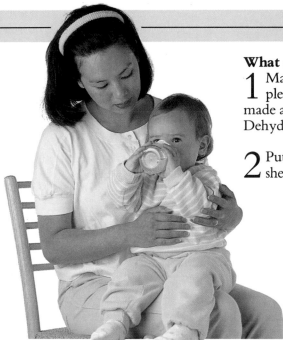

> ### ■ CALL THE DOCTOR ■
>
> Call your doctor now if your child:
> ▲ has had diarrhea for more than six hours
> ▲ has blood in her stool
> ▲ shows any signs of dehydration (see page 214).

What can I do?

1 Make sure that your child has plenty to drink. A sugary drink, made as described for vomiting (see Dehydration, page 214), is ideal.

2 Put your child in a diaper again if she has just outgrown them.

3 Pay careful attention to hygiene: wash your hands after changing your baby's diaper and before preparing her food, and make sure that your child always washes her hands after using the toilet and before eating.

What the doctor might do

The doctor will examine your child to find out the cause of her diarrhea, and will treat her according to the diagnosis. If your child has become dehydrated, the doctor may prescribe an oral rehydration product for her to drink. If she is very dehydrated, he might arrange for her to be admitted to the hospital, where she can be given the extra liquid she needs intravenously.

> ## ABNORMAL-LOOKING BOWEL MOVEMENTS
>
> Changes in the color of your child's bowel movements are probably caused by a change in her diet, so check whether she has eaten anything unusual. Sometimes an underlying illness accounts for the different appearance.
> ■ **Very pale, bulky BM's** that smell very offensive and float when you try to flush them away may mean that your child cannot properly digest gluten, a protein found in cereals (celiac disease). Consult your doctor.
> ■ **Frothy stool** may indicate that your child can't digest milk properly (lactose intolerance). Consult your doctor.

> ### ■ CALL THE DOCTOR ■
>
> Call your doctor now if your child:
> ▲ is under two and may have gastroenteritis
> ▲ is over two and has had symptoms of gastroenteritis for more than two days.

What the doctor might do

The doctor will probably treat your child for dehydration and may advise you to give him only liquids for a few days. He may ask for a sample of your child's stool.

> ### Q**UESTION** & A**NSWER**
>
> *"What steps can I take to prevent gastroenteritis?"*
> Clean all your baby's feeding equipment thoroughly for as long as he drinks formula or milk from a bottle (see pages 100–101). Put prepared bottles in the refrigerator—never store them warm in an insulated container, since bacteria thrive in warm conditions.
>
> Pay careful attention to hygiene when preparing food. If you store any cooked food, don't keep it in the refrigerator for longer than two days, and make sure it is thoroughly heated when you serve it, because heat kills the bacteria that could cause gastroenteritis.
>
> Wash dishes and glasses in very hot water. Dry them on paper towels, not a dish towel.
>
> If you are traveling in a foreign country with a baby or small child, ask your doctor about any precautions you should take, particularly with water, fruit, and salads.

BLADDER, KIDNEY, AND GENITAL PROBLEMS

Most urinary tract infections are caused by bacteria entering the urethra (see diagram below) and spreading up into the bladder. They are reasonably common in young children, and are usually not serious. Some children are born with minor abnormalities of the urinary tract, which make them prone to such infections. Minor infections of the genitals are also quite common, and in babies and young children they are often part of the symptoms of diaper rash (see page 176).

The urinary tract
Your child has two kidneys which filter his blood. The clean blood returns to his bloodstream, while the waste product (the urine) drains into his bladder, where it collects until he is ready to urinate.

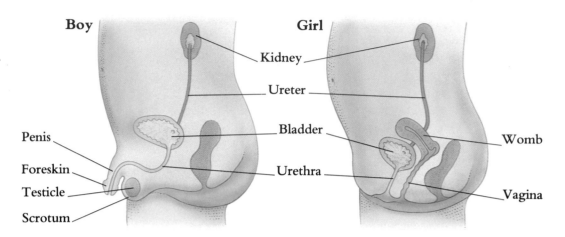

Boy

Girl

Kidney

Ureter

Bladder

Penis

Foreskin

Testicle

Urethra

Scrotum

Womb

Vagina

URINARY TRACT INFECTIONS

What are they?
Any part of the urinary tract—the kidneys, the bladder, and the connecting tubes—can become infected with bacteria. Infections are more common in girls, because the tube from the bladder (the urethra) is shorter in a girl than in a boy, and its opening is nearer to the anus, so germs can spread to it more easily.

What can I do?

1 If your child seems sick, check to see whether her urine looks pink or cloudy. Note whether she is urinating more frequently than usual and whether it seems to hurt when she goes to the bathroom. If your child is still in diapers, you probably won't be able to tell that urination is frequent or painful, but you will probably notice a change in odor.

2 Make sure that your child has plenty to drink, to keep her kidneys flushed.

3 If your child has a fever give her a dose of aspirin-free children's medication with acetaminophen to reduce it.

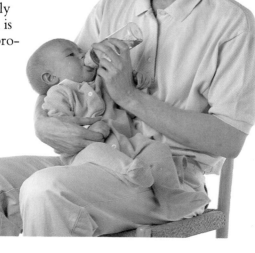

■	SYMPTOMS	■
▲ Urinating more often than usual
▲ pain when urinating
▲ pink, red, or cloudy urine
▲ change in odor of the urine
  ▲ fever
    ▲ listlessness
      ▲ loss of appetite
        ▲ abdominal pain.

■ CALL THE DOCTOR ■
Consult your doctor as soon as possible if you think your child has a urinary tract infection.

What the doctor might do
The doctor will examine your child and may ask you to take a sample of her urine (ask your doctor how you should collect this). He may prescribe an antibiotic.

GENITAL PROBLEMS IN GIRLS

What can go wrong?
A little girl's vagina can become sore due to diaper rash (see page 176), an infection such as thrush (see page 206), or pinworms (see page 224). If your daughter has a blood-stained or smelly discharge from her vagina, she may have pushed something into it. Newborn girls often produce a white or blood-stained discharge for a few days, and this is nothing to worry about. After this age until just before puberty, a discharge is abnormal.

What can I do?
1 If your daughter's bottom is sore or red, don't use soap when you wash it—just use water, and dry it thoroughly. Always wipe from front to back, so that germs can't spread forward from her anus.

2 Don't put rubber pants over your daughter's diapers, since they prevent air from circulating to her bottom. Dress an older child in 100% pure cotton underpants.

3 If your daughter has a discharge from her vagina, make sure that she hasn't pushed something into it. If she has, **consult your doctor as soon as possible**.

What the doctor might do
The doctor will examine your daughter and may take a sample of the discharge. If she has something lodged in her vagina, he will remove it gently. If she has an infection, he may prescribe antibiotics to be taken by mouth, or a cream to be applied to the affected area, depending on the cause of her symptoms.

> **■ SYMPTOMS ■**
> ▲ Soreness or itching in or around the vagina
> ▲ redness around the vagina
> ▲ discharge from the vagina.

> **■ CALL THE DOCTOR ■**
> Consult your doctor as soon as possible if your daughter:
> ▲ has a discharge from her vagina
> ▲ still has symptoms after two days of home treatment
> ▲ has pushed something into her vagina.

GENITAL PROBLEMS IN BOYS

What can go wrong?
In an uncircumcised boy, the foreskin, which covers the tip of the penis, can become inflamed or infected (balanitis), often as part of diaper rash (see page 176).

If a swelling develops in your son's groin or scrotum, he may have a hernia (intestines bulging through a weak area in the abdomen).

What can I do?
If your son's foreskin is inflamed, wash it without using soap and dry it thoroughly at each diaper change, or at least once a day. Change to a mild laundry soap and rinse his diapers or underpants thoroughly.

How can I prevent inflammation?
Don't try to pull your son's foreskin back—it won't retract until he is at least four. If you try to force it, you may make his foreskin inflamed.

> **■ SYMPTOMS ■**
> **Inflamed foreskin**
> ▲ Red, swollen foreskin
> ▲ discharge of pus from the penis.
>
> **Hernia**
> ▲ Soft, painless bulge in the groin or scrotum, which may disappear when your child lies down and get bigger when he coughs, sneezes, or cries.

What the doctor might do
If your son's foreskin is inflamed, the doctor may prescribe an antibiotic cream. If your son has a hernia, he may need no treatment, but if he is under six months old, or if the lump feels hard or does not disappear when he lies down, your doctor may recommend surgery to repair the hernia in his groin or scrotum.

> **■ CALL THE DOCTOR ■**
> Consult your doctor as soon as possible if:
> ▲ your son's foreskin looks red or swollen, or if there is any discharge
> ▲ your son's hernia becomes painful, or changes in any other way.
> Consult your doctor if you think your son may have a hernia.

> **CIRCUMCISION**
> This is a surgical procedure to remove the foreskin. If you want to have your son circumcised, discuss it with your doctor. Once considered routine for newborn boys, it is done now only for religious or specific medical reasons.

SKIN PROBLEMS

Minor skin problems are common in childhood. Most clear up quickly, but some are very contagious, and must be treated promptly. If your child has a rash combined with other signs of illness, he may have an infectious illness (see pages 197–99). For other problems, see the guide below.

QUICK DIAGNOSIS GUIDE

One or more red spots, or a rash, see Spots and boils, Hives, Heat rash (below and opposite), Insect stings (page 244) or, if dry and scaly, see Eczema (page 220).

Raw, cracked areas, usually on or around the lips, or on the cheeks or hands, see Chapped skin (page 221).

Small blisters or crusty patches on or around the mouth, see Cold sores or Impetigo (pages 222–23).

Hard lump of skin, usually on the hands or feet, see Warts (page 222).

Itchy head, see Lice and nits (page 224).

Intense itching around the anus, see Pinworms (page 224).

DEALING WITH ITCHING

Many skin problems cause itching, and since scratching can make the skin infected, it is important to relieve your child's itchiness.
- Dress him in cotton clothes, since cotton is less irritating to the skin than wool or other fabrics.
- Gently dab the area with cotton balls soaked in calamine lotion, to soothe inflamed or irritated skin.
- Dissolve a handful of baking soda in your child's bathwater and let him have a good soak.
- Put cotton socks on his hands when he is in bed.

SPOTS AND BOILS

What are they?

A spot is a small red swelling, usually on the face. A boil is an infection in the skin that causes a large, painful lump, which then festers to produce a head of pus in the middle. Boils are most likely to occur on the face or on pressure points such as the buttocks, but they can appear anywhere on the body.

Don't worry if your child gets occasional spots, but recurrent boils may be a sign of illness.

SYMPTOMS

Spot
▲ Small, red, painless lump.

Boil
▲ Painful, red lump that gradually gets larger
▲ white or yellow center of pus appearing after a day or two.

CALL THE DOCTOR

Consult your doctor as soon as possible if:
▲ your child has a spot that looks inflamed
▲ your child has a boil in an awkward or painful place
▲ the center of pus does not appear three days after the boil first developed
▲ red streaks spread out from the boil.
Consult your doctor if your child often gets boils.

What can I do?

1 If your child gets occasional spots, simply ignore them. They will clear up in a few days without treatment. If she tends to dribble, and the spots appear around her mouth, smear a barrier cream over the area.

2 If your child has a boil, or a spot that looks inflamed, gently clean it and the skin around it with a cotton ball dipped in antiseptic.

3 Cover it with an adhesive bandage. If it is rubbed by clothing, or is in a painful place such as the buttocks, cushion it with a large adhesive bandage or sterile gauze pad and surgical tape.

4 The boil will come to a head and burst of its own accord in a few days. Don't squeeze it—this may spread the infection. After it has burst, clean it gently with a cotton ball dipped in antiseptic, and keep it covered with a bandage or gauze pad until it has healed.

What the doctor might do

The doctor may lance the boil and drain away the pus, to reduce the pain and swelling, and might prescribe a cream. If your child has a lot of boils, the doctor may prescribe a course of antibiotics.

HIVES

What are they?
Hives (also known as urticaria) are itchy red patches on the skin. They usually fade after a few hours, but new ones may appear. In a child, they may be caused by a prickly, or nettle, plant, harsh sunshine or an allergy to certain foods or drugs.

■ SYMPTOMS ■
▲ Itchy rash of raised red patches (welts), sometimes with a pale center
▲ welts varying in size from $\frac{1}{16}-\frac{1}{2}$in. (1mm. to 1cm.) across
▲ larger welts joining together.

What can I do?
1 Dab your child's rash with cotton balls dipped in calamine lotion.

2 If the rash is caused by an allergy, try to find out what your child is allergic to, so that you can help her avoid it in the future. Such a rash usually develops a few hours after contact with an allergen, so try to remember whether, for example, she has recently eaten a new food.

■ CALL THE DOCTOR ■
Call your doctor now if your child's face or neck is swollen.

Consult your doctor as soon as possible if:
▲ the rash does not disappear within four hours
▲ your child has frequent attacks of hives.

What the doctor might do
The doctor may prescribe an antihistamine cream or medication for your child. He might also test her to find the cause of the allergy. If your child's face or neck is swollen, she might require an injection to reduce the swelling.

HEAT RASH

What is it?
Heat rash is a faint rash caused by overheating. It is more common in babies than in children, and usually appears on the face or in skin creases, where sweat can gather. It is not a serious disorder, and you can treat it yourself at home.

■ SYMPTOMS ■
▲ Pink rash on the face or in skin creases.

■ CALL THE DOCTOR ■
Consult your doctor as soon as possible if the rash has not faded 12 hours after your child cools down.

What can I do?
1 Take off any heavy bedding and remove a layer of your baby's clothing. Let him sleep dressed in just a T-shirt and diaper.

2 Give him a bath in lukewarm water. Pat his skin dry gently, leaving it slightly damp so that he cools down as his skin dries. When he is dry, apply a little baby powder to absorb new sweat.

3 Take your baby's temperature; if it is raised, give him an aspirin-free children's medication with acetaminophen or sponge bathe him (see page 188).

How can I prevent heat rash?
Dress your baby in light clothes when the weather is hot, with cotton next to his skin rather than wool or a manmade fiber. Make sure he's well protected from the sun.

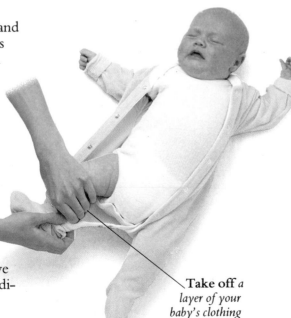

Take off *a layer of your baby's clothing*

What the doctor might do
The doctor will check that the rash is just a heat rash. If it is, your baby needs no medical treatment. If the rash has another cause, the doctor will treat that.

ECZEMA

What is it?

Eczema is an allergy resulting in areas of itchy, red, scaly skin. It most commonly affects the face and skin creases such as the inside of the elbows and the back of the knees, but it can be more widespread.

It usually first appears between the ages of three months and two years, then improves as the child grows older. About half of all children with eczema grow out of it by the age of six, and nearly all of them grow out of it by puberty. Your child is more likely to develop eczema if other people in the family suffer from allergies such as eczema, asthma, and hay fever.

What can I do?

1 When you give your child a bath, clean the affected areas by wiping them with baby oil, rather than washing with soap. Rinse the oil off with plenty of water.

Use cotton balls *to apply the baby oil*

■ SYMPTOMS ■

▲ Itchy, red, scaly, dry patches, usually on the face or in skin creases
▲ clear fluid oozing from the affected areas.

2 After a bath, apply an unscented moisturizing cream to your child's skin, since it may be very dry. Babies' brands are ideal.

3 Dress your child in cotton, rather than wool. In cold weather, put cotton clothing under warmer layers.

4 Try to stop your child from scratching the affected areas—put cotton socks on his hands at night and keep his fingernails short.

5 Try to discover the cause of the allergy. Common allergens include foods (especially dairy products and wheat), animal fur, woolen clothes, and laundry detergents.
Anxiety can also trigger eczema.

6 When your child's eczema is bad, keep him away from anyone with chicken pox or cold sores because of a greater infection risk.

■ CALL THE DOCTOR ■

Consult your doctor as soon as possible if:
▲ your child's eczema is very widespread or very itchy
▲ fluid is oozing from the eczema.
Consult your doctor if you think your child has eczema.

What the doctor might do

The doctor may prescribe a cream, and if the area is infected, an antibiotic. Most importantly, he'll try to determine the exact allergen and advise you on how to eliminate it from your child's daily environment, if at all possible.

SUNBURN

What is it?
Sunburn is sore or reddened skin caused by exposure to the sun. Babies and young children, especially those with fair hair and blue eyes, have very sensitive skin, so they are particularly vulnerable to it.

SYMPTOMS
- ▲ Red, sore areas of skin
- ▲ blisters appearing on badly affected areas
- ▲ flaking or peeling skin a day or two later.

What can I do?
1 Take your child inside or into the shade as soon as her skin begins to look red. Bear in mind that the worst symptoms of sunburn are likely to be delayed for a few hours.

2 Cool down any reddened areas of skin with cold water, then apply a soothing after-sun lotion or dab on some calamine lotion.

PREVENTING SUNBURN
Never let your baby sleep in the sun and, unless your child has been regularly exposed to the sun, don't allow her to spend more than 15 minutes uncovered at first. Gradually increase the exposure time by five minutes each day. Apply a sunscreen or block every hour. (Choose a water-resistant one with a sun-protection factor of at least 10.) Dress her in a T-shirt and a sun hat. Make her keep the T-shirt on when she is swimming or playing near water. If her skin is red the next day, keep her out of the sun.

CALL THE DOCTOR
Consult your doctor as soon as possible if:
- ▲ your child has a fever and seems sick
- ▲ blisters appear over a large area.

What the doctor might do
The doctor may prescribe a soothing and healing cream.

CHAPPED SKIN

What is it?
Chaps are small cracks in the skin that occur when the skin becomes dry after being exposed to cold or hot, dry air. Chapping is not serious, but it can be painful.

What can I do?
1 Moisturize lips with lip salve or apply moisturizing cream or petroleum jelly to the skin.

2 Use baby oil or lotion to wash the area, and keep his hands warm and dry.

3 If the cracks bleed, put a bandage or gauze pad over them.

SYMPTOMS
- ▲ Tiny cracks in the skin, usually on or around the lips or on the cheeks or hands
- ▲ bleeding if the cracks are deep.

CALL THE DOCTOR
Consult your doctor as soon as possible if:
- ▲ the cracks do not heal after three days
- ▲ the cracks become red, sore, or pus-filled.

What the doctor might do
If the chapped area has become infected, the doctor may prescribe an antibiotic. Otherwise, there is no treatment.

COLD SORES

What are they?

Cold sores are small blisters, usually on or around the lips but they sometimes develop inside the mouth or elsewhere on the face.

They are caused by a virus which, once it has infected a child, lies dormant in the skin and tends to flare up occasionally, so if your child has had a cold sore, he is liable to get others in the future. Strong sunlight can trigger a recurrence, and so can a minor illness, such as a cold (which is why they are called cold sores).

SYMPTOMS

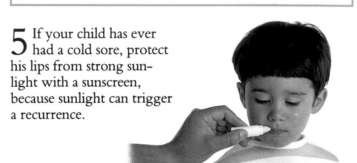

- ▲ Raised, red area that tingles or itches, usually around the mouth
- ▲ small, painful yellow blisters forming about a day later
- ▲ blisters crusting over after a day or two
- ▲ fever and general illness during the first attack.

What can I do?

1 At the first sign of a cold sore, hold an ice cube against the affected area for ten minutes. This may prevent the blister from developing.

Wrap an ice cube *in a cloth and hold it against your child's lip*

2 If your child develops a blister, apply a cream such as petroleum jelly.

3 Keep his hands clean, and stop him from touching the sore, which could spread infection.

4 Since cold sores are very contagious, don't let your child kiss other people, and if he tends to put toys into his mouth, don't let him share them with other children until the sore has gone.

5 If your child has ever had a cold sore, protect his lips from strong sunlight with a sunscreen, because sunlight can trigger a recurrence.

CALL THE DOCTOR

Consult your doctor as soon as possible if:
- ▲ your child has a cold sore for the first time
- ▲ your child's cold sore starts to ooze or spread
- ▲ your child has a cold sore near his eyes.

What the doctor might do

The doctor will probably prescribe a cream to be spread over the affected area several times a day, which will help the blister to heal.

WARTS

What are they?

A wart is a lump of hard, dry skin; a plantar wart (verruca) is a wart on the sole of the foot. Warts are caused by a virus that invades the skin, and most children get them occasionally.

Warts are not painful, and disappear spontaneously, usually after a few months, so treatment is not necessary. Plantar warts tend to be painful because of the pressure put on them whenever your child walks or wears shoes, so they should be treated promptly.

SYMPTOMS

Wart
- ▲ Hard lump of dry skin.

Plantar wart (verruca)
- ▲ Hard, painful area on the sole of the foot, perhaps with a tiny black center.

What can I do?

1 If your child has a wart, simply ignore it, unless it is on his genitals or near his anus; in that case call your doctor. It will disappear on its own after a few months, though some last for a year or more.

IMPETIGO

What is it?
Impetigo is a bacterial skin infection that may develop when a rash such as eczema or a cold sore becomes infected, though healthy skin can sometimes become infected with impetigo. It usually affects the skin around the mouth and nose, but it can occur anywhere on the body. Impetigo isn't a serious disorder in children, but in a young baby it can spread over a large area and make him seriously ill. It is very contagious, so it is important to have it treated promptly.

What can I do?
1 Keep your child's washcloth and towel separate from those of the rest of the family, and wash them frequently, so the infection doesn't spread.

2 Try to keep your child from touching the affected area—don't let him suck his thumb or pick his nose, because this could spread the infection.

3 Remove the scabs each day by wiping them with warm soapy cotton balls. Don't rub hard, but persevere until they loosen.

Wipe the scabs gently *with cotton balls dipped in warm soapy water*

SYMPTOMS

- ▲ Rash of small red spots
- ▲ blisters forming over the spots
- ▲ the spots burst, then form large brownish-yellow scabs
- ▲ fever and general malaise in a young baby.

4 Pat the area dry with a tissue or paper towel and throw it away immediately, so that the infection can't spread.

5 Keep your child away from other children, especially young babies, until he is better.

CALL THE DOCTOR
Call your doctor now if your baby is under three months old and suddenly develops widespread impetigo. Consult your doctor as soon as possible if you think your child has impetigo.

What the doctor might do
The doctor may prescribe a cream and tell you to wipe the scabs away (see left) before applying it. If the infection is still there after five days, consult your doctor again.

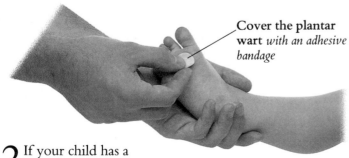

Cover the plantar wart *with an adhesive bandage*

2 If your child has a plantar wart, keep it covered with an adhesive bandage and don't let him go barefoot until it has cleared up. It may disappear spontaneously. Keep his towel and washcloth separate.

CALL THE DOCTOR
Consult your doctor if:
- ▲ your child's warts multiply
- ▲ your child has a wart on his genitals or anus
- ▲ your child has a plantar wart, or verruca.

What the doctor might do
Your doctor may prescribe a lotion to be applied regularly to the wart until it disappears. Alternatively, he may refer your child to a podiatrist or dermatologist to have it burnt or frozen off under local anesthesia.

LICE AND NITS

What are they?

Lice are tiny insects that infest the hair, and make the child's head itchy. Their minute white eggs (nits) cling to the hair roots. Lice spread very easily from one head to another, so treat the whole family if your child picks up lice, and tell your friends to check their children's heads.

Use cotton balls *to apply the lotion*

SYMPTOMS

- ▲ Itchy head
- ▲ tiny white grains firmly attached to the hairs near the roots
- ▲ red bite marks on the scalp.

What can I do?

1 Ask your pharmacist for a lotion or shampoo to kill the lice and nits. Apply it all over your child's head, and leave it on his hair for as long as the instructions specify.

3 Clean your child's brush, comb, and hats, thoroughly. Try sealing his hats in a plastic bag for at least ten days—the lice and nits will all have died by then.

2 Wash and rinse his hair, then comb it thoroughly with a special fine comb to remove the dead lice and nits. Though some new products boast of one-step eradication, you may need to repeat this treatment.

4 If your child goes to a toddler group, nursery school, or child care center, inform the staff that he has lice, and keep him home until they have been completely eradicated.

PINWORMS

What are they?

Pinworms are tiny, white thread-like worms, about $\frac{1}{2}$in. (1cm.) long. They can enter the body in contaminated food, and then live in the bowels, coming out at night to lay eggs around the anus, and causing intense itchiness. They are common in children, and are harmless, though the itching may be extremely uncomfortable. In little girls, the worms may crawl forward to the vagina.

SYMPTOMS

- ▲ Intense itching around the anus, which is usually worse at night
- ▲ intense itching around the vagina
- ▲ tiny white worms in the stool.

What can I do?

1 Try to prevent your child from scratching, because she might inflame the skin around her anus.

2 Keep her fingernails short so that, if she scratches, she doesn't pick up any eggs under her nails, which could reinfect her or other people.

3 Make sure that the whole family washes their hands thoroughly after going to the bathroom and before eating. Use a nail brush to clean the nails properly.

CALL THE DOCTOR

Consult your doctor as soon as possible if you think your child has pinworms.

4 If your child no longer wears diapers, make sure she wears pajamas, or cotton underpants under a nightgown. Change her pants and pajama bottoms every day and sterilize them in boiling water to kill any worms or eggs on them. Change her sheets every day and wash and rinse them thoroughly in very hot water.

5 When she feels itchy, lay her across your lap and look for tiny white worms near her anus. Remove any you see with a damp wad of toilet paper and flush them away.

What the doctor might do

The doctor will probably prescribe a medication for the whole family, which will kill the worms. He may also prescribe a cream for your child to soothe any inflammation around the anus or vagina.

FAINTING, DIZZINESS, AND CONVULSIONS

Even children under three occasionally feel faint or dizzy. Ordinarily this simply means they need food or to be calmed down after a period of intense excitement or anxiety. A convulsion, however, is worrisome and should send you straight to the telephone for a professional opinion.

FAINTING AND DIZZINESS

What is it?
Fainting is a brief loss of consciousness that is usually preceded by your child feeling lightheaded and looking pale. It may follow a bout of dizziness.

> ■ **CALL THE DOCTOR** ■
>
> Call your doctor now if your child loses consciousness.

1 If your child faints, lay him down with his legs higher than his head. Loosen any tight clothing.

2 As he begins to recover, put him into the recovery position (see page 233). If you are outside under hot sun, find a cooler spot. Let him rest for a few minutes. Once he's fully conscious and recovered, offer him something sweet to drink, such as orange juice.

A CONVULSION

What is it?
A convulsion, seizure, or fit is caused by a departure from normality in the electrical activity of the brain. When it accompanies a high fever, it's called a fever convulsion (see page 188); a tendency to have convulsions when there is no fever is known as epilepsy.

What can I do?
1 Put your child on his side on the floor. Stay with him to make sure he doesn't injure himself, but don't try to restrain him.

2 After it's over, put your child into the recovery position (see page 233). Don't wake him, but check his breathing. Reduce any fever.

> ■ **CALL THE DOCTOR** ■
>
> Call your doctor now if your child has a convulsion.

> ■ **SYMPTOMS** ■
>
> **Convulsions (also known as major seizures or grand mal convulsions)**
> ▲ Sudden unconsciousness
> ▲ eyes rolling back into the head
> ▲ clenched teeth
> ▲ shaking spasms in the muscles
> ▲ wetting the pants, or loss of bowel control
> ▲ sleeping, or gradual return to consciousness, when the twitching movements stop.
>
> **Absence attacks (also known as petit mal convulsions)**
> ▲ Sudden lack of movement
> ▲ dazed expression
> ▲ complete recovery in a few seconds.

MENINGITIS

What is it?
Meningitis is an inflammation of the tissues that cover the brain. It is a very serious disease, and must be treated promptly. Inflammation of the brain itself (encephalitis) causes similar symptoms.

> ■ **CALL THE DOCTOR** ■
>
> Call your doctor now if you think your child may have meningitis or encephalitis.

> ■ **SYMPTOMS** ■
>
> ▲ Fever
> ▲ listlessness and drowsiness, or sudden irritability
> ▲ change for the worse in a child who has recently had an infectious illness such as measles or mumps
> ▲ vomiting
> ▲ loss of appetite
> ▲ headache or, in babies, slightly bulging fontanelle
> ▲ reluctance to bend the neck forward
> ▲ convulsions.

225

YOUR CHILD'S SAFETY

Accidents—especially the ones that happen at home—are a major threat to your child. But there are a number of ways you can make your home safer. The best precaution of all is to keep your child under your own watchful eye. Remember that the chances of an accident happening are greatest when your child is tired, hungry, or sick, or when you are busy or preoccupied. The risks are also high when the family is in a different environment—on vacation or away from home. When you buy equipment or toys for your child, read all manufacturers' directions and safety precautions carefully and make sure you use them only for the age of child they are designed for. Secondhand items should be sturdy and all the parts, including safety harnesses and brakes, should be in good working condition.

SAFETY IN YOUR HOME

ALL CHILDREN are accident prone, because their desire to explore and experiment far outstrips their common sense and forethought. Many accidents can easily be prevented, and it is your responsibility to make sure that your child can't injure himself. However, keeping him safe should not mean restricting his activities, but simply making sure that his world is safe for him to play in and explore.

Store plastic bags *and wrap out of his reach*

Keep a fire *extinguisher in a handy location*

Push hot drinks *to the back of kitchen counters*

Keep him away *from the stove when it's in use. Turn your saucepan handles to the rear. Use back burners as much as possible*

Fit a child-resistant *lock on your refrigerator and/or freezer*

Buy coiled electrical cords *for your appliances, or make sure that the cords are short*

Keep all *household cleaners and bleaches, and your waste basket, in a cabinet with a child-resistant catch*

Don't let *your child touch the oven door while it is hot*

Have nonslip flooring *and wipe up any spills immediately*

KITCHEN

Your kitchen is full of potential hazards for your child and these dangers are increased if you are preoccupied. So keep him away from the immediate cooking area when you are cooking—an infant seat or a playpen is ideal. Remember that stovetops, burners, kettles, and irons stay hot long after you have turned them off. At mealtimes, keep hot food and drinks near the center of the table, so that your child can't grab them. Don't use a tablecloth, because he could pull it and spill hot things on himself. Make sure that your child can't get into your waste basket.

Keep sharp utensils *such as kitchen knives in a drawer with a child-resistant catch or lock*

KEEPING YOUR BABY SAFE

With each new skill your baby develops, he will find ways of running into danger, so anticipate the possible hazards. He will learn to roll over when he is very young, so if you need to lay him down for a moment, put him on the floor. He will be able to grasp an object at about two months and reach for and grab things by about three months. Make sure that anything he can reach is safe and too large for him to swallow or choke on. Don't eat, drink, or carry anything hot, and don't smoke, while you are holding your baby. Never leave him alone with a bottle because he could choke. Always use safety belts or a harness when he is in his carriage or stroller as well as in the high chair and infant seat, and don't put him in an infant seat on a high surface because it could easily fall off.

Don't leave a young child alone with your baby: he might pick him up and drop him, or give him dangerous objects to play with.

BEDROOM

Your child will spend a lot of time in his bedroom, so make sure he can explore it safely. Don't put a pillow in his crib until he is at least two, and don't use loose plastic sheeting as a waterproof mattress cover—it could become loose and smother him. Never attach his toys to the crib with cords or ribbons—they might wind around his neck. Keep large toys and pillows out of the crib—he could use them to help him climb out. Don't string toys across the crib once he can stand. His toys should be nontoxic and nonflammable, and have no sharp edges, snags, or small pieces.

Fix locks on the windows *so that they can be opened only a little way. Open sash windows from the top*

Cut any strings *or ribbons on crib bumpers short, so that they can't wind around his neck*

Always use *a safety belt when changing your baby's diapers; don't leave him alone on a changing table*

Make sure *that the furniture is sturdy and has rounded edges*

Put a few *small toys in the crib*

Use flame-resistant *sleepwear and bedding*

Set the crib mattress *on its lowest position before your baby can pull himself to standing*

Cover hot *radiators with towels*

Store your child's toys *in a low cabinet or shelf so that he can reach them without climbing*

BATHROOM

Never leave your child alone in the bathroom, even for a few seconds, until he is at least two and a half, and use nonslip bath mats and rugs. Set your water heater lower than 130°F (55°C), and run cold water into your child's bath before hot. Test the temperature before putting your child in.

Other accidents that may occur in the bathroom can easily be prevented:
■ Keep all medicines out of your child's reach in a cabinet with a lock or a child-resistant catch.
■ Put razors and cosmetics out of your child's reach.
■ Cover radiators and any dangerous heating vents with towels.

■ If you have a portable electric heater, it should not be used anywhere your baby might be able to reach.
■ Keep cleaning products and the toilet brush in a cupboard with a child-resistant catch or lock.
■ If you have a shower with a glass door, make sure it's safety glass.

ELECTRICITY

Electric shocks from any power source can be very serious, so minimize the chances of your child receiving a shock:

■ Turn off electrical appliances when you are not using them.
■ Never leave a socket switched on with nothing plugged into it.
■ Cover unused sockets with childproof socket covers, or mask them with heavy insulating tape.
■ Check electrical cords regularly, and repair any with exposed wires.
■ Don't let your child play with electrically powered toys until he is at least four.

LIVING ROOM

When you buy upholstered furniture, ask the salesperson about the fabric content. You don't want it to give off toxic fumes if you have a fire. Always use a fireplace screen. Don't let your child touch the back of your television.

Don't leave cigarettes, matches, alcohol, sewing equipment, or coins lying around. Keep indoor plants out of his reach, as some are poisonous.

If you have low glass panels in doors or windows, use toughened, laminated, or wire-net glass, apply a transparent safety film, or put colored stickers on them, so that your child can see where the glass is. Avoid glass-topped tables.

HALL AND STAIRS

Put safety gates at the top and bottom of the stairs before your child can crawl or climb. Make sure that the hall, stairs, and landings are well lit and that your banisters aren't so wide apart that your child could fall through. Don't leave toys, piles of laundry, or anything else on steps. Make sure that the door knobs and locks are out of his reach or not easily opened. Install smoke detectors.

Repair loose tiles or tears in rugs or flooring, and, if your floors are polished, put a nonslip backing on any rugs. On polished floors, don't let your child wear socks without shoes, and if you let him go barefoot, make sure there are no splinters.

IN THE YARD

Keep an eye on your child when he is playing in the yard, and if you put your baby to sleep outside, have a mosquito net handy to slip over the carriage. Never let your child play in or near a wading pool without an adult supervising him, and empty the pool after use. If you are near a stream or a pond, fence your yard securely. Keep all your walks in good condition—remove weeds regularly so that they don't become slippery in wet weather, and repair walks if they are uneven. Don't let your child play in an area of your yard where you have recently used pesticide, weedkiller or fertilizer, as these can be poisonous.

CARS

Your child should always travel in a car seat that is officially approved for his age and weight. Use the locks on car doors and don't let your child lean out of the window or put his hand out while the car is moving. Don't ever leave your child alone in the car, even if it is only for a moment.

Check where your child is before closing the car door. When you are backing out of a driveway, always make a note of where your child is. Don't take any chances when he is playing outside in the yard. If he is just behind the car, you won't see him in the rearview mirror.

Lock up *all your gardening tools and equipment, and any weed-killer, fertilizer, or pesticide*

Teach your child *not to eat any berries*

Fix child-resistant *locks on all fence gates*

Make sure *that the plants in your garden aren't poisonous, and pull up mushrooms or fungi as soon as they appear*

Put your child's *play equipment on grass or sand, not on a hard surface*

Make sure *that the sand in your child's sandbox is too shallow for him to bury himself and teach him not to throw sand. Cover the sandbox when he is not playing in it*

FIRST AID

If your child is injured, always treat the most serious injury first. If he is unconscious, check his breathing, and resuscitate him if necessary (see pages 230–32), before giving first aid for any other injury. If he is breathing, first treat anything that might prevent him from breathing properly, such as choking, suffocation, or drowning (see pages 234–35), then control any heavy bleeding (see page 238). If your child is badly injured or in shock, he will need urgent medical treatment, but you should give first aid before calling for medical help. The instructions in this chapter explain how to cope with various injuries and tell you when help is necessary. If you need to get your child to the hospital quickly, it may be faster to take him there yourself, rather than to call for an ambulance, but check this page for occasions when you must call an ambulance.

GETTING YOUR CHILD TO A HOSPITAL

Call for an ambulance, or ask someone else to phone if:
- you think your child might have a spinal injury
- you think he'll need special treatment on the way to the hospital
- you have no suitable transportation of your own.

If you take your child to a hospital yourself, have someone else drive while you sit with your child and continue to give first aid.

If your child is unconscious, don't leave him alone for more than a minute or so while you call for help. If he is not breathing, resuscitate him before phoning for an ambulance. Don't stop until he is breathing again, but shout to other people between breaths if necessary.

■ WARNING ■

If there is a chance that your child has injured his neck or spine—for example, after a bad fall—don't move him unless it is absolutely essential. Leave him in whatever position you found him while you check to see if he is breathing. If you need to perform artificial respiration, get someone to help you if possible. Turn your child on his back very gently without twisting his spine—try to hold his head, shoulders, and hips so that his body turns as a single unit.

FIRST AID KIT

Keep a supply of first aid equipment in a clean, dry container, and replace anything you use as soon as possible. Take some antiseptic wipes with you on outings, to clean cuts and scrapes.

Surgical tape This is useful for sticking on bandages, and drawing together the edges of large cuts.

Cotton

Calamine lotion Soothes sunburn, insect bites, and any stings.

Eye bath

Nonadherent, absorbent, sterile gauze bandages These peel easily off a wound.

One gauze bandage

Scissors

Tweezers

Triangular bandage This can be used to make a sling or secure a dressing.

Safety pins

Gauze bandage rolls

Assorted adhesive bandages Use these for dressing minor cuts and scrapes.

Prepared wound dressings These consist of a pad attached to a bandage, and are easy to put on.

LIFESAVING TECHNIQUES

FAMILIARIZE YOURSELF with these instructions so that you can act quickly in an emergency. Every second counts. If your child seems to be unconscious, follow these procedures before treating any injuries. If he has stopped breathing, it is vital to get air into his lungs quickly, so that he doesn't suffer brain damage. By breathing your own air into his lungs, you can prevent this, and revive your child. If his heart has stopped beating, you can pump it manually to keep his blood circulating through his body. Don't give up—children have been revived after several hours of resuscitation.

> ### ■   EMERGENCY   ■
> Call for emergency help if your child becomes unconscious, even if this is only for a few seconds.

CHECKING FOR UNCONSCIOUSNESS
Tap the soles of your child's feet, and call his name. Note whether he responds.
Don't shake him, since this could worsen any injuries he may have.

Tap *the soles of his feet*

✚ **If he doesn't respond,** he is unconscious, so check his breathing immediately.

✚ **If he responds,** check for injury and treat any he may have (see pages 234–45).

CHECKING BREATHING

Pull his chin
down gently to open his mouth

2 Place your ear close to his mouth and nose, looking toward his feet. Listen for any sound of breathing, note whether you can feel any breath against your ear, and watch his chest to see whether it rises and falls as he breathes.

1 Lay your child on his back on a firm surface and stand or kneel beside him. Place one hand on his forehead and press gently to tilt his head back slightly. Open his mouth.

✚ **If there are no signs of breathing,** turn your child on to his side, or put him on his front over your lap. Sweep one finger around inside his mouth to clear any obstruction that might be blocking his breathing, but be very careful not to push anything down his throat. Check again for any signs of breathing.

✚ **If there are still no signs of breathing,** start artificial respiration right away (see opposite).

✚ **If your child is breathing,** put him on his side in the recovery position (see page 233) and call for emergency help immediately.

ARTIFICIAL RESPIRATION FOR A BABY

2 Take a deep breath, place your lips around your baby's mouth and nose, making as good a seal as you can, then breathe out gently.

3 Watch your baby's chest to see whether it rises as you breathe out.

1 Slide one hand under your baby's neck, cupping the base of his head, to support him and keep his head tilted back. Leave your other hand on his forehead.

✚ **If his chest doesn't rise,** he probably has something blocking his windpipe. Treat him for choking (see page 234), then continue with artificial respiration if necessary.

✚ **If his chest rises,** remove your mouth from his face and let his chest fall. Give two quick, gentle breaths, then check his heartbeat (see next page).

ARTIFICIAL RESPIRATION FOR A CHILD

Pinch *his nostrils as you breathe into his mouth*

2 Take a deep breath and seal your lips around your child's mouth. If he is still very small, seal your mouth over his mouth and nose, as for a baby (see above). Blow gently into his mouth.

3 Watch your child's chest to see whether it rises as you breathe out.

1 Lift your child's chin to pull his jaw forward. Open his mouth and pinch his nostrils together.

✚ **If his chest doesn't rise,** he probably has something blocking his windpipe. Treat him for choking (see page 234), then continue with artificial respiration if necessary.

✚ **If his chest rises,** remove your mouth from his face and let his chest fall. Give two quick breaths, then check his heartbeat (see next page).

LIFESAVING TECHNIQUES *continued*

CHECKING HEARTBEAT

Listen *for a heartbeat*

Your child *has strong pulses here*

Voice box

For a baby
Put one ear gently against his chest and listen carefully for about five seconds to check whether you can hear a heartbeat.

For a child over two
Place the pads of two fingers over the voice box at the front of his neck, then slide them into the slight hollow beside this. Feel for five seconds.

For a baby or a child

✚ **If you can't feel a pulse or hear a heartbeat,** his heart has stopped. Start external chest compression immediately (see below).

✚ **If his heart is beating,** continue breathing gently into his lungs at a rate of about one breath every three seconds, until he starts to breathe on his own, or until emergency help arrives. As soon as he starts to breathe again, turn him on his side in the recovery position (see opposite).

EXTERNAL CHEST COMPRESSION
For a baby

Bottom of the breastbone

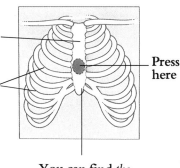

Breastbone

Ribs

Press here

You can find *the bottom of the breastbone by feeling where the rib cage forms an inverted V-shape*

1 Slide one hand under your baby's shoulders and grasp the top of his arm. With your other hand, find the bottom of his breastbone (see right), then measure halfway up to his neck.

2 Place two fingers just below the middle of his breastbone and press down to a depth of about $\frac{1}{2}$–1in. (1.5 to 2.5cm.), then release the pressure.

For a child over two

Bottom of the breastbone

1 Find the bottom of your child's breastbone (see diagram above), then measure halfway up to the base of his neck.

2 Place the heel of one hand just below the halfway point and press down to a depth of about 1–1$\frac{1}{2}$in. (2.5 to 3.5cm.), then release the pressure.

For a baby or a child

3 Give five compressions at a rate of about two per second, then give a breath into his lungs. Continue with five compressions followed by one breath until his heart starts to beat, or emergency help arrives. Every two or three minutes, check whether he is breathing and whether his heart has started to beat.

4 When his heart starts to beat, stop giving compressions, but continue artificial respiration until he begins to breathe by himself, or help arrives.

THE RECOVERY POSITION

PUT YOUR child into this position if he is unconscious, but breathing. This is the safest position because it prevents his tongue falling back into his throat and obstructing his airway, and avoids the risk of him choking if he vomits.

1 Turn your child's face toward you, keeping his chin pulled forward. Place the arm nearest to you by his side, and tuck his hand under his buttocks, with the palm up. Fold the arm farther from you over his chest, and cross his farther leg over his near leg.

> ### ■ WARNING ■
> Do not use the recovery position if there is a possibility that your child's neck or spine is damaged, for example, after a bad fall or a car accident.

His head must be turned to one side and tilted well back with the chin jutting forward

2 Lay a coat or blanket in front of your child, if available. Put one hand by his face to protect it, then grasp his hip with your other hand. Roll him toward you on to the coat or blanket.

3 Make sure that his nose and mouth aren't obstructed, then bend his top arm and leg up to a right angle, so that they support him. Gently pull his lower arm out from under his hip, and leave it by his side.

4 Cover him with a coat or blanket, then call for emergency help. Stay with him until help arrives, and every three minutes check his breathing and his heart-beat (see opposite), if his heart had stopped.

CHOKING

This happens when a small object or piece of food gets lodged in the windpipe, causing a coughing fit. It is important to dislodge the object quickly, so that your child can breathe properly again. Choking is common in very young children, who tend to put everything they get hold of into their mouths. They may find it hard to swallow dry, crumbly foods, so avoid them if possible.

HELPING A BABY

1 Hold your baby face down with his head lower than his body: either support him along your forearm, or hold him upside down by his ankles. Strike him between the shoulder blades up to four times.

Breastbone

Ribs

Press here

Navel

2 If he is still choking, lay him on his side and tilt his head back slightly. Support his back with one hand, and place two fingers of your other hand about halfway between his navel and the point where the bottom of his ribs forms an inverted V-shape (see diagram). Press inward and upward with a quick, thrusting movement.

3 If your baby does not start breathing normally when the blockage is removed, carry out artificial respiration immediately (see pages 231–32).

HELPING A CHILD

1 Sit down or kneel on one knee and lay your child on her front over your knee, with her head hanging down. Support her chest with one hand and strike her between her shoulder blades several times.

2 If this fails to dislodge the obstruction, sweep around your child's mouth with a finger and try to hook it from the back of her throat. Be very careful not to push anything further down her throat.

3 If she is still choking, sit her on your lap, facing forward. Support her back with one hand and hold the other in a fist, thumb inward, halfway between her navel and the V-shape at the bottom of her ribs (see diagram, left). Press sharply inward and upward up to four times.

Tuck your thumb *in when you make a fist*

4 If your child does not start breathing normally when the blockage is removed, carry out artificial respiration (see pages 231–32).

SUFFOCATION

Anything lying across your child's face may block her mouth and nose, and prevent her from breathing.

What can I do?

1 Pick your child up or remove whatever is covering her face.

EMERGENCY

Call for emergency help immediately if your child:
▲ becomes unconscious
▲ stops breathing, even if only for a few seconds
▲ shows any symptoms that worry you.

---

2 Check to see if your child is conscious and breathing (see page 230).

If she is not breathing, start artificial respiration immediately (see pages 231–32) and ask someone to call for emergency help.

If she is breathing but unconscious, place her in the recovery position (see page 233), then call for emergency help.

If she is conscious, simply comfort and reassure her.

DROWNING

Babies and children can drown in very shallow water. When a young child's face is submerged, his automatic reaction is to take a deep breath to scream, rather than to lift his face up out of the water.

What can I do?

Make sure that your child is conscious and breathing (see page 230). If he is coughing, choking, or vomiting, he is still breathing. If there is any chance that he has injured his neck or back, lift him very gently and be careful not to twist his spine.

If he is not breathing, don't waste time trying to drain the water from his lungs. Clear any debris, such as mud or seaweed, from his mouth and start artificial respiration (see pages 231–32) right away— if possible while he is still being carried from the water—and **call for emergency help.** Continue artificial respiration until help arrives or until he starts to breathe again. When he starts to breathe again, put him in the recovery position (see page 233).

Clear any debris
from his mouth with your finger

EMERGENCY

Call for emergency help immediately if your child was rescued from drowning, even if he didn't become unconscious.

If he is breathing but unconscious, place him in the recovery position (see page 233) so that water can drain from his mouth and lungs, and **call for emergency help immediately.** Cover him with a coat or blanket to keep him warm. Get him to a warm room as soon as you can, because he may have become dangerously chilled after even a short period of immersion in cold water.

If he is conscious, simply comfort and reassure him, and make sure he keeps warm.

SHOCK

A life-threatening state of collapse, when blood pressure falls dangerously low, shock is a reaction to any severe injury, especially one in which your child has been badly burned or suffered heavy bleeding.

What can I do?

SYMPTOMS

▲ Pale, cold, sweaty skin
▲ blue or grayish tinge inside the lips or under the fingernails
▲ rapid and shallow breathing
▲ restlessness
▲ drowsiness or confusion
▲ unconsciousness.

EMERGENCY

Call for emergency help immediately if your child is in shock.

1 Lay your child down on her back, if possible on a coat or blanket. Turn her head to one side, then raise her feet about 8in. (20cm.) and rest them on something, such as a pile of clothes or a bag.
Don't raise her legs if she has a broken leg or a poisonous bite on her leg.

2 Cover her with a blanket or coat, or cuddle her, to keep her warm.
Don't try to warm her up with a hot water bottle or an electric blanket—this only draws blood away from the vital body organs to the skin.

3 If she complains of thirst, moisten her lips with a damp cloth.
Don't give her anything to eat or drink. There is one exception to this—you can give sips of water to your child if she has been badly burned.

4 If she becomes unconscious, check her breathing (see page 230).

✚ **If she is not breathing,** start artificial respiration (see pages 231–32).

✚ **If she is breathing,** put her into the recovery position (see page 233).

POISONING

Poisoning is one of the most common emergencies in young children. Keep poisonous substances locked up, and post the number of the nearest Poison Control Center by your telephone. Never hesitate to call.

What can I do?
1 If your child is unconscious, check his breathing (see page 230).

✚ **If he is not breathing,** start artificial respiration immediately (see pages 231–32), but wipe his face first (see above) or place a fine cloth over his mouth and breathe through that, to avoid getting any poison into your own mouth.

✚ **If he is breathing,** put him into the recovery position (see page 233).

SYMPTOMS

Your child's symptoms will depend on the type of poison he has swallowed. You may notice any of these signs:
▲ stomach pain
▲ vomiting
▲ symptoms of shock (see above)
▲ convulsions
▲ drowsiness
▲ unconsciousness
▲ burns or discoloration around the mouth if your child has swallowed a corrosive poison
▲ poison or empty container nearby.

EMERGENCY

Call for emergency help immediately if you think your child has swallowed something poisonous.

2 If you see signs of burning around your child's mouth, or think he has swallowed a chemical product, wash his skin and lips with water. If he is conscious, give him some milk or water to drink. Try to find out what he has taken, and when.

3 If the doctor recommends that you induce vomiting—**always check first**—use one tablespoon of ipecac syrup for a baby or young child and two for your older child.

4 If your child vomits, save a sample for medical personnel. If he isn't able to vomit, he may have his stomach emptied at the hospital.

BURNS AND SCALDS

A small, superficial burn that causes reddening of the skin over an area of about 1in. (2 to 3cm.) is a minor burn, and can safely be treated at home. A burn that affects an area greater than this is a major burn, and is dangerous for your child, since fluid is lost from the damaged area and infection can enter it. For sunburn, see page 221.

For sunburn, see page 221.

MINOR BURNS
What can I do?

1 Cool the burn immediately, by holding it under cold, slowly running water until the pain decreases. This will help to prevent blisters from developing.

2 If a blister develops, put a pad of clean, non-fluffy material over it and hold it in place with adhesive bandages or surgical tape.
Don't burst the blister – it protects the damaged area underneath while the new skin is growing.
Don't put any cream or lotion on the burn.

BURNING CLOTHES
What can I do?

1 Lay your child on the ground with the burning area up. Avoid touching the burning area with your hands or your own clothes, if possible.

2 Put out the fire by throwing water on it or smothering the flames with a rug, blanket, or heavy curtain, keeping this away from your child's head if possible.
Don't throw water over him if he is near an electrical appliance that is turned on.
Don't try to smother the flames with nylon or any other flammable fabric.
Don't let him rush outside —air will only fan the flames.

3 When the flames are out, treat your child for a major burn (see right).

treat your child for a major burn (see right).

> ■ **EMERGENCY** ■
>
> Get your child professional medical help as soon as you have given first aid if:
> ▲ the burn covers an area of more than about 1in. (2 to 3cm.)
> ▲ the burn was caused by an electric shock (see page 243).

MAJOR BURNS
What can I do?

Cut his undershirt *down the front and remove it with his stretchsuit*

1 Remove any loose clothing that has been soaked in boiling water, fat, or corrosive chemicals, taking care not to let it touch your child's skin anywhere else. Cut his clothes off rather than pull them over his face.
Don't remove dry, burned clothing, or any clothing that is sticking to the burn.

2 Cool the burn immediately by drenching it with cold water: put your child in a cold bath or soak a sheet or towel in cold water and cover the burn with this.
Don't rub his skin.

✚ **If chemicals have burned his skin,** wash them off with plenty of cold water, but **don't** let the water run onto unharmed areas.

3 Cover the area very loosely with a clean, non-fluffy material. If you don't have a sterile dressing, an ironed handkerchief or pillowcase will do.

4 Check for symptoms of shock, and treat your child for this if necessary (see opposite). If he complains of being thirsty, give him sips of water.

treat your child for this if necessary (see opposite).

HEAVY BLEEDING

If blood spurts forcefully from a wound, or bleeding continues for more than five minutes, try to stem the flow so that the blood has a chance to clot.

What can I do?

1 Raise the injured part above the level of your child's heart, to reduce the amount of blood flowing through it. Check for embedded objects in the wound; if there are any, treat them as described below.

2 Place a pad of clean, non-fluffy material over the wound—a clean handkerchief or dishtowel is ideal—then press hard on it for about ten minutes. If there is no clean material available, press with your fingers, drawing the edges of the cut firmly together.

3 Leaving the original pad in place, bind a clean pad or dressing firmly over the wound so that the pressure is maintained. If this becomes soaked with blood, don't remove it, just bandage another pad over it, maintaining the pressure all the time.

4 Check for symptoms of shock (see page 236), and treat your child for this if necessary.

> ■ **EMERGENCY** ■
>
> Get your child professional medical help as soon as you have given first aid if he's been bleeding heavily.

EMBEDDED OBJECTS

Small pieces of dirt in a cut will probably be washed out by bleeding, and larger pieces may wipe easily off the surface of the wound. However, if your child has something embedded in a wound, treat it as shown below.

What can I do?

1 If your child's wound is bleeding heavily, raise the injured part above the level of his heart and apply pressure around the embedded object, not directly on it. If this seems to make the bleeding worse, release the pressure. **Don't** try to pull the object out and don't probe or try to clean the wound.

Lightly cover *the embedded object and the fabric ring with a piece of gauze*

2 Release the pressure for a moment, and roll up a small piece of material such as a clean handkerchief into a sausage shape, then twist this into a ring.

3 Place the ring of material round the cut and cover it with gauze, then bandage it in place firmly. **Don't** bandage tightly *over* the embedded object.

> ■ **EMERGENCY** ■
>
> Get your child professional medical help as soon as you have given first aid if he has an embedded object.

CUTS AND SCRAPES

Cuts and scrapes are common through-out childhood, and you can treat most of them yourself at home. Keep your child's tetanus injections up to date (see page 196), since tetanus can result from dirt entering a wound. Treat an animal bite as a cut, but if your child has a poisonous bite or sting, see page 244.

(see page 196)

see page 244

■ EMERGENCY ■

Call your pediatrician and get your child professional medical help as soon as you have given first aid if:
▲ the cut is large or deep
▲ the cut has gaping edges
▲ your child has cut his face badly
▲ the cut or scrape is very dirty
▲ your child has a puncture wound (a deep cut with only a small opening in the skin) caused by something like a rusty nail or animal's tooth.
Consult your doctor as soon as possible if the area around the wound later becomes tender and red—it may be infected.

What can I do?

1 Wash your hands first, if possible. Clean the cut by holding it under running water, or wiping gently around it with an antiseptic swab or cotton soaked in warm water. Use a clean ball or piece of cotton for each stroke.
Don't remove anything that is embedded in the cut (see opposite).

✚ **If your child has been bitten by an animal,** wash the wound thoroughly with soap and water.

2 If the cut is still bleeding after five minutes, press a pad such as a clean handkerchief firmly on it for a few minutes.

3 Put an adhesive bandage or dressing over it, to help protect it and keep it clean. **Don't** put any antiseptic ointment on your child's cut.

4 Keep the cut covered with an adhesive bandage or a dressing until it has completely healed. This ensures that the area remains moist, and helps the cut heal more quickly. Change the bandage every day.

NOSEBLEEDS

Nosebleeds can result from a bump on the nose, nose-picking, or excessive nose-blowing. Sometimes there is no apparent reason for them. A few children seem prone to nosebleeds, probably because they have unusually fragile blood vessels in their noses.

■ CALL THE DOCTOR ■

Call your doctor now if your child's nose is still bleeding just as badly after half an hour. Consult your doctor if your child has frequent, severe nosebleeds.

What can I do?

1 Help your child to lean forward over a bowl or sink, and pinch her nostrils firmly together for about ten minutes. Try to stop her from sniffing or swallowing the blood—encourage her to spit it out into the bowl instead.

Pinch your child's nostrils firmly

2 If her nose is still bleeding, hold a cloth wrung out in very cold water, or an ice pack wrapped in a cloth, over her nose for about two minutes, then pinch her nose again.

3 Don't have your child blow her nose for about four hours after the bleeding has stopped.

HEAD AND FACE INJURY

Bumps on the head are common in young children, and may raise a sizeable bruise, but are seldom serious. A cut on the forehead or scalp, even a very small one, is likely to bleed profusely.

If your child has had a severe blow to her head, she may suffer from a concussion, which results when the brain is shaken within the skull, or from bleeding inside the skull. However, this is not always apparent for several hours. Signs of these injuries are listed below.

EMERGENCY

Call for emergency help immediately if your child has injured her head and shows any unusual behavior or has any of these symptoms up to 24 hours later:
▲ unconsciousness, however brief
▲ vomiting
▲ noisy breathing or snoring, if your child doesn't normally snore
▲ difficulty in waking, or abnormal drowsiness
▲ discharge of clear or blood-stained fluid from her nose or ear
▲ unusual crying
▲ severe headache
▲ dislike of bright light.

BROKEN TEETH
If your child has broken a tooth, or one has become dislodged, cover the tooth or broken piece with milk, and take your child and her tooth to your dentist or to a hospital immediately.

What can I do?

1 If your child's head is bruised, hold a cloth wrung out in very cold water, or an ice pack wrapped in a damp cloth, over the bruise. This may stop it from swelling. Check the skin underneath every minute, and remove the pack if a red patch with a white waxy center develops.

2 If your child's head is bleeding, place a clean cloth over the cut and press on it, just as you would for bleeding anywhere else on the body (see page 238).

3 Watch your child carefully for the next 24 hours, in case she develops any of the emergency signs listed in the box, left. If she bumped her head badly, wake her every three hours. If she won't wake up, **call for emergency help immediately**.

4 If a discharge of clear or blood-stained fluid trickles from your child's nose or ear, put her into the recovery position with a pad of clean material placed under her nose or ear. If the fluid is coming from her ear, lay her on the injured side, so that the fluid can drain away. **Don't** stop it from trickling out.

BRUISES AND SWELLING

A bruise appears when a fall or blow causes bleeding into the tissues beneath the skin, which produces swelling and discoloration. Bruises normally fade gradually, and disappear after about a week.

CRUSHED FINGERS AND TOES
If your child has crushed his fingers in a door or window, or dropped something heavy on his foot, hold the injured area under cold running water for a few minutes. If it is very swollen, or still painful after half an hour, get professional medical help.

What can I do?

1 Hold a pad wrung out in very cold water, or an ice pack wrapped in a damp cloth, over the bruise for about half an hour. This should help to reduce pain and swelling.

2 If your child seems to be in great pain or if it hurts him to use a bruised limb, especially if the swelling is severe, check for any signs of a sprained joint or a broken bone (see opposite).

SPRAINED JOINTS

When a joint is sprained, the ligaments (tough fibers that support the joint) are damaged. This can cause symptoms very much like a broken bone: if you are not sure which it is, treat it as a broken bone (see below).

What can I do?

1 Gently take off your child's shoe and sock, or anything else that might constrict swelling around the injured joint.

Rest *the injured joint on some soft material*

2 Support the injured joint in the most comfortable position for your child, then hold a cloth wrung out in ice-cold water, or an ice pack wrapped in a damp cloth, on the joint, to reduce swelling and pain.

3 Wrap a thick layer of cotton or a clean cloth around the joint, then bandage it firmly, but not so tightly that the beds of his toenails (or fingernails if you have bandaged his wrist or elbow) turn white or pale blue.

FRACTURES AND DISLOCATED JOINTS

Broken bones are unusual in babies and young children: their bones have not yet hardened, so they are flexible and tend to bend rather than break. Sometimes there may be a partial break, which mends easily (often called a "greenstick" fracture). A joint is dislocated if one or more bones have slipped out of place.

If you think your child's neck or back might be broken, do not move him or change his position unless he stops breathing (see pages 229–30).

What can I do?

1 Gently take off your child's shoe and sock, or anything else that might constrict swelling around the injured area.
Don't move him unless it is absolutely essential.

2 Support the injured part in the most comfortable position for your child.
For a broken wrist, arm or collarbone, put padding around the injured area and, if your child will let you, gently fold his arm across his chest, then support it in a sling. Don't try to force his arm into this position.

Tie *the bandages on the uninjured side*

For a broken leg or ankle, lay your child down and put padding around the injured area and between his knees and ankles. Bandage the injured leg to the uninjured one, securing it above and below the injury. Put some padding under the knots.

3 Check for symptoms of shock and treat him for this if necessary (see page 236). If you think he has a broken leg, don't raise his legs.

FOREIGN BODY IN THE EYE

Eyelashes or particles of dust can easily get into the eye. If your child's eye seems irritated but you can't see anything in it, she may have an eye infection (see page 202).

SYMPTOMS

▲ Pain in the eye
▲ red, watering eye
▲ your child may rub her eye.

CHEMICALS IN THE EYE
If your child has splashed any chemicals or corrosive fluids in her eyes, wash her eyes out immediately under cold running water, keeping her eyelids apart with your fingers. If only one eye is affected, tilt her head so that the injured eye is lower, and the chemical cannot wash over into the uninjured one. Then cover the eye with a pad and take your child to a hospital. If possible, take the chemical bottle with you.

What can I do?

1 Wait a few minutes to see if the natural watering of the eye washes the foreign body away. Try to stop your child from rubbing her eye.

2 If the object is still there, examine your child's eye under a good light. Ask her to look up while you pull her lower eyelid gently down with your thumb.

3 If you can see the object on the white part of your child's eye, try to remove it by sweeping across it very gently with the corner of a clean handkerchief or a piece of damp, twisted cotton.

4 If you can't see anything, hold the eyelashes and draw the upper lid gently outward and down over the lower lid. If the object is under the upper lid, this may dislodge it.

5 If your child's eye still feels gritty or painful, or if the object is not on the white of the eye, or not easily removable, cover the eye with a pad of cotton secured with a bandage and seek professional medical care. Try to stop her from rubbing her eye.
Don't try to remove anything on the central colored part of the eye, or anything that is embedded in the white of the eye.

FOREIGN BODY IN THE EAR

Insects may crawl into your child's ear, and children sometimes push small objects into their ears. Don't let your child play with beads, marbles or similar small objects until he is old enough to understand that they should not be put into his ears.

SYMPTOMS

▲ Tickling in the ear
▲ partial deafness
▲ your child may rub or tug at his ear.

What can I do?

Tip the container
very gently, so just a few drops go into his ear

1 Put a towel around your child's shoulders, then hold his head on one side, with the affected ear on top, and pour a few drops of lukewarm water into his ear.

2 Tip his head the other way, so that the affected ear is underneath. The water may wash out whatever was in his ear. If this doesn't work, seek professional medical attention for him.

FOREIGN BODY IN THE NOSE

Children sometimes stuff small pieces of food or other objects such as beads up their noses.

SYMPTOMS

▲ Smelly, blood-stained discharge from the nose.

What can I do?
If your child can blow his nose, help him to blow it, one nostril at a time. If this does not dislodge the object, don't try to remove it yourself—get professional medical help right away.

ELECTRIC SHOCK

A mild electrical shock gives only a brief pins and needles sensation. A severe one can knock your child down, render her unconscious, and stop both breathing and heartbeat. Electric current can also burn.

If your child touches a faulty appliance with wet hands, she will get a worse shock than touching it with dry hands.

EMERGENCY

Get your child to the hospital as soon as you have given first aid if:
▲ she was unconscious, even if only for a few seconds
▲ she has any electrical burns.

What can I do?

1 Turn off the electricity, at the source.

✚ **If you can't do this,** stand on an insulating material—such as a rubber mat or a pile of dry newspaper. Separate your child from the electrical source by pushing the cable or your child away, using some dry, nonconducting object such as a wooden chair or broom handle.

✚ **If nothing is available,** drag your child away, insulating your hand as much as you can by wrapping it in a dry cloth or newspaper. Grasp your child's clothes, and avoid touching her skin.

Move *the cable rather than your child's arm*

ELECTRICAL BURNS

Electricity can burn where the current enters the body and where it leaves, so your child may have burns where she touched the electrical source and anywhere that was in contact with the ground. Although these burns may look small, they are often very deep.

2 Check to see if your child is conscious (see page 230).

✚ **If she is unconscious,** check her breathing: start artificial respiration immediately if necessary (see pages 231–32). If she is breathing, put her in the recovery position (see page 233).

✚ **If she is conscious,** comfort and reassure her. Look for symptoms of shock (see page 236).

3 Examine her for any burns: check areas that were in contact with the electrical source or the ground (burns will look red or scorched, and may swell up). If you find any, treat them as major burns (see page 237).

INSECT BITES AND STINGS

Most plants, insects and jellyfish cause only minor stings which, while they may be painful, are not dangerous for your child. However, a few people develop a serious allergic reaction to stings, and therefore need urgent medical treatment.

■ SYMPTOMS ■
▲ Sharp pain
▲ redness
▲ slight swelling
▲ itching.

■ EMERGENCY ■

Get your child to a hospital emergency room as soon as you have given first aid if he:
▲ has difficulty breathing
▲ develops a widespread rash
▲ feels dizzy or faints
▲ develops symptoms of shock (see page 236)
▲ has a sting inside his mouth.

What can I do?

1 If your child has been stung by a bee, see if the stinger has been left in the skin. Scrape it off with a fingernail, or pull it out with tweezers. If the tiny sac of poison is visible and still intact, try not to squeeze it.

2 Hold a cloth wrung out in ice-cold water over the sting.

✚ **If he has been stung in his mouth,** give him a cold drink or, if he is over two, let him suck an ice cube. This helps to reduce swelling.

3 Soothe the area around the sting, which will quickly become red, swollen and itchy, by dabbing it gently with cotton balls dipped in calamine lotion or by applying a little antihistamine ointment to the area around the sting.

SNAKE AND SPIDER BITES, SCORPION STINGS

Bites from snakes and poisonous spiders, and scorpion stings are always serious for young children. Snake bites carry a risk of tetanus, but your child can be vaccinated against this.

Ask your pediatrican for information about local varieties of snakes, spiders or scorpions.

What can I do?

1 Calm your child, and help him to sit down. Keep the bitten or stung part still, and position it below the level of his heart.

2 Wash thoroughly around the area, but **don't** suck out any poison.

3 Check for shock, and treat your child for this if necessary (see page 236). If he was bitten or stung on his leg or foot, don't raise his legs.

4 If he becomes unconscious, check his breathing (see page 230).

✚ **If he is not breathing,** start artificial respiration (see pages 231–32).

✚ **If he is breathing,** put him into the recovery position (see page 233).

5 Try to identify the snake, spider or scorpion. If it has been caught, show it to the doctor.

■ SYMPTOMS ■
Your child's symptoms will depend on what has bitten or stung him; some symptoms may not appear for a few hours:
▲ severe pain
▲ one or two puncture marks
▲ swelling
▲ nausea or vomiting
▲ difficulty breathing
▲ shock (see page 236)
▲ convulsions
▲ drowsiness
▲ unconsciousness.

Keep *the bitten part lower than his heart*

■ EMERGENCY ■

Get your child to a hospital as soon as you have given first aid if he has been bitten by a snake or spider, or stung by a scorpion.

SEVERE JELLYFISH STINGS

The type of jellyfish most likely to give you or your child a severe sting is the Portuguese man-of-war. This gelatinous, pale marine creature has tentacles that can be as long as 50 feet and doesn't just live in waters near Portugal. Its sting feels like a hot iron and will make your child very sick.

■ SYMPTOMS ■
▲ Burning pain
▲ redness
▲ shortness of breath
▲ fainting.

What can I do?

1 If your child still has any tentacles stuck to her skin, wash the area with fresh water and then scrape it with wet sand. Avoid touching any tentacles yourself.

2 Put your child into the recovery position (see page 233) and cover her with something dry.

■ EMERGENCY ■
Get professional medical help as soon as you have given first aid if she has a severe jellyfish sting.

THORNS AND SPLINTERS

Thorns or tiny splinters in a child's hands or feet are quite common. Those on your child's feet may not hurt, but splinters in the tips of his fingers will.

■ CALL THE DOCTOR ■
Consult your doctor as soon as possible if:
▲ the area around a splinter becomes red, swollen or tender up to 48 hours later
▲ you cannot remove a large or painful splinter
▲ your child has a splinter of glass or metal.

What can I do?

Grip the end of the splinter

1 If the end of the splinter is sticking out, sterilize a pair of tweezers in a flame, then pull the splinter straight out gently. Wash the area thoroughly with soap and water.

2 If there is no loose end, but you can see the splinter clearly, it is probably lying just below the surface of the skin. Sterilize a needle in a flame and let it cool, but don't touch the point. Then, starting where the splinter entered, gently tear the skin a little way along the line of the splinter. Carefully lift up the end of the splinter with the needle point and pull it out with tweezers, then wash the area thoroughly with soap and water.

3 If a small splinter has gone straight down into the skin, and is not painful, leave it alone. It will probably work its own way out in time. If your child is in pain, call your pediatrician.

BLISTERS

Blisters form when burns, scalds, or friction damage the skin. The fluid-filled blister protects the new skin forming underneath. It will peel off of its own accord in a few days.

What can I do?

1 Don't burst or prick the blister. Dress your child in clothes that will not rub against it.

Cover the blister with an adhesive bandage to prevent your child's shoe from rubbing it

2 If the blister bursts, leave it uncovered, unless it is likely to be exposed to further friction (for example, if it is on your child's foot). In this case, protect the blister with an adhesive bandage.

GROWTH CHARTS

GIRLS

THE CHARTS BELOW show average growth in children (the solid line), and the range of normal measurements. You can check your baby's progress by weighing and measuring her regularly. The pediatrician will do this, but you too can mark her growth curves on the charts. A healthy rate of growth is indicated by the shape of the "average" curve.

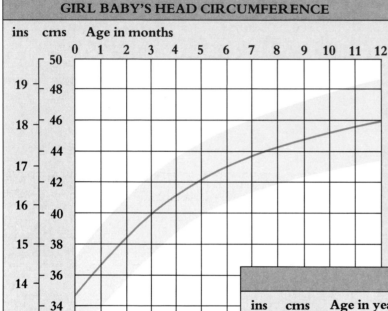

GIRL BABY'S HEAD CIRCUMFERENCE

HEAD CIRCUMFERENCE

Your pediatrician will measure this for you (see page 81). During the first year of life, head circumference is an easier yardstick of healthy growth to measure than length.

ROUGH GUIDE TO CLOTHES SIZES

Size	Weight
0 to 3 months, infant	up to 13lbs
3 to 6 months	14 to 18lbs
6 to 12 months	19 to 22lbs
12 to 18 months	23 to 25lbs
18 to 24 months	26 to 28lbs

Buy clothing according to the weight marked on it, rather than the age, if you can. After age two, manufacturers often call sizes Toddler, or "T".

/ average

range of measurements likely in a normal child; 94% of girls fall within this area

GIRL CHILD'S HEIGHT

YOUR CHILD'S HEIGHT

About every six months measure your child standing up against the same wall. She should stand close to it, without shoes and with feet together. Use a ruler at right angles to the wall to mark her height lightly in pencil, then measure from mark to floor. Don't worry if she has periods of slow growth interspersed with spurts; but if two consecutive measurements seem low, ask your doctor about it.

GIRL BABY'S WEIGHT

YOUR BABY'S WEIGHT

Your baby's weight gain is a vital indicator of her general health and well being throughout the first year. Your pediatrician will weigh her once a month, wearing just a clean diaper, and more often if you are at all worried that she might not be gaining normally.

GIRL CHILD'S WEIGHT

YOUR CHILD'S WEIGHT

After her first birthday, your child won't put weight on steadily, but the periods of slow and rapid growth should balance out. She shouldn't *lose* weight: even if she looks fat to you, it won't be long before her height catches up to her weight and she slims down. Ask your doctor for advice if your child's weight drops, or if you are worried about her gaining too much too fast.

BOYS

THE CHARTS BELOW show average growth in children (the solid line), and the range of normal measurements.. You can check your baby's progress by weighing and measuring him regularly. The pediatrician will do this, but you too can mark his growth curves on the charts. A healthy rate of growth is indicated by the shape of the "average" curve.

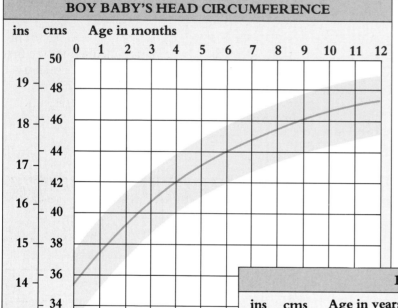

BOY BABY'S HEAD CIRCUMFERENCE

HEAD CIRCUMFERENCE
Your pediatrician will measure this for you (see page 81). During the first year of life, head circumference is an easier yardstick of healthy growth to measure than length.

ROUGH GUIDE TO CLOTHING SIZES

Size	Weight
0 to 3 months, infant	up to 13lbs
3 to 6 months	14 to 18lbs
6 to 12 months	19 to 22lbs
12 to 18 months	23 to 25lbs
18 to 24 months	26 to 28lbs

Buy clothing according to the weight marked on it, rather than the age, if you can. After age two, manufacturers often call sizes Toddler, or "T".

⟋ average

▢ range of measurements likely in a normal child; 94% of boys fall within this area

BOY CHILD'S HEIGHT

YOUR CHILD'S HEIGHT
About every six months measure your child standing up against the same wall. He should stand close to it, without shoes and with feet together. Use a ruler at right angles to the wall to mark his height lightly in pencil, then measure from mark to floor. Don't worry if he has periods of slow growth interspersed with spurts; but if two consecutive measurements seem low, ask your doctor about it.

BOY BABY'S WEIGHT

YOUR BABY'S WEIGHT

Your baby's weight gain is a vital indicator of his general health and well being throughout the first year. Your pediatrician will weigh him once a month, wearing just a clean diaper, and more often if you are at all worried that he might not be gaining normally.

BOY CHILD'S WEIGHT

YOUR CHILD'S WEIGHT

After his first birthday, your child won't put weight on steadily, but the periods of slow and rapid growth should balance out. He shouldn't *lose* weight: even if he looks fat to you, it won't be long before his height catches up to his weight and he slims down. Ask your doctor for advice if your child's weight drops, or if you are worried about him gaining too much too fast.

INDEX

A

A & D ointment, 148, 153
  applying on a boy, 151
  applying on a girl, 150
abdomen: abdominal pain, 212
  examination, 36, 69, 81, 184, 212
abnormalities, congenital, 19
abscess, breast, 96
absence attacks, 225
accidents: first aid, 229-45
  lifesaving techniques, 230-33
  safety precautions, 226-28
acetaminophen, 188, 190, 197
activity centers, 121
AFP test, 19, 37
afterpains, 71
age of mother, 10
aggression, in children, 171
alcohol: alternatives to, 53
  and breast-feeding, 93
  and conception, 11
  in pregnancy, 12, 13
allergies: asthma, 210-11
  breast-feeding and, 87
  diaper rash, 176
  eczema, 220
  hives, 219
  milk, 102
  stings, 244
alpha fetoprotein (AFP) test, 19, 37
ambulances, 229
American Academy of Pediatrics,
  102, 112
American College of Nurse
  Midwives, 32, 33
American College of Obstetricians
  and Gynecologists, 33
amniocentesis, 19, 37
amniotic fluid, 23
anemia, 34, 35, 38, 52
anesthetics: children, 185
  epidural, 64, 67
  general, 65, 67
  local, 64-65
animal bites, 239
ankles: fractures, 241
  swollen, 36, 42
anti-colic nipples, 99
antibiotics, 189, 196
antibodies: from breast milk, 87, 92
  and immunization, 196
  in newborn babies, 174
anxiety: in children, 119, 170
  and missed period, 12
  in pregnancy, 19
  separation, 163
  and stomach pain, 212
Apgar score, 63
appendicitis, 212
appetite: adjusting bottle-feedings
  to, 102, 106
  letting child control, 87, 108, 115,
    116
  loss of, 174, 180
  in pregnancy, 18, 19
  premature babies, 80
  sick children, 192
  stimulating breast milk, 92
apron, 134
areola, 90
  expressing milk, 94-95

areola continued
  positioning baby on, 91, 96
  in pregnancy, 22
  swollen, 93
  see also breasts; nipples
arms: development of fetus's, 15, 17,
  19, 21, 23
  fractures, 241
artificial respiration, 229, 230-31
aspirin, 13, 190, 197
assisted delivery, 66
asthma, 210-11
  and eczema, 220
  and frequent chest infections, 208
attention lapses, 180

B

baby carriage, *see* carriage
baby food: commercial, 110
  home-made, 109, 110-11
baby walker, 161
baby wipes, 134, 148
babysitters, 163
back injuries, 229
backache: and bathing, 138
  in labor, 59
  preventing in pregnancy, 44
  using an infant carrier, 85
  see also posture
backpack, 156
bacteria: in formula milk, 87, 102,
  215
  see also gastroenteritis
bacterial infections, 189
bad behavior, 170-71
balanitis, 217
balls, 161, 162
bandages, 229
barrier creams, 148
  applying on a boy, 151
  applying on a girl, 150
  and runny nose, 195
  and spots, 218
bassinet, 27, 120, 122
bath liquid, 135
bath mats, 134
bathing babies, 134-43
bathrooms, safety, 227
bathtub, baby, 134, 138
bed: birthing, 32
  for night feedings, 125
bed rest, sick children, 193
bedding, crib, 120, 121
bedrooms, safety, 227
bedtime: routines, 120, 124-25, 126
  unsettled, 126
bedwetting, 155
bee stings, 244
behavior problems, 170-71
bibs, 108
bilirubin, 70
birth, *see* labor
birthing bed, 32
birthing centers, 32
birthing rooms, 32
birthmarks, 68, 69
  in pregnancy, 21
bites, 239, 244
biting: in breast-feeding, 97
  dealing with, 171

bladder: after labor, 71
  infections, 216
  in labor, 61
  in pregnancy, 28, 41
  toilet training, 154-55
blankets: buying for newborn, 27,
  120
  security, 163
  swaddling baby in, 123
bleeding: after labor, 71
  from cord stump, 136
  emergencies, 238
  gums, 20, 40
  miscarriage, 39
  nosebleeds, 239
  vaginal, 39, 71
blepharitis, 202
blisters, 245
  burns and scalds, 237
  cold sores, 222
blood: in pregnancy, 16, 31
  in stools, 146, 174, 213
  tests, 35
blood groups, rhesus negative, 38
blood pressure, 35
  after birth, 73
  low, and faintness, 40
  raised, and preeclampsia, 38
blue patches, 69
blues, postnatal, 71
blurred vision, 38
bodysuits, 128
  taking off, 132
boiling, sterilizing bottle-
  feeding equipment, 100
boils, 218
bones, fractures, 241
booster seats, 109
bootees, 129
bottle brushes, 99
bottle-feeding, 98-107
  adding sugar, 213
  advantages and disadvantages, 87
  away from home, 87, 101
  burping, 107
  changing to, 97, 106
  diluting feedings after
    gastroenteritis, 179
  formula milk, 88, 101, 102, 103-5,
    179
  gas and burping, 88
  giving a feeding, 106-7
  making up formula, 102-5, 179
  nipples, 98, 99, 101
  ready-to feed formula, 102, 103
  sterilizing equipment, 99-101,
    215
  and thirsty babies, 113, 117
  weaning, 113
bottles, 98, 105
bottoms: cleaning, 150-51
  genital problems, 217
  sore, 118, 150, 176
  wiping, 155
  see also diaper rash
"bouncer", 162
bowels: contents at birth, 31, 69, 146
  in labor, 61
  moving after birth, 71
  normal movements in children,
    213
  in pregnancy, 16, 40
  toilet training, 154-55

bowels continued
  see also constipation; diarrhea;
    stools
bowls, spillproof, 108
brain: concussion, 240
  development of fetus's, 15, 23, 25
  encephalitis, 225
  epilepsy, 225
  meningitis, 225
bras: for breast-feeding, 29, 55, 96
  for pregnancy, 17, 23
Braxton Hicks contractions, 24, 30,
  31, 56
bread, 51, 52
  for children, 110, 116, 213
breast abscess, 96
breast-feeding, 90-97
  advantages and disadvantages, 87
  after birth, 63
  changing to bottle-feeding, 97,
    106
  and contraception, 73
  expressing milk, 94-95
  latching on, 90, 91
  let-down reflex, 91
  milk production, 92
  night feedings, 87, 88, 97, 126
  problems, 96
  routine, 97
  weaning, 97, 113
breast milk, 87, 88, 92, 93, 97
breast pads, 55, 91, 96
breasts: after breast-feeding, 93
  baby's at birth, 68
  blocked duct, 96
  care of, 96
  engorged, 93, 96
  leaking, 96
  mastitis, 96
  nursing bras, 29, 55
  in pregnancy, 12, 16, 18, 20
  pregnancy bras, 23
  stopping breast milk, 97
  see also areola; nipples
breathing, 208
  after birth, 63
  artificial respiration, 230-31
  checking, 230
  emergencies, 174, 208
  exercises, 19, 23, 49, 56
  in labor, 59, 60
  wheeziness, 208, 210
breathlessness, 26, 28, 40
  see also asthma; bronchitis
breech birth, 67
broken bones, 241
bronchitis, 210
  and flu, 195
bruises, 240
brushes: hair, 135
  treating lice and nits, 224
bumper, crib, 121
burns, 237
  electrical, 243
burping, 88, 92, 107
"butterfly mask", 21

C

C-section, *see* Cesarean section
caffeine: and breast-feeding, 93
  in pregnancy, 53
calcium, 50
carriage, 21, 27, 120
  advantages and disadvantages,
    156
  choosing, 156
  for daytime sleep, 120, 122
  for soothing baby, 78, 125
carrier, infant, *see* infant carrier
cars: car seats, 156, 157, 228
  putting babies to sleep, 125
  safety, 157, 228
  traveling in, 157
cat nets, 228
catch, playing, 162
caudal anesthesia, 64
celiac disease, 215
cervix, 14
  after birth, 73
  examination of, 36, 73
  incompetent, 38
  in labor, 57, 60
  pap smear, 36
Cesarean section, 67
  anesthesia, 65
  exercising after, 72
chairs, high, 109, 116
changing mat, 146, 147, 148,
  156, 227
chapped skin, 221
checkups: prenatal clinics, 19, 34–37
  six-week, 73, 80–81
cheese, snacks for children, 116
chemicals: burns, 237
  in eyes, 242
chest: antibiotics to clear infections,
    189
  external compression, 232
  infections, 195, 208
chicken pox, 199
  and antibiotics, 189
chilling, 178
chocolate, 53
  see also sweets
choking, 123, 234
chorionic villus sampling
  (CVS), 37
circulation: checking, 232
  in pregnancy, 21
  see also blood
circumcision, 217
clinics, prenatal, 19, 34–37
cloth diapers, 146, 148, 149, 153
clothes: baby, 27, 128–33
  burning, 237
  children dressing themselves, 133
  dressing up, 166
  in pregnancy, 18, 25
  sizes, 246, 248
coffee: and breast-feeding, 93
  in pregnancy, 12, 53
cold sores, 206, 222
colds, 118, 194–95
  and antibiotics, 189
colic, 118, 174
collar-bones, fractures, 241
coloring, painting, 166
colostrum, 20, 87, 92, 93

combs, 135
  treating lice and nits, 224
comforters, 120, 121
conception, 13, 14
  planning for, 10
concussion, 240
conjunctivitis, 177, 202
constipation: in children, 213
  in pregnancy, 16, 17, 38, 40, 51
contraception, 73
contraceptive pill, 10
  and breast-feeding, 73
contractions: afterpains, 71
  Braxton Hicks, 24, 30, 31, 56
  coping with, 58–61
  first stage of labor, 56
  second stage of labor, 60
  timing, 56
  transition stage of labor, 60
convenience foods, 53
convulsions: epilepsy, 225
  feverish, 188
  and immunization, 196
corpus luteum, 14
cotton balls, 134, 148
cotton swabs, 135
cough, 208, 209
  fetus in womb, 23
  medication, 201, 209
  whooping cough, 196, 201
cracked nipples, 96
cradle, 120, 122
cradle cap, 138, 177
cramps, 24, 40, 71
cravings, 12, 53
crawling, 160
crayons, 165
crib, 21, 27, 120–21, 122
  crib bumper, 121
  safety, 120–21, 123, 227
croup, 208
cruising, 161
crushed fingers and toes, 240
crying, 117–19
  and demand-feeding, 88
  as emergency sign, 174
  in first six weeks, 78
  and sleeping problems, 126
cuddling babies, 117
cups: giving drinks in, 108, 113, 114
  mixing formula milk in, 104
  training, 192
curl-downs, 72
curl-ups, 73
cuts and scrapes, 239
CVS test, 37
cystic fibrosis, 10

D

D. and C. (dilation and curettage),
  39
dandruff, 138
dark, fear of, 170
daytime sleep, 120, 122
deafness, partial, 204, 205
decongestants, 194
dehydration, 214
  in babies, 179
  in children, 192, 214–15
delirium, 188

delivery, *see* labor
delivery date, calculating, 13
demand feeding, 88, 102
Demerol, 64
dentists: for children, 144
  in pregnancy, 17
depression: postnatal, 71
  in pregnancy, 19
development: of child, 158–71
  of fetus, 14–31
diabetes, 10, 34, 38
diagnosing illness, 174–75, 180–84
diaper bag, 156
diaper rash, 146, 150, 175, 176
  avoiding, 149, 150
  cause of crying, 118
  coping with, 150, 176, 217
  and infection, 176, 217
diapers, 146–55
  changing, 138, 143, 146, 147,
    150–53, 176, 227
  cloth, 146, 148, 149, 153
  diaper services, 146, 148
  disposable, 146, 148, 149, 152, 156
  equipment, 148
  giving up, 154–55
  types, 146
diaphragm, contraceptive, 73
diarrhea: babies, 146, 179
  bottle-feeding and, 87
  children, 215
  gastroenteritis, 214–15
  in pregnancy, 38
diet: babies, 108, 110–11
  while breast-feeding, 92
  fiber, 51, 116, 213
  for older children, 116
  pre-pregnancy, 11
  in pregnancy, 50–53
digestive system: baby's, 88
  fetus's, 15
digital thermometers, 186–87
dimmer switches, 121
diphtheria, immunization, 196
discharges: in babies and children,
    217
  vaginal, 20, 42, 68
discipline, 168, 170–71
dishwashers, 100
dislocated joints, 241
disposable diapers, 146, 148,
  149, 152, 156
disposable liners, bottle-
  feeding, 105
dizziness, 225
doctors: examining sick children,
    184
  group practices, 33
  prenatal care, 32, 33
  when to call, 174, 182
dolls, 166
Down's syndrome, 10, 37
DPT immunization, 196
drawing, 165
dreams, in pregnancy, 24
dressing babies, 130–31
dressing children, 133
dressing up, 166
drinking, fetus in womb, 23
drinks: at bedtime, 97
  and bottle-fed babies, 113
  encouraging sick child, 192
  in pregnancy, 52, 53

drinks continued
  to prevent dehydration, 179, 214,
    215
  and weaning, 113
  what to give, 116
droppers, medicine, 189
drops: ear, 191, 204
  eye, 191
  nose, 190, 194
drowning, 235
drugs and medications, 189–91
  and breast-feeding, 93
  for children, 189–91
  and colic, 118
  drops, 190–91
  giving to babies, 189
  giving to children, 190
  in labor, 64
  in pregnancy, 13
  and teething, 119
drying babies, 139
drying cord stump, 136

E

ears, 204
  development of fetus's, 15
  drops, 191, 204
  foreign bodies, 242
  glue ear, 205
  infections, 204, 205
  lying baby down, 123
  wax in, 204
eclampsia, 38
eczema, 220
  and ear infections, 204
edema, 42
EFM (electronic fetal
  monitoring), 65
egg, conception, 14
eggs, for children, 110, 115
electric shocks, 243
electrical burns, 243
electricity, safety, 168, 228
electronic fetal monitoring (EFM),
  65
embedded objects, 238
embryo: development of, 15
  implantation, 14
  see also fetus
emergencies, accidents, 229–45
emergency signs: babies, 174
  children, 182
  in pregnancy, 38
emotional problems: after birth, 71,
    76–77
  and breast-feeding, 96
  in pregnancy, 12, 16
encephalitis, 225
enemas, 57
engaging of fetus's head, 27, 28, 29
engorged breasts, 93, 96
entertainment: in cars, 157
  sick children, 193
epidural anesthesia, 64, 67
epilepsy, 10, 225
  and immunization, 196
episiotomy, 62, 65, 66, 71
equipment: baby clothes, 128–29
  for bathing and washing, 134
  for bottle-feeding, 98–99

equipment continued
buying for newborn, 27, 129
car safety, 157
carriages etc., 156-57
for children in the hospital, 185
clothes for pregnancy, 25
for diaper-changing, 148-49
for expressing milk, 94-95
for feeding solid foods, 108-9
for first aid, 229
for labor and birth, 54-55
for sleep, 120-1
for toilet training, 154-55
for traveling, 156
exercises: before pregnancy, 11
breathing, 19, 23, 49, 56
classes, 17
pelvic floor, 27, 41, 45, 71, 72, 73
postnatal, 71, 72-3
in pregnancy, 40, 43-49
relaxation, 29, 43, 48-49, 56
expressing milk, 94-95
external chest compression, 232
eye contact, 78, 86, 159
eyes: baby's, 68
blepharitis, 202
conjunctivitis, 202
development of fetus's, 15, 17, 22, 23, 24
drops, 177, 191
foreign bodies in, 242
and measles, 198
ointment, 191
problems, 202-3
squints, 68, 80, 203
sticky eye, 177
styes, 203
watering, 175
eyesight, 68, 80, 159

F

face injuries, 240
fainting, 40, 225
Fallopian tubes, 14
family-centered births, 32
family practitioners, 33
fathers, in labor, 29, 57, 58, 59, 60, 61, 62
fears, 170
feces: and toxoplasma, 13
see also stools
feeding, 87-116
at bedtime, 97, 113, 125, 126
bottle-feeding, 87, 88, 98-107, 179
breast-feeding, 87, 88, 90-97
demand feeding, 88, 102
gas and burping, 88, 107
after gastroenteritis, 179
night feedings, 125, 126
older children, 116
premature babies, 80, 88
self-feeding, 114-15
sick children, 192
solid foods, 108-15
to sooth babies, 117
twins, 88
feet: baby's, 68
checking at birth, 69
exercising after birth, 72

feet continued
plantar's warts, 222-23
and walking, 133, 164
see also shoes
fertility, 15
fertilization, 14
fertilizers, safety, 228
fetus: development of, 15-31
heartbeat, 19, 36, 57, 63, 65
movements, 21, 23, 25
fever, 186-88
aspirin and, 197
bringing down, 188
convulsions, 188
delirium, 188
reading a thermometer, 186
signs of, 180
taking temperature, 184, 187
fiber, 51, 52, 116, 213
fighting, 171
finger foods, 110-11, 114, 160
fingernails: at birth, 68
care of baby's, 135, 145
fetus's, 29, 30
in pregnancy, 21
fingerprints, 18
fingers: crushed, 240
fetus's, 15, 16, 18, 29
first aid kit, 229
fish, in pregnancy, 50
fits, *see* convulsions
flu, 194, 195
fluid, retention, 22, 42
see also drinks
fluoride: supplements, 102, 144
toothpaste, 116, 135, 144-45
folic acid, 19, 52
fontanelle: at birth, 68, 69
bulging, 225
as emergency sign, 174, 225
handling baby, 68, 82
sunken, 179, 214
symptom of dehydration, 214
symptom of meningitis, 225
food, *see* diet
food cravings, 53
food fads, 115
food mills, 108
food poisoning, *see* gastroenteritis
foods, top, 52
foods to avoid: for children, 110, 111
in pregnancy, 53
foot pedaling exercise, 72
forceful vomiting, 179
forceps delivery, 66
foreign bodies: in ear, 242
embedded in wounds, 238
in eye, 242
in nose, 243
foremilk, 92
foreskin, 135, 137, 151
inflamed, 217
formula milk, *see* bottle-feeding
fractures, 241
fraternal twins, 15
freckles, 18, 21
freezing baby food, 111
friends, 166, 167
fruit: baby food, 110-11
and constipation, 213

fruit continued
purées, 110
vitamins, 51, 116
frustration, 119, 170

G

games, 162
gas, burping, 88, 107
gastroenteritis, 193, 212, 214-15
in babies, 179
bottle-feeding hygiene, 100, 101, 179, 215
prevention, 100, 101, 179, 215
gates: stair, 161, 228
yard, 168, 228
general anesthesia, 65, 67
genetic counseling, 10
genitals: at birth, 68, 69
cleaning, 135, 137, 150-51
playing with, 170
problems, 217
German measles (rubella), 194, 197
immunization, 10, 196
in pregnancy, 10, 35, 197
glands: feeling for, 183, 184
swollen, 180
glue ear, 205
gluten, 215
good behavior, 170-71
grand mal convulsions, 225
grasp reflex, 81
greenstick fractures, 241
group practices, doctors, 33
gums, bleeding, 20, 40

H

hair: at birth, 68
brushing baby's, 135
fetus's, 21, 28
lanugo, 19, 31, 69
lice and nits, 224
in pregnancy, 21
shaving pubic hair, 57
washing baby's, 138, 141, 142
hairbrushes, 135
treating lice and nits, 224
halls, safety, 228
hallucinations, 188
handling babies, 82-86
hands: baby's, 68
and chilling, 178
and clothing, 128, 131
fetus's, 15, 20
learning to use, 128, 131, 166
swollen, 36, 42
harness, safety, 109, 157
hats, 128, 129, 221
to prevent chilling, 178
treating lice and nits, 224
hay fever, 220
head: baby's, 68, 69
cradle cap, 138, 177
engaging of fetus's, 27, 28, 29
injuries, 240
lice, 224
measuring circumference, 81, 246, 248

headache, 38
hearing, 15, 204
baby in womb, 21, 23, 24
partial deafness, 204, 205
heart: baby's, 63, 65, 69, 81
checking for beat, 232
development of fetus's, 15
fetal heartbeat, 19, 25, 31, 36, 57
irregular heartbeat, 69
in pregnancy, 16
resuscitation, 230, 232
heartburn, 24, 28, 41
heat rash, 219
height, measuring, 246, 248
hemophilia, 10
Hemophilus (Hib) infections, immunization, 196
hemorrhoids, 41
herbal teas, 53
hernia, 175, 217
hiccups, 175
fetus in womb, 23
hide-and-seek, 162
high chairs, 109, 116
hindmilk, 92
hips, dislocated, 69, 81
hives, 219
home, safety in, 168, 226-28
home birth, 32
hormones: after labor, 71
in pregnancy, 12, 16, 42
hospitals: admission in labor, 57
children in, 185
emergencies, 229
hospital birth, 32, 33
hunger, 88, 108, 114, 117, 119
see also appetite
hygiene: bottle-feeding, 99, 100, 101, 215
and diarrhea, 215
and gastroenteritis, 214-15
keeping skin clean, 134
solid food, 215
and toxoplasma, 13
vaginal, 42

I

ice cubes, 192
of puréed food, 111
to prevent cold sores, 222
ice popsicles, 192
identical twins, 15
identity, developing a sense of, 171
illness: caring for a sick child, 192-93
diagnosing, 174-75, 180-84
imaginary friends, 166
imagination, 166
imitating adults, 165
immunity: and breast-feeding, 87, 174
to German measles, 10, 35
to infections, 21, 174, 197
immunization, 38, 196
against flu, 195
impetigo, 223
implantation, 14
incompetent cervix, 38
incubators, 70
independence, 114, 133, 164, 170, 171
indigestion, 24, 28

induced labor, 66
infant carrier, 85, 156
    soothing babies, 124
infant seat, 120, 158
infectious illnesses, 197-201
    immunization, 196
    in young babies, 174
influenza, 194, 195
inherited diseases, 10
insect nets, 122, 228
insect stings, 244
insects, in ears, 242
intensive care units, 70
internal examinations, 36, 57, 60, 73
iron: dietary sources, 52
    supplements, 19, 38, 40, 52, 102
itchiness: and chicken pox, 199
    in children, 218
    in pregnancy, 30, 41
IUD, 73

jaundice, 70
jellyfish stings, 245
jigsaw puzzles, 166
joints: development of fetus's, 15, 19
    dislocated, 241
    in pregnancy, 20, 26
    sprained, 241
jumping, 166

kidneys, 216
    infections, 216
    in pregnancy, 16, 34
kitchens, safety, 168, 226
kneeling, in labor, 60, 61

L

labor: birth, 62-63
    breathing exercises, 49
    father and companion, 29, 57, 58,
      59, 60, 61, 62
    first signs, 56
    first stage, 57-59
    home birth, 32
    in the hospital, 32, 33
    learning about, 17, 19
    monitoring, 65
    pain relief, 64-65
    positions, 58-59, 61
    preparation for, 54-55
    second stage, 60
    special procedures, 66
    third stage, 63
    transition, 60
lactose intolerance, 215
lambskins, 121, 125
lanugo, 19, 31, 69
latching on, 90, 91
lavatory, using, 155
laxatives, 40, 213
leaking breasts, 96
leaking urine, 27, 38, 41, 61, 72, 73

leaving children, 163
legs: checks on, 69, 81
    development of fetus's, 15, 17, 19,
      20, 21, 23
    fractures, 241
    swollen, 36, 42
    varicose veins, 29, 36, 42
let-down reflex, 91, 96
lice, 224
lifesaving techniques, 230-33
lifting, in pregnancy, 44
likes and dislikes, 112, 115, 116
linea nigra, 18, 21, 26
liners: diaper, 149
    disposable for bottle-feeding, 105
lips, chapped, 221
living rooms, safety, 228
local anesthesia, 64-65
lotion, baby, 135, 148
love: and babies, 78, 80
    and children, 168, 171
    fears about, 19
    making, 27, 73
lullabies, 125
lungs, 210
    asthma, 210-11
    bronchitis, 210
    development of fetus's, 15, 25
    pneumonia, 211
    see also cough

major seizure, 225
massage, 17, 58, 59
mastitis, 96
masturbation, 170
mattresses, 121
mealtimes, 108, 113, 114-15, 116
measles, 198
    and antibiotics, 189
    and colds, 194
    immunization, 196
meat, 13, 50, 52, 110-11
meconium, 31, 69, 146
medications, *see* drugs
meningitis, 225
menstrual periods: after
      contraceptive pill, 10
    after miscarriage, 39
    and fertility, 15
    first after birth, 73
    missed, 12
meperidine, 64
mercury thermometers, 186-87
microwave ovens, 111
midwives, 32, 33, 57
milia, 175
milk: cow's, 102, 114, 192
    expressing, 94-5
    lactose intolerance, 215
    soy, 102
    see also bottle-feeding; breast-
      feeding
milk spots, 175
milk teeth, 144
mineral supplements, 102
miscarriage, 19, 37, 38, 39
mittens, 128
mobiles, 121
moisturizers, 21, 42, 135, 174

moles, 18, 21
monitoring in labor, 65
morning sickness, 12, 16, 18, 41
mouth: fetus's, 15, 17, 23
    infections, 176, 206
    stings in, 244
multiple pregnancy, 15, 39, 67
mumps, 200
    and antibiotics, 189
    immunization, 196
music, 23, 125

nails, *see* fingernails; toenails
names, learning, 165
naps, 120, 122
    staying dry, 155
nausea: in labor, 60
    in pregnancy, 12, 16, 18, 19, 38, 41
navel, 26, 76, 136, 175
nets, cat/insect, 122, 228
nettle stings, 219
neural tube defects, 37
night: feedings, 87, 88, 97, 125, 126
    giving up diapers, 155
    night waking, 126
    sleep, 122, 124-25
night-lights, 121, 170
nightwear, 27, 55, 129
nipple cream, 55, 96
nipples: breast-feeding, 88, 90-93
    cracked, 96
    expressing milk, 94-95
    feeding premature babies, 88
    flat, 23, 93
    inverted, 23
    in pregnancy, 18, 20, 22, 23
    sore, 55, 78, 96
    see also areola; breasts
nipples (bottle-feeding), 98, 105, 107
    care of, 101
    enlarging holes, 101
    types, 99
nits, 224
noses: drops, 190, 194
    foreign bodies in, 243
    nosebleeds, 239
    wiping, 194
nursery schools, 166
nursing, *see* breast-feeding
nursing bras, 29, 55, 96
nursing sick children, 192-93
nutrition, *see* diet
nuts, 50, 51, 52, 111

obstetric stethoscope, 36, 65
obstetricians, prenatal care, 32, 33
    see also doctors
oil, baby, 135, 148
ointment, eye, 191
operations, children, 185
overheating, 175, 178
    cause of crying, 118
overtiredness, 119
ovulation, 13, 14
oxytocin, 63

pacifiers, 117, 118, 124
pails, diaper, 148, 149
pain: abdominal, 212
    afterpains, 71
    babies and children, 119, 183
    as emergency sign, 38, 174, 182
    in labor, 56, 64-65, 66, 67
    self-help in labor, 59
pain medication, 71, 183
    acetaminophen, 188, 190, 197
    aspirin, 13, 190, 197
    in labor, 64-65
painting, 166
panting, 49, 62
pants: for after birth, 55
    and genital infections, 217
    rubber, 149, 153, 176, 217
    training, 154
paracervical block, 64
"pat-a-cake", 161
patting, soothing babies, 117
peanuts, 50, 52, 111
peek-a-boo, 162
pelvic floor, 45
    and episiotomy, 66
    exercise, 27, 41, 45, 71, 72, 73
pelvic tilt, 45
pelvis, size of, 34
penis: aiming, 155
    avoiding zips, 133
    changing diapers, 151, 152
    playing with, 170
    problems, 217
periods, *see* menstrual periods
personality, 23, 168
pertussis, *see* whooping cough
pesticides, safety, 228
petechial rash, 176, 194
petit mal convulsions, 225
petroleum jelly, 148, 195, 221
pets, 13, 122, 167, 211
phenylketonuria (PKU), 69
phobias, 170
phototherapy, 70
physicians, *see* doctors
picking babies up, 82-84
pigmentation, skin, 18, 20, 21
pinworms, 217, 224
PKU (phenylketonuria), 69
placenta, 23
    bleeding, 39
    delivery, 63
    development of, 14, 18
    food crossing, 53
    placenta previa, 39
    placental abruption, 39
    proportion of weight gain, 31
    "small for dates" babies, 39
plantar warts, 222-23
play, 82, 86, 158-62, 165-67
    bathtime, 141, 142
    before sleep, 124
    diaper-changing, 78, 147
    early morning wakers, 122
    teeth-cleaning, 144
playgroups, 167
playpen, 161, 226
pneumonia, 211
    and flu, 195
poisoning, 236

polio, immunization, 196
popsicles, 192
port wine stains, 69
Portuguese man-of-war stings, 245
postnatal depression, 71
postnatal exercises, 71, 72-73
postpartum checkup, 73
posture, in pregnancy, 16, 21, 24, 28, 44
potty chair, 154-55
powder, baby, 135, 136, 139
preeclampsia, 34, 35, 36, 38
pregnancy, confirming, 12
premature babies: chilling, 178
 development, 159
 feeding, 88
 first weeks, 80
 health care, 174
 special care, 70
prenatal care, 32-42
prenatal checkups, 19, 34-37
prenatal classes, 17, 26, 27
processed foods, 53
protein: in diet, 50
 in urine, 34
pubic hair, shaving, 57
pudendal block, 64-65
pulling up, 161
pulse, 184, 232
pumps, expressing milk with, 95
punishments, 116, 170
purées, 109, 110, 113
pus, sticky eye, 177
puzzles, 166
pyloric stenosis, 179

quilts, 121

R

rashes, 175, 176, 181, 183
 allergies, 101, 102
 chicken pox, 199
 diaper, 118, 146, 149, 150, 175, 176, 217
 as emergency sign, 182
 German measles, 197
 heat rash, 219
 hives, 219
 impetigo, 223
 measles, 198
 newborn baby, 69, 176
 in pregnancy, 41
recovery position, 233
recycling disposable diapers, 149
reflexes: grasp, 81
 let-down, 91, 96
 rooting, 90
 sucking, 107
relaxation exercises, 23, 29, 43, 48-49, 56
rest: after labor, 79
 in pregnancy, 23, 25, 26, 27, 29, 31, 40, 42
 see also sleep
resuscitation, 229, 230-32
rewards, 116, 170

Reye's syndrome, 190, 197
rhesus blood groups, 35, 38
rice cereal, 110
rocking, 86, 117, 124
rolling over, 159
rooting reflex, 90
rubber pants, 149, 153, 176, 217
rubella, see German measles
running, 166

S

saddle block, anesthesia, 64
safety, 119, 168, 226-28
 bathtime, 141
 carriages and strollers, 157
 in cars, 157, 228
 crawling babies, 160
 medicines, 190
 nuts, 111
 pets, 122
 sleeping babies, 120, 121, 123, 227
 stairs, 161, 228
 in the yard, 168, 228
safety diaper pins, 149
safety harnesses, 109
salt: in pregnancy, 38, 52
 in sugar drink, 214
sandboxes, 167, 228
scalds, 237
scans, ultrasound, 19, 37
scars, 21, 67
scissors, nail, 135
scorpion stings, 244
scrapes and cuts, 239
scratching, 218
 and chicken pox, 199
seat belts, 157
seats: booster, 109
 car, 156, 157, 228
 infant, 120, 158
security blanket, 163
sedatives, in labor, 64
seizures, see convulsions
separation anxiety, 163
sex of baby, 15, 19, 37
sexual intercourse: after pregnancy, 73
 in pregnancy, 27
 timing for conception, 15
sexually transmitted diseases, 35
shampoos, 135, 141
shapes, learning, 165
sharing play, 166, 167, 171
shaving pubic hair, 57
sheets, 120, 121
shock, 229, 236
shocks, electric, 243
shoes: for children, 133, 164
 in pregnancy, 21, 25
show, sign of labor, 56
sickle cell trait, 35
sickness, see morning sickness; nausea; vomiting
side bends, 73
sight, see eyesight
sinusitis, 194
sitting: for bathing, 138
 for breast-feeding, 90
 in labor, 61

sitting continued
 learning to sit, 159, 160
 tailor posture, 46
six-week checkup, 80-81
skin: at birth, 63, 69
 birthmarks, 68, 69
 blisters, 245
 boils, 218
 bruises, 240
 burns and scalds, 237
 chapped, 221
 chilling, 118, 178
 cold sores, 222
 cuts and scrapes, 239
 diagnosing problems, 218
 dry, 174
 eczema, 220
 fetus's, 19, 21, 22, 23, 24, 25, 28, 31
 heat rash, 219
 hives, 219
 impetigo, 223
 jaundice, 70
 keeping clean, 134
 milk spots, 175
 overheating, 118, 175, 178
 pigmentation, 18, 20, 21
 in pregnancy, 18, 20, 21, 30, 41
 spots and boils, 218
 stretch marks, 24, 42
 stroking, 130, 132, 159
 sunburn, 221
 tearing in labor, 62
 thorns and splinters, 245
 warts, 222-23
 yellow, see jaundice
 see also itching; rashes
sleep, 120-27
 amount, 76, 122
 baby in womb, 23
 during bottle feedings, 107
 during breast-feedings, 92
 in pregnancy, 27, 41
 problems, 126
 sick children, 193
sleepsuits, 129
slings, for fractures, 241
"small for dates" babies, 39, 70
smiling, 80, 159
smoking, 11, 13, 19, 39
 and asthma, 211
 and chest infections, 208
smothering, 123
snacks, 116
snake bites, 244
soap, 135, 138, 140, 142
socks, 129, 133
solid food, introducing, 108-15
soothing babies, 78, 79, 87, 88, 117, 124-25
sore nipples, 55, 78, 96
sore throats, 207
soy milk, 102
spanking, 170
special care units, 70
speech development, 165, 170
sperm, 14, 15
spider bites, 244
spillproof bowls, 108
spina bifida, 37
spinal anesthesia, 64
spinal injuries, 229

splinters, 245
spoiling children, 168
sponge bathing, 134, 135, 136-37, 142-3
sponges, 135
sponging, bringing down a fever, 188
spoons: feeding babies, 108, 112, 114, 115
 medicine, 189
spots, 218
 milk spots, 175
 newborn babies, 69, 176
 see also rashes
sprained joints, 241
squatting: in labor, 61
 in pregnancy, 47
squints, 68, 80, 203
stairs: climbing, 161, 164
 gates, 161, 228
 safety, 161, 228
sterilizing, bottle-feeding equipment, 87, 99-101
stethoscope, 81, 184
 obstetric, 36, 65
sticky eye, 177
stillbirth, 10, 70
stings, 244-45
stitches: Cesarean section, 67
 children, 185
 coping with, 71
 episiotomy, 66, 71, 73
stomach: doctor's check, 69, 81
 gastroenteritis, 179, 214-15
 muscles, 72
 pain, 38, 212
 upsets, 179, 214-15
stools: abnormal, 212, 215
 baby's, 69, 146
 blood in, 146, 174, 213
 emergencies, 174
 see also constipation; diarrhea
storage: baby food, 110-11
 formula milk, 102, 105
stories, bedtime, 125
strawberry birthmarks, 69
straws, drinking, 192
 and mumps, 200
 and sore mouth, 206
stretch marks, 24, 42
stretchsuits, 27, 128, 129
 putting on, 130-31
 taking off, 132
stroller, 120, 122, 156-57
stye, 203
sucking: after birth, 63
 baby in womb, 17, 19, 23
 breast-feeding, 87, 91, 92, 93, 96, 97
 for comfort, 87, 92, 97, 107, 117, 124
 mouthing, 160
 nipples, 99
sucking reflex, 63, 107
suction, assisted delivery, 66
suffocation, 235
sugar: adding to bottle-feedings, 213
 drink for dehydration, 214
 in pregnancy, 53
 in urine, 34
suits, 128, 129
sun hats, 128, 129, 221
sunburn, 178, 221

supplements, dietary: for babies, 102, 115
for pregnant women, 19, 38, 40, 52
surfactant, 25
surgery, children, 185
swaddling, 117, 122, 123
sweaters, for newborn, 27, 128, 129
sweating: babies, 118, 178
fevers, 188
heat rash, 219
overheating, 118, 178
in pregnancy, 22, 42
sweets, 116
swellings, first aid, 240
swimming, 43
swollen glands, 183, 184
swollen legs and hands, in pregnancy, 36, 38, 42
symptoms, 174-75, 180-84
syphilis, 35

T

tailor sitting, 46
talking, 158, 165
tantrums, 119, 168, 170
taste: fetus's sense of, 23, 25
first sign of pregnancy, 12
not liking, 112
tea, 53, 93
tear ducts, blocked, 175
teeth: broken, 240
care of child's, 116, 135, 144-45
decay, 144, 190
fetus's, 21
medications and, 190
in pregnancy, 17, 40
teething: and illness, 182
order of appearance, 144
soothing pain, 119
temper tantrums, 119, 168, 170
temperament, 168
temperature: baby's room, 118, 121, 178
bath water, 227
bringing down a fever, 188
chilling, 178
emergencies, 38, 174
fever, 180, 184, 186-88, 197
overheating, 118, 178
in pregnancy, 38
regulating in womb, 23
of solid food, 110
taking a child's, 183, 186-87
temperature indicator strip, 186-87
testicles, 68, 69, 151, 216
fetus's, 29
tests: alpha fetoprotein (AFP), 19, 37
amniocentesis, 19, 37
Apgar, 63
blood, 35
chorionic villus sampling (CVS), 37
pregnancy, 12
for syphilis, 35
urine, 34
tetanus, 239, 244
immunization, 196
texture, of solid food, 110-11
thalassemia, 35

thermometers, 186-87
thigh strengthener, 46
thorns, 245
throat: checking for infection, 183, 184
infections, 207
tonsillitis, 207
thrush, 176, 206, 217
thumb sucking, 118, 124
thyroid deficiency, 69
tiredness: first sign of pregnancy, 12
and napping, 122
in pregnancy, 28, 29, 42
in young children, 119
tissues, 148, 150, 151
toenails: care of baby's, 135, 145
fetus's, 29
toes: crushed, 240
fetus's, 15, 16, 29
toilet training, 154-55
toiletries, 135
tongue: baby's, 68
development of fetus's, 15
tonsillitis, 207
toothbrushes, 135, 144-45
toothpaste, 116, 135, 144-45
towels, 135
toxoplasma, 13
toys, 158-63, 165-67
bathtime, 141
crib, 121
for sick children, 193
training pants, 154
tranquilizers, in labor, 64
transition stage, labor, 60
traveling: bottle-feeding, 87, 101, 156
breast-feeding, 87
in cars, 157
in pregnancy, 21
tuberculosis, immunization, 196
twins: conception, 15
delivery, 67
feeding, 88
pregnancy, 39
ultrasound scans, 37

U

ultrasound scans, 19, 37
umbilical cord, 14, 23
cleaning stump of, 136
delivery of baby, 62, 63
separation from navel, 68, 76
umbrella-style folding stroller, 157
unconsciousness, 229, 230-33
undershirts, 128
putting on, 130
taking off, 132
undressing babies, 132
universal nipples, 99
urinary system, 216
urinary system infections, 216
and antibiotics, 189
and stomach pain, 212
urination: after labor, 71
frequent, 12, 16, 26, 41, 216
painful, 38, 216
urine: leaking, 27, 38, 41, 61, 72, 73
odd-coloured, 216

urine continued
passing in womb, 17, 23
tests, 12, 34
urticaria, 176, 219
uterus, see womb

V

vaccination, see immunization
vacuum extraction, 66
vagina: baby's, 135
bleeding, 38, 39, 71
discharges, 20, 42, 68, 217
in labor, 63
problems in babies and children, 217
varicose veins, 29, 36, 42
VDTs (visual display terminals), 10
vegetables: baby food, 110-11
fiber, 51, 213
likes and dislikes, 115
purées, 110, 112
sources of nutrients, 51, 52
vegetarian diet, 52
vernix, 21, 24, 31, 68, 69
verrucas, 222-23
virus diseases: and antibiotics, 189
developing resistance, 194
see also infectious illnesses
vitamin C, 51, 52
vitamin K, 63
vitamin supplements, 52, 102, 115
vomiting, 214
babies, 87, 179
emergencies, 38, 174
in labor, 60
in pregnancy, 12, 16, 18, 38, 41
sick children, 192, 193

W

waking, night, 126
walking, 133, 164, 165
warts, 222-23
washcloth, baby, 135, 148
washing: babies, 134-43
baby clothes, 128
bottles, 100
breasts, 96
diapers, 149, 176
hair, 21
water: for bottle-fed babies, 102, 113, 117
drinking in pregnancy, 22, 38, 42, 52
drowning, 235
fear of, 142
formula milk, 102
playing with, 142, 161
retention in pregnancy, 22, 42
safety, 228
to avoid constipation, 17, 40
watering eye, 175
waters, breaking, 56
wax in ears, 204
weaning, 93, 97, 113
weedkillers, safety, 228
weight, baby's/child's, 76, 81, 115, 247, 249

weight continued
bottle-feeding, 106
breast-feeding, 93
slow weight gain, 106, 174
weight, fetus's, 16, 18, 20, 22, 24, 26, 28, 29, 30, 31
weight, mother's: before pregnancy, 11
gain in pregnancy, 16, 18, 20, 22, 24, 26, 28, 30, 31
prenatal checks, 34
wheeziness, 208, 210
whining, 170
whooping cough, 201
immunization, 196
windpipe, choking, 234
womb: after labor, 73
afterpains, 71
implantation of fertilized egg, 14
pressing upward, 26
proportion of weight gain, 31
see also contractions
work: and breast-feeding, 97
hazards, 10
in pregnancy, 25
worms, pinworms, 217, 224
wounds: cuts and scrapes, 239
embedded objects, 238
heavy bleeding, 238
wrists, fractures, 241

Y

yard: gate, 168, 228
safety, 228
sleeping in, 122
yeast infections, 42

ACKNOWLEDGMENTS

DORLING KINDERSLEY would like to thank **Elizabeth Fenwick**, the author of the English edition, for all the work she put into writing the book; and the following for their design and editorial work: Rowena Alsey, Carole Ash, Tina Hill, Tanya Hines, Claire Le Bas, Sarah Pearce, and Daphne Razazan.

Special photography

(numbers indicate pages; t = top, b = below, c = center, l = left, r = right)

Antonia Deutsch assisted by Pamela Cowan: 2tl, 6: 1st column, 11–14, 16–22, 24–31, 33–42, 43t, 44–49, 53t, 56t and br, 57–61, 64, 67, 70, 71–73, 90tr and br, 91tl, tc, and cr, 92bl and br, 94, 95 all except bl, 96, 97;

Dave King: 2cl, 4: 1st column pictures 2–4, 2nd column pictures 1–4; 6: 2nd column t and lower c, 7: 1st column, 2nd column all except bl, 8–9, 32t, 50–52, 53b, 54 tr and c, 55 all except tr, 74–75, 76–81, 83tr, 85, 88tl, 95bl, 98, 99t, l, and tc, 100bl, 101, 104, 105 all except bl, 108 all except t and br, 109br, 110–11, 112tl, 114–16, 117t, 2nd row r, 119, 121 all except t and tl, 124bl, 125tr and b, 128–33, 134t, 138–41, 142tr, 145t, cl, and bl, 146t, 149 bl and c, 154, 158bl and bc, 159–167, 169, 171–73, 174t and l, 176b, 177tr, cr, and br, 178–96, 197r, 198t, cr, and b, 199tr and br, 200–1, 202br, 203tr and b, 204–5, 206tl, tr, and cr, 207t, 209–17, 218c and r, 219t and bl, 220cl, cr, and b, 221tl, tr, and bl, 222tl and cr, 223tl, cr and b, 224c and r, 226t, 229, 246b, 247b, 248–49;

Ray Moller: 6: 2nd column upper cr, 100, 106cl, cr, bl, and br, 107, 136t, cr, and br, 137 all except br, 142bl and br, 143, 146bl, 175c;

Stephen Oliver: 4: 1st column pictures 1 and 5; 10, 15, 54l and b, 55tr, 56bl, 99bc and br, 103, 105bl, 108t and bl, 109l and tr, 120bl and br, 121t and tl, 125tl, 134 all except t, 135, 146br, 148, 149tl, box tr, cl and cr, 153, 155, 156bl and br;

Susanna Price: 1, 2–3 main picture, 6: 2nd column upper cl and b, 7: 2nd column bl, 68–69, 82, 83tl and c, 84, 86–87, 88tr, bl, and br, 89, 90tl and c, 91tr and bl, 92tl and tr, 93, 106t, 112tr, c, and br, 117 2nd row l, 3rd row l and r, 4th row l, c, and r, 118, 120t, 123, 124 all except bl, 125 c, 127, 136bl and bc, 137br, 142tl, 144, 145cr, bc, and br, 147, 150–52, 158t and br, 168, 246t, 247t;

Steve Shott: 2: 2nd column picture 5; 157–9;

Anthea Sieveking: 65.

Picture credits

The publishers would like to thank the following for their kind permission to reproduce photographs:

(numbers indicate pages; t = top, b = below, c = center, l = left, r = right)

Genesis Film Productions Ltd/Neil Bromhall: 23; Lupe Cunha: 62; Lesley Howling: 43b; Ron Sutherland: 67c; Sue Ford, Western Ophthalmic Hospital: 175tr, 177bl, 202r; National Medical Slide Bank: 175br, 198l, 202tl, 206bl, 218l, 219cl, 224l; St. John's Institute of Dermatology: 220tl, 223tr; St. Mary's Hospital: 177tl, 199tl, 199bl; Dr. I. Williams: 174br, 175cr, 176t and cr, 197r, 203l, 207b, 219bl, 221br, 222t, bc, and b; ZEFA: 63.

Loan or supply of props

Baby B's, Fulham, London, England; The Nursery Collection, Watford, England. Special thanks to: Mary Snyder at Snugli, Inc.; Gerry Baby Products Company, Denver, Colorado; Judi's Originals, Scottsdale, Arizona.

Illustrators

Coral Mula: all line artwork except pp. 226–28; Jim Robins: 226–28.